Dr. Vinod Verma

AYURVEDIC FOOD CULTURE AND RECIPES

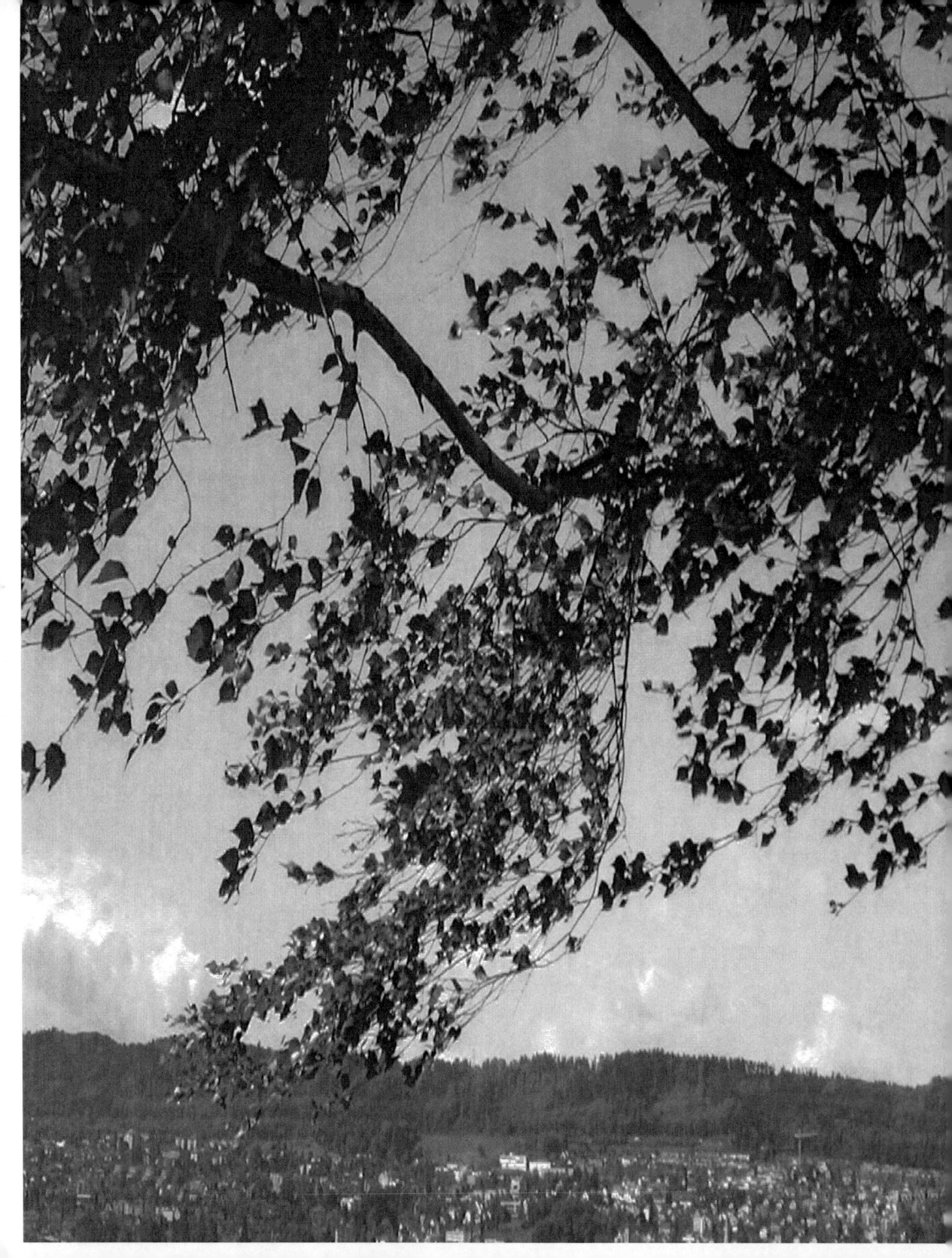

Dr. Vinod Verma

AYURVEDIC FOOD CULTURE AND RECIPES

Gayatri Books International

The information provided in this book is not intended to replace the services of a physician. Suggestions for a healthy Ayurvedic diet are given in this book for the purpose of self-help and education. The author and the publisher are in no way responsible for any medical claims regarding the material presented in this book. For using methods and recipes provided in this book at commercial level requires the prior permission from the author. For more information, write to the author directly at ayurvedavv@yahoo.com.

© Dr. Vinod Verma 2001
First published by Penguin India in 2001, in German 2002 and subsequently in other languages.

Revised Edition in colour: 2009

Present B&W edition: 2013
All Rights Reserved

Visit Dr. Vinod Verma at www.ayurvedavv.com and www.drvinodverma.com to find out about her other publications and activities like seminars, lectures, consultations, etc. Look for more information on the last pages of the book.

Published by : Gayatri Books International, Village Astal, Tehsil Dunda, District Uttarkashi, India

The contents of this book may not be reproduced, stored or copied in any form—printed, electronic, photocopied, or otherwise—except for excerpts used in review, without the written permission of the publisher.

Book and cover design: Vanaja Vishal
Consultant: Mohit Joshi

ISBN: 978-81-89514-23-5

This book is dedicated to the following persons:

- To Charaka, the great Ayurvedic sage who wrote the timeless wisdom about Ayurvedic food culture two thousand six hundred years ago.
- To my Ayurvedic Guru, Acharya Priya Vrat Sharma for providing the detailed pharmacology of all the food products.
- To all those Indian women and vaidyas (Ayurvedic physicians) who kept this tradition alive until today.

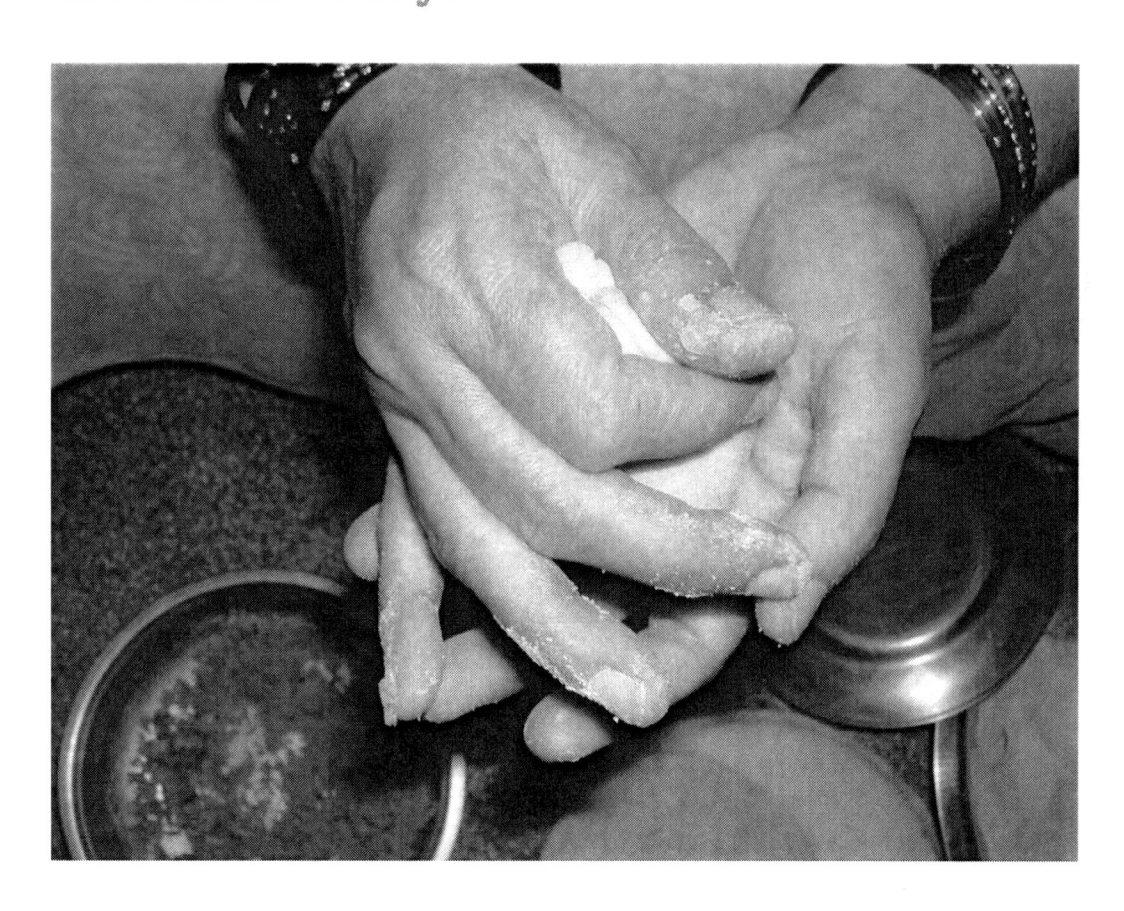

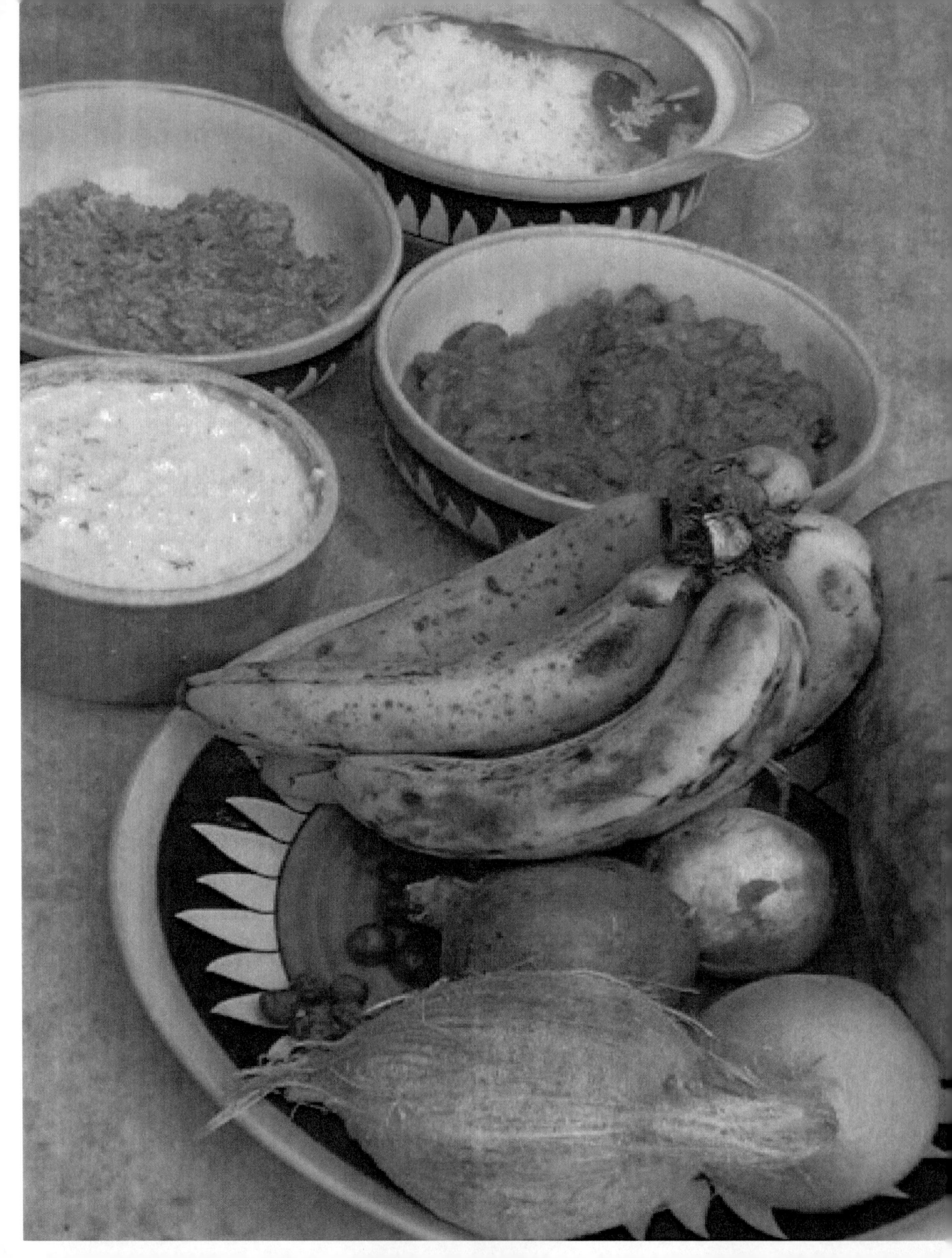

Contents

Dedication	5
Foreword	9
Preface	11
Acknowledgement	15

SECTION I
THE AYURVEDIC FOOD CULTURE — 17

Introduction to the Ayurvedic food culture — 19
What is Ayurvedic Food? 19; Body, 19: The Three Energies of the Body, 20; Prakriti or the Individual Constitution, 21; Importance of Prakriti, 22; Influence of Mind on Prakriti, 23; Five Elements in Food: The Rasa Theory, 24; Essential Features of Ayurvedic Food Preparation; 26; Basic Understanding of the Ayurvedic Food Culture, 28; The Eight Golden Principles of Ayurvedic Food Culture, 35

The Practical Aspects of Ayurvedic Food Preparations — 37
Rasas in Practice, 38; Methods for Balanced Food Preparation, 40; Discovering the Rasas in Cosmos, 41; Alcohol and Tobacco, 42; Food as Nectar or Poison, 44; Your Menu in Case of Vikriti, 45

Prana in your food — 47
Six Dimensions of Food, 50; Our Relationship with Food, 51; Enriching your Food, 52

Preparation of the Basic Ayurvedic Cuisine — 55
Herbs and Spices, 55, Cleaning and Storage of Spices, 69; Collection of Ingredients, 69; Equipment, 72
Some Fundamental Preparations, 73
Spice Mixtures, 73; Preparations with Milk Products, 77

SECTION II
AYURVEDIC FOOD RECIPES   83

Introduction to the Recipes	85
Beverages	89
Breakfast Recipes	105
Main Meals	115
Soups	115
Warm Starters	125
Main Course	129
Cheese	177
Salads	181
Breads	189
Beans and lentils	205
Small Meals	217
Side-dishes	221
Dessert	231

APPENDIX   241

About the Author   255

Foreword

Etymologically, the term Ayurveda stands for science of life—wisdom to live life in a holistic manner. According to the Upanishads, life is like a chariot. Its structure is the body, its reins the mind, its charioteer the intellect. The owner of the chariot is the soul or the *atman*. A span of life is sustained by the union of the body, senses, mind, intellect and soul. Sushruta defines health as the joy experienced by the soul, mind and senses when they are in a state of cosmic harmony.

Ayurveda is the science to live and understand life in a holistic way and maintain an optimum state of well-being. It is not merely an art of healing but a comprehensive medical system whose goal is to enable human beings to remain healthy in all respects and be disease-free (arogya). According to Charaka, without the optimum state of health, one cannot achieve the other goals in life like virtue, wealth, gratification and emancipation. An unhealthy state hinders the achievements of these goals and destroys well-being and even life itself.

Charaka counts food, sleep and oneness with the cosmic energy as three means of attaining health. Amongst these three, food is the first and the principal means to attain health. The word for food is *aahar* in Sanskrit and it literally means—that which eradicates disease (*aharo rogaharah*). According to *Kashyapa Samhita*, 'there is no medicine comparable to food. Human beings can remain healthy only by a balanced intake of food products. One cannot cure a sick person simply by medication and without paying attention to the diet. That is why, the health specialist call food as best of all the medicines'.

In *Taittiriya* Upanishad food is said to be a boon of nature for living beings. It is said that food is greatest medicine of all the medicines. An ancient book on Ayurvedic nutrition and cooking called *Pakadarpana* states that the combination of the six principal rasas (the tastes in the cosmos) in all edible products along with five types of grains, cooked in a specific manner and eaten at proper timings keep the fundamental balance in human constitution. This is done by maintaining equilibrium in the three principal energies of the body (vata, pitta and kapha), and this balance keeps one healthy and free of disorders.

The great Ayurvedic scholar Vagbhatta in 6 Century AD formulated a simple three step programme (Three-Aphorism Principle) for maintaining health and remaining disease free. These are: 1) to live with natural principles for maintaining one's constitution; 2) diet intake in a limited manner; 3) food bought with money earned with righteous means.

Foreword

The Bhagavad-Gita suggests that human beings should adopt yogic ways, and those who do not do that are frequently sick. Yoga means balance and harmony. A systematic balance between the following factors is yoga: 1) food and lifestyle; 2) virtuous conduct and pious thoughts; 3) imaginative and vigilant state of mind. It is stated that the first step to yoga is nutrition. The purity of diet leads to the purity of mind and a pure mind leads to a higher level of consciousness (buddhi). In Chandogya Upanishad, it is written that pure food leads to a sattva state of mind and that leads to mental lucidity.

In this stressful and competitive age, we have forgotten the value and importance of appropriate food. Food is being replaced with junk and toxic chemicals are added to it. Food is no more that which takes away the ailments (*ahara*). On the contrary, it has become the cause of the ailments. Toxins in food in our times lead to an amazing number of new and unheard of ailments.

Dr. Vinod Verma's book, which is based upon the ancient scientific principals of Ayurveda and is presenting modern methods of preparation is like a ray of hope in this age of darkness and confusion when our food is little better than poison. It is not only a recipe book but describes also the Ayurvedic food culture, which can help many people heal their digestion-related ailments. Besides, there are modern ways of preparing rejuvenating foods with all the ancient wisdom of using specific spices, herbs and food combinations for balanced preparations. The use of modern equipments to shorten the time and systematic preparations of numerous spice combinations make the book a valuable gift to humanity. This book is a commendable and extraordinary attempt to present the ancient wisdom in a modern way for the benefit of humanity.

Professor Dharmanand Sharma
Philosophy Department
Panjab University, Chandigarh

January 2001

Preface

I am writing this book on the popular demand of my students and readers from all over the world. I have been writing about the Ayurvedic life-style and have also provided some recipes in my previous three books on the subject. However, in my previous books, my purpose has been to give you some ideas about cooking according to the Ayurvedic principles which you may adapt into your own specific recipes. These ideas are for making your food preparations in equilibrium in relation to the specific nature of your body (your basic constitution or *prakriti*), weather, climate and place etc. Thus, before learning Ayurvedic recipes, it is essential to know the fundamentals of Ayurveda. Ayurveda is the wisdom about life and it deals with all aspects of life. It is truly a holistic science that visualises the cosmic unity and holds the view that any change in our universe leads to a chain reaction, as all what exists is interrelated, interconnected and interdependent. Therefore, to write a book exclusively on Ayurvedic recipes without talking about the fundamentals of Ayurvedic food culture sounds ridiculous to me. In this book, in the first Section, I explain the basic principles of Ayurvedic food culture and the second Section has the Ayurvedic food recipes.

Ayurvedic food means a harmonious combination of food products prepared with various seeds, herbs and spices in order to create equilibrium in your body and to rejuvenate you. This food should increase 'ojas' (immunity and vitality) in the body. The preparation of the food, the way it is consumed and its quantity also play a significant role. The quality of the food should be according to the place, weather, climate, specific situation (like fatigue, sickness, stress etc.) and the fundamental nature of an individual. The food preparation should be balanced in relation to the five fundamental elements (ether, air, fire, water and earth) of which the whole universe is made and in addition the equilibrium should be sought in the above-described factors. It is essential to know all these basic factors to comprehend properly about the Ayurvedic food preparations.

Ayurvedic cooking does not mean 'Indian cooking' and Ayurvedic cooking preparations do not have to be Indian. Ayurvedic principles are largely followed in many traditional homes in India. Nevertheless, not all Indian foods are prepared according to the principles of Ayurveda. Most existing books on Ayurvedic cooking are simply Indian cookbooks and those too at times are westernised. For example, the wheat bread eaten in most Indian homes is made with dough prepared simply with flour and water and this flat bread is baked on an iron pan. It is called *chapati* and it is freshly made for each meal. There is no salt or fat in the *chapatis*. They may be slightly smeared with ghee (clarified butter) on the top after they are ready. The *chapatis* are eaten with various vegetable or meat preparations, which are salted. However, to my utter surprise,

Preface

many of the so called Ayurvedic cookbooks had instructed to add salt in the dough for *chapatis*, obviously to make the taste comparable to the salted bread eaten in the West. There are also many deep-fried, oily and fatty recipes written under the name of Ayurvedic cooking. In the ancient texts of Ayurveda, these foods are specifically prohibited and when eaten, they should be made with particular spices that promote digestion. However, these spices are not mentioned in the recently published books.

I have written this book to give you an over all understanding of the Ayurvedic concepts of food preparation by illustrating the scientific reasons for using particular spices in particular preparations. This way, you will not only learn the limited Ayurvedic recipes but will also be able to use the specific products in your own recipes at an appropriate time in order to make them according to the Ayurvedic principles of balance and harmony.

Many recipes described in this book are specifically designed and are invented by me to suit our modern way of life, available equipment and time constraint. Since I have spent a substantial part of my adult life in Europe and also three years in the USA, and have travelled around the world, my recipes are very often cross-cultural but modified according to the principles of Ayurveda.

I grew up in an extended family where I assimilated the wisdom about the fundamentals of Ayurvedic food culture and preparations. This knowledge included what to eat when, with what and in which situations, etc. While living in foreign countries when I encountered different kinds of foods and food preparations, I naturally could apply the same principles to those. If one grows up with the Ayurvedic culture of balance and harmony, it comes naturally and effortlessly to feel the effect of the food on one's being and to create harmony and balance in the food one consumes. For this book, most of my hard work was required to figure out the exact measures of the ingredients, as I am not used to cooking with weights and measures. I rather cook with intuitive wisdom.

The Ayurvedic herbs and spices not only help to make our food healthy and rejuvenating but they also serve as a little apothecary. However, I will limit the present book only to the preparation of food products and various other aspects of Ayurvedic food culture. I hope you will enjoy these recipes as much as my students have been enjoying in our Ayurvedic cooking classes for many years in different parts of the world.

Ayurveda basically does not tell you to be vegetarian for good health. According to the Ayurvedic food culture, whether it is meat or vegetables, the equilibrium of the food based upon certain cosmic principles is essential. Ayurveda is the science of life and takes a morally neutral point of view. Milk has a great importance in Ayurveda as a source of animal fat and protein. Personally, I do not eat any kind of meat or eggs because I was born in a family with centuries of vegetarian tradition. I find eating meat barbaric. I am also very much influenced by the yogic tradition of ahimsa (not killing and paining others). In some parts of the world, meat eating could be a need. But with the rapid modes of transportation these days, this is also fast disappearing. There are two other reasons for which I am against meat eating. One is that we are biologically too close to animals and somehow eating the similar flesh and blood is not appetising and appealing. Secondly, meat does not look appealing to me. Fresh vegetables of diverse colours and form are bubbling with prana energy. Meat is something that is obtained after killing and is a dead food. To end this discussion, I will give the point of view of one of the famous Ayurvedic physician from Delhi, Vaidya Brihaspati Dev Triguna. According to him, the animals, which are led to the slaughterhouses, know about their end and leave behind their flesh with the negative energy of fear, pain, anger and frustration. In contrast to that, the milk can be only produced with the feeling of love.

Vinod Verma
March, 2000
www.ayurvedavv.com
ayurvedavv@yahoo.com

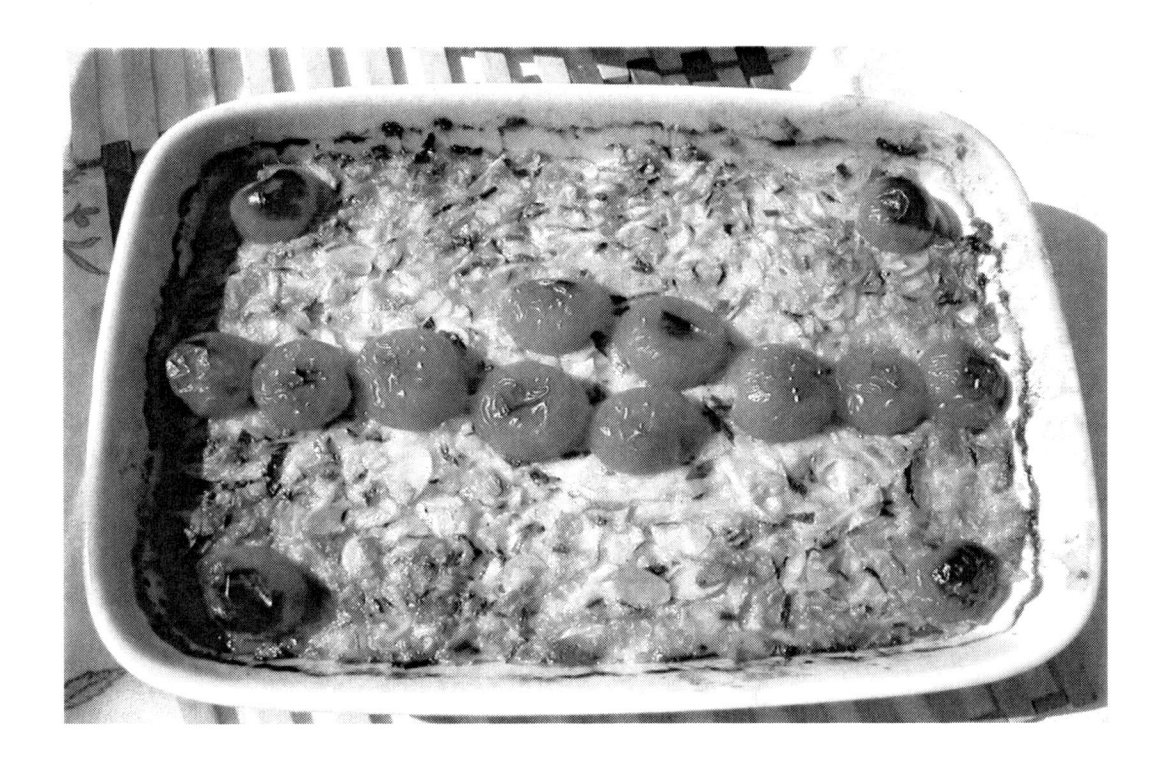

Preface to the 2009 and the Present 2013 Editions

This book was first published in India by Penguin as paperback in 2001 and then in German a hard bound edition in colour with beautiful pictures in 2002. Both the editions were very well received. They got very good reviews, which went as far as saying—*the only authentic book on Ayurvedic recipes and food culture.*

I was not happy with the paperback edition in English which was without pictures. I feel that a book on Ayurvedic food cultures and recipes needs demonstrative, as well as inspiring pictures. Being over-worked with research on new themes and publication of books on Companionship and Sexuality, Ayurvedic concepts of Beauty, Losing Weight, and so on; I did not find time to arrange the proper English publication for this book. The problem is that the moment a book becomes a little old, the author likes to revise it. That is where time is needed and delays take place.

I very much hope that this edition will benefit many people in the English-speaking world, as it has done in Germany, Switzerland and Austria.

This B&W edition is principally to bring the sale price of the book down. Since we do not produce in bulk, the colour prints cost us very high and we sell them only one dollar more than the printing costs. This edition will be at a lower price and will also allow people in India to buy it.

Vinod Verma
January 2008

www.ayurvedavv.com   www.drvinodverma.com
ayurvedavv@yahoo.com

Acknowledgements

I am indebted to my grandmother and aunts from whom I assimilated the fundamentals of Ayurvedic food culture and cooking. My grandmother was an encyclopaedia of Ayurvedic wisdom and we were always told what to eat when and how and the reasons behind all this.

I am extremely grateful to my Ayurvedic teacher and Guru Acharya Priya Vrat Sharma who provided me the scientific aspects about the wisdom of Ayurvedic food culture. Without his detailed books on Ayurvedic pharmacology, it would not have been possible for me to develop the international recipes of Ayurvedic food. I also express my gratitude to Professor Dharmanand Sharma for writing the foreword for this book. With the profound understanding of the Vedic culture, Professor Sharma is the most appropriate person I could think of for the appraisal of this work.

I express my gratitude to my French friends for teaching me the fine art of French cuisine during my student days in Paris. I learnt the French food culture and cooking particularly from Dr. Gisèle Nicolas, Prof. Jean André and Lucile Wyllie. This knowledge was very helpful for writing international recipes with Ayurvedic principles. I thank my friend Gisela Binder from Basel for the pictures of some of her wonderful food preparations.

All my students in Europe who attended my Ayurvedic classes or who came to our centres in Delhi and in the Himalayas were a great source of inspiration to develop new recipes. They also helped me to comprehend the difficulties foreigners face in understanding Ayurvedic food culture and cooking.

Dr, Heinrich Heyne (HH) was a constant source of inspiration for making new recipes, as he loves to eat delicately prepared good food with diverse flavours. His critical comments and valuable suggestions were always very helpful. I am extremely indebted to him for editing this book extensively.

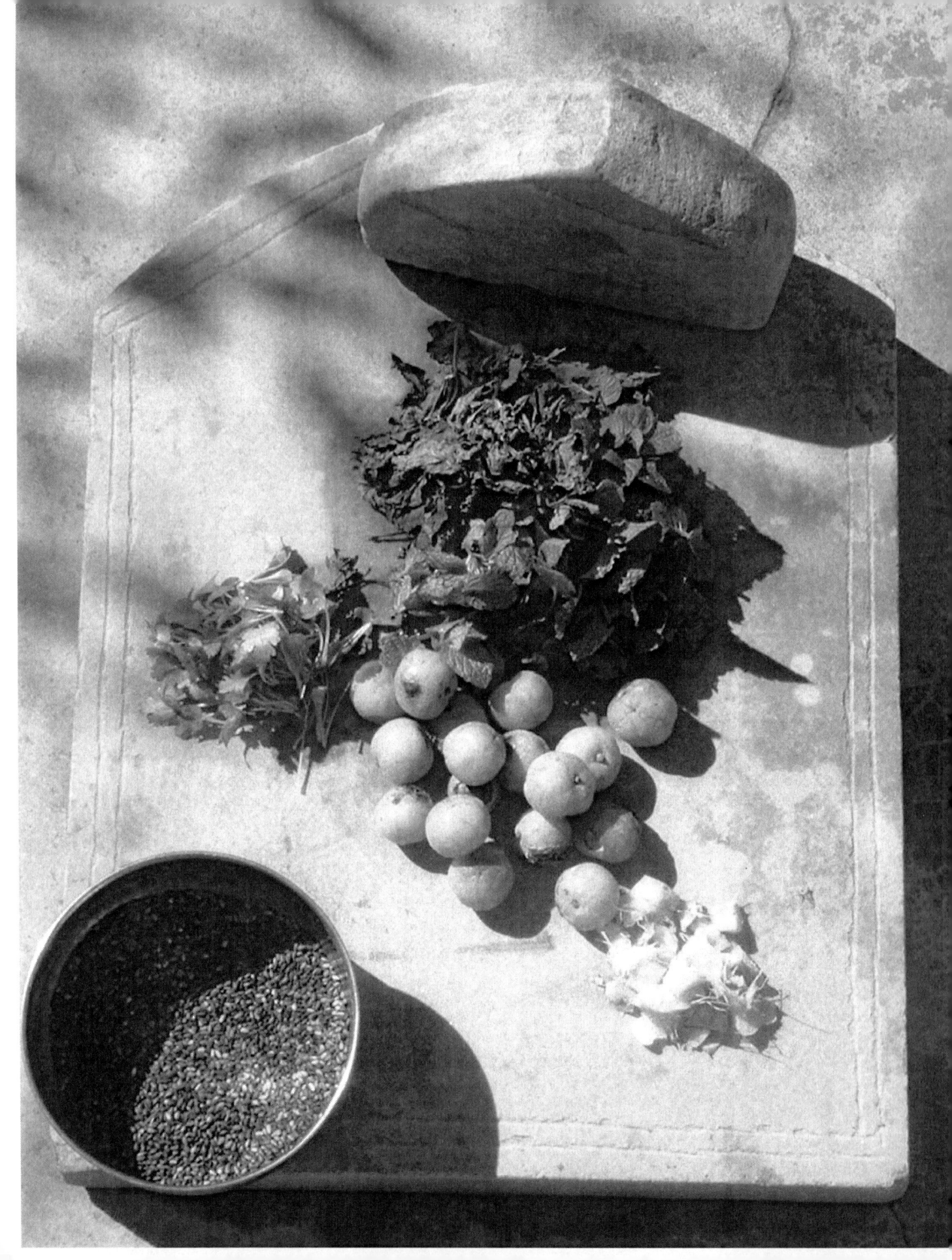

SECTION I

THE AYURVEDIC FOOD CULTURE

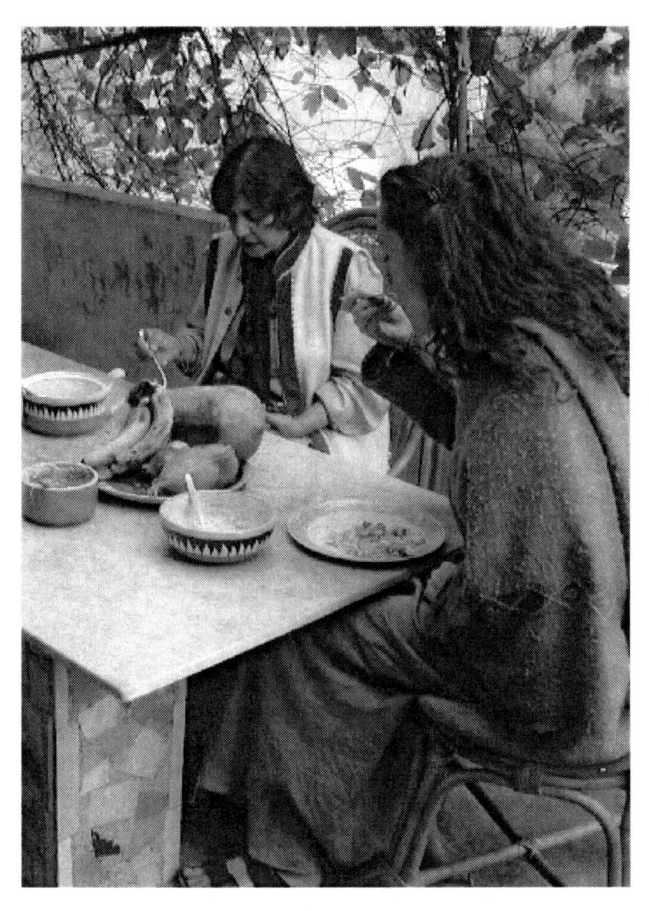

"Food or any other thing that is not wholesome and that has unpleasant consequences should not be used out of ignorance and carelessness. One should eat warm, unctuous and non-antagonistic food in proper quantity, after the previous food is digested, in a favourable place with all the favourable accessories, not too fast, not too slow, not while talking or laughing, with full concentration, and after due consideration to one's age and constitution"

Charaka Samhita
Sixth Century BC

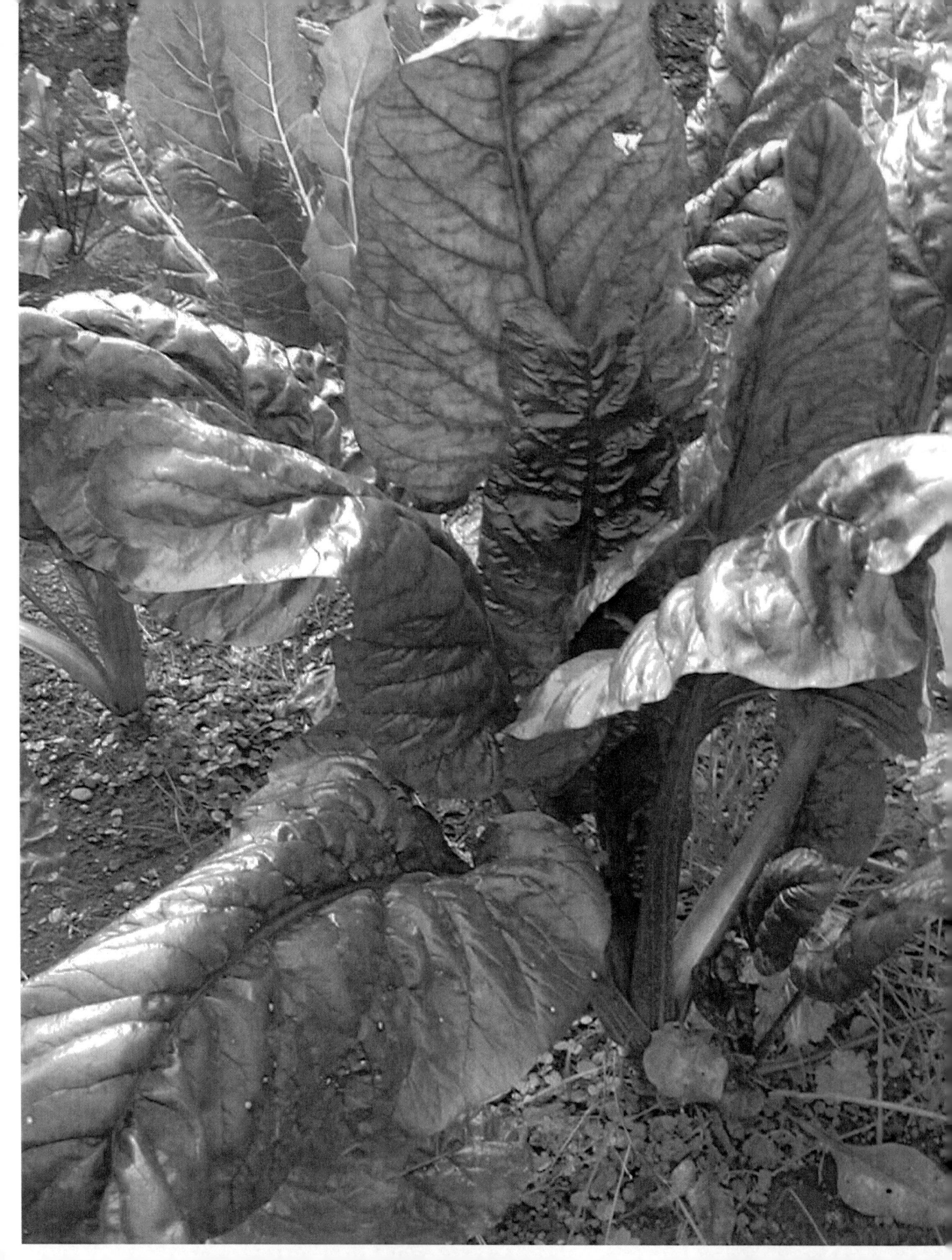

Introduction to the Ayurvedic Food Culture

What is Ayurvedic Food?

The concept of Ayurvedic food is based upon the principle of the basic unity in all that exists. Everything in the universe is interconnected, interrelated and interdependent.

All that exists is made of five fundamental elements. These are:

> **Ether**
> **Air**
> **Fire**
> **Water**
> **Earth**

Since everything is made of these five elements, so is our body and so is our food.

Ether is the first element. Ether is space and without space nothing can exist. Air exists in ether and it is the second element of the order. The third element is fire and its existence is dependent upon both ether and air. Water is the fourth element and its existence depends upon the previous three. Earth is the last and the heaviest of all the elements and it has the previous four elements.

The Body

To perform all the physical and mental functions of the body, the five elements are present in the form of three principal energies or energies, namely *vata*, *pitta* and *kapha*. Vata is constituted from ether and air, pitta from fire and kapha from water and earth.

ETHER AND AIR ⟶ **VATA**
FIRE ⟶ **PITTA**
WATER AND EARTH ⟶ **KAPHA**

The equilibrium of the three energies or the five elements constitutes good health; whereas their imbalance leads to loss of energy, ailments and diseases. From the Ayurvedic point of view, health means well-being in all respects, be they physical, mental, social or cosmic. These different levels cannot be separated, as they are interrelated and interdependent. For good health, it is essential to make a constant effort to maintain equilibrium of vata, pitta and kapha. Food, weather, climate, place, age, and mental state are some of the major factors that affect this balance constantly. In the present context, we are dealing with food to maintain our equilibrium as it relates to our mental and physical energy. Energy is constantly being used for performing various functions. Food and breathing keep replenishing it throughout our lives. In the box on the next page, I present a very precise description of the three principal energies (called dosha), which manage our bodily systems and their relationship with the three states of mind, as well as the fundamental human constitution or prakriti. For more details, please refer to my several previously written books on Ayurveda*.

The Three Energies of the Body

All that exists is made of five elements, so is the human body. The same cosmic principles apply to it. But the body has soul in it, which is the cause of consciousness and makes it a vital organism. For the performance of vital functions, the five elements form three principal energies referred to as energies in English (*dosa* in Sanskrit), and these are– *vata* from ether and air, *pitta* from fire and *kapha* from water and earth. These energies perform various mental and physical functions of the body and the nature of those functions depends upon the nature of the element they originate from.

Vata is the wind and space energy and is responsible for entire body movements, blood circulation, respiration, excretion, speech, sensation, touch, hearing, feelings like fear, anxiety, grief, enthusiasm etc., natural urges, formation of foetus, sexual act and retention.

Pitta is responsible for vision, hunger, thirst, heat regulation, softness and lustre, cheerfulness, intellect and sexual vigour.

Kapha constitutes all the solid structure of the body and is responsible for binding, firmness, heaviness, sexual potency, strength, forbearance and restraint.

Each person differs from another because of a slight difference in his or her fundamental constitution called **prakriti**. This difference is due to the variation in the proportion of the three main energies. This variation is in terms of

---

*
1. *Ayurveda, A Way of Life,* 1990, 1995, 2008
2. *Ayurveda for Inner Harmony, Nutrition, Sexual Energy and Healing,* 1990,1997 2007
3. *Programming Your Life with Ayurveda,* 2002

All these books are available at www.Amazon.com and at Pilgrims Publications.

dominance of a particular energy or the combination of two energies. This is what makes us different from one another and unlike machines, as the system of modern medicine tends to make us. The prakriti not only describes the variations in physiological features of individuals but also their personality types. (See box for the description of *prakriti*).

For good health and long life, these three vital forces or energies should be in a state of equilibrium within their individual organisation as well as with respect to each other. However, if there is disturbance in one of the energies and it deviates from its quality, quantity or place or the three energies are not in a balanced proportion to each other, it leads to **vikriti**, which is a state of being unwell. When the state of vitiation is left unattended for a long time, it may give rise to serious disorders.

Prakriti or the Individual Constitution

A mother observes differences in the personality traits of her two babies from the beginning and the siblings differ in their likes and dislikes of food products, their reaction to weather and climate, the effect of drugs, the fundamental way of reacting to situations and other personality traits. According to Ayurveda, each one of us has an individual constitution from birth. It is the basis of our physiological and psychological reactions. For maintaining good health and equilibrium, it is essential to take the individual constitution into consideration.

Prakriti of an individual is due to the dominance of one or more energies, which attribute the individual, the characteristics of that particular energy in slightly more predominance than the others. For example, the pitta prakriti individuals will be more sensitive to heat, they sweat more and eat and drink more. The vata prakriti ones are more agile and swift in their movements. The kapha prakriti persons are slow and stable in their movements and are more tolerant than the previous two. In the mixed prakriti, the person may experience different attributes at different times.

Seven types of prakriti

VATA	**VATA-PITTA**	**SAMADOSHA (equilibrium of energies)**
PITTA	**PITTA-KAPHA**	
KAPHA	**VATA-KAPHA**	

Introduction to the Ayurvedic Food Culture

> The difference in the proportion of the energies is one factor of variation. Their degree is another factor. For example, one may be slightly vata dominating or in various upwards grades. The proportion of the two energies may vary in the mixed prakriti. The fundamental presence of the grade of these three energies is another varying factor. For example, there are some individuals with plenty of energy, tremendous stamina and vitality, very good immune system and a brilliant mind. These persons have basically all the three energies or energies in high grade. Then comes the domination of one or more of the energies and forms their prakriti.
>
> If we imagine the fundamental presence of the three energies on a scale of 10 and then multiply them with seven types of prakriti, we get a large number of human types. Further on, in each case, the degree of dominance is also considered and in mixed prakriti, the proportion of the two energies is also taken into consideration, we will find numerous variants of prakriti.

Importance of Prakriti

Since all in this cosmos is made of five elements including our body and everything is interconnected and interdependent, the outer factors influence us constantly. To maintain the equilibrium of five elements in the body, which are present in the form of three energies, it is essential that an individual knows his or her constitution. If a person with predominant fire element (pitta prakriti) does actions or consumes foods with the dominance of the same element, he or she may end up in getting this energy vitiated and thus, may fall ill. Therefore, it is essential for you to know your prakriti for benefiting from Ayurvedic wisdom. For nutrition, weather, geographical location as well as remedies, prakriti or the fundamental constitution is taken into consideration.

With external factors like nutrition, geographical location and lifestyle, one can alter the vitiation and proportion of the energies but the basic individual constitution does not alter. However, in pathological conditions like due to an illness or accidental injuries, one may temporarily acquire different traits than one's prakriti, but upon getting cured, the usual features by which one is characterised, come back. For example, if you have vata prakriti and due to some sickness, you sleep a lot, become slow in your movements and so on, after getting cured, you will automatically acquire your usual swiftness.

The basic human nature does not change, the variations may occur due to life situations. Imagine someone pitta dominating who is impatient and gets angry very quickly, and has also a pitta-dominating partner. This couple may have fights, confrontations and disputes. Being similar, both these individuals will tend to enhance and aggravate each other's anger. Later in life, imagine one of them living with a kapha predominant person with patience and tolerance. Gradually, this pitta dominant person will lessen his anger. The other person's patience gives time to think and reflect and not to react.

Besides being important for health and healing, the knowledge of the Prakriti of individuals can lead us to better understanding of each other in family life, at the work place and in other aspects of social interaction. For more details on these themes see my books *Stress-Free Work with Yoga and Ayurveda, Companionship and Sexuality,* and *The Kamasutra for Women.* The book list is given at the end of this book.

Influence of Mind on Prakriti

Time, place, situation, nutrition, emotions, etc., constantly influence energies or the vital forces and learning about the influence of these factors on your particular constitution, you can learn to maintain their equilibrium. These three vital forces are also related to our thought process and therefore it is foremost to keep equilibrium in **the three qualities of the mind**. The **rajas** quality of mind includes thinking, planning and taking decisions. The **tamas** quality is that, which hinders motion (state of sleep) and expansion of the mind (greed, anger, jealousy, laziness and so on). The **sattva** quality of mind includes equilibrium, goodness, truth, compassion, stillness and peace. Balance of *sattva, rajas* and *tamas* influences the equilibrium of the energies and their imbalance can cause mental ailments. Thus, for maintaining good health and longevity, a six dimensional equilibrium is essential as these three dimensions at two levels mutually influence each other. The imbalance of these three qualities of mind also influences the equilibrium of the energies and vice versa.

Figure 1. The six dimensional human equilibrium

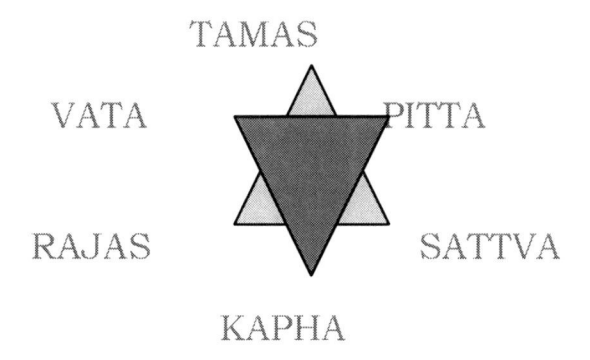

```
              TAMAS
VATA                   PITTA

RAJAS                  SATTVA
              KAPHA
```

It should be understood that the three energies of the body and the three qualities of the mind, which form six dimension of the human being are not compartmentalised. They are fluid entities and they change constantly in proportion. Their proportion is subjected to our way of life and thinking. In addition, the three energies and the three qualities of mind influence each other. For example, if you are leading a hectic life and are living in a state of mind of 'too much to do', you have too much rajas and that may lead to vata vitiation. Similarly, if your vata is vitiated due to windy weather or dry and cold food or any other reason, you may attain a hectic state of mind or imbalance of rajas. Excessive sleep or lack of movements causes imbalance of tamas and that may vitiate kapha. Pitta and sattva are related to each other because pitta is body's energy and sattva is the Inner Light, which is obtained after having achieved stillness of mind.

Five elements in Food: The Rasa Theory

Like the body, food is also constituted of five elements and gives us vitality by providing these elements to our body. The five elements in right proportion in our food give us the balance of vata, pitta and kapha and thus, we are blessed with good health and longevity. It is also possible to cure minor disorders through dietary measures if we have the wisdom of Ayurvedic food culture. It is not possible to estimate the proportion of the five elements in the food we consume, therefore it is essential to learn the Ayurvedic methods which provide us an analysis of these cosmic mysteries. The five elements are traced in the form of different tastes in our food. There are six *rasas* or tastes and each one of the *rasas* is derived from two elements. Let us see what a *rasa* is and how the *rasas* affect in diverse manners our bodily energies and thus our health.

Rasa literally means taste but in the present context, it is the total effect of a particular taste on our body. Our tongue deduces taste, and it is like a doorkeeper. A substance with a particular taste as sweet, sour, pungent etc. has an effect on the body and is called rasa. Just as our sense of sight perceives a particular colour or other events that ultimately create physiological and emotional reactions in us, similarly the tongue indicates specific taste but that particular taste also has its effect on our system when it is consumed.

There are six rasas in Ayurveda:

Sweet
Sour
Saline
Pungent
Bitter
Astringent

In modern biology, only four tastes are recognised according to the presence of the taste buds on the tongue. Pungent and astringent are not recognised. In fact, pungent and astringent are recognised by other parts of the body directly and it is not exclusively the tongue that detects them.

According to Ayurvedic principles, each rasa is composed of two fundamental elements. It has its influence on our body's three principal energies as it brings us the elements it is composed of. For example, the **sweet** rasa is composed of water and earth. It is obviously kapha promoting and it pacifies vata and pitta. The **sour** rasa is from fire and water and it enhances pitta and kapha, whereas it pacifies vata. The **saline** rasa is from fire and earth and has a similar character to sour. Thus, the first three rasas, the sweet, sour and saline are kapha promoting and vata-pacifying.

The fourth rasa is **pungent**, and it is constituted from air and fire. It is vata and pitta promoting and kapha decreasing. The picture that emerges is that **sour**, **saline** and **pungent** are pitta-promoting. The fifth rasa is a **bitter** rasa, which is from ether and air. Obviously, it promotes vata but pacifies pitta and kapha. The sixth rasa is **astringent,** which is from air and earth and it enhances vata but pacifies pitta and kapha. Thus, the last three rasas– the **pungent**, **bitter** and **astringent** enhance vata, but pacify kapha. I have summarised below in Table 1 the total picture that emerges from the six rasas.

Table 1. The Relationships of the Rasas and the Energies

Energy	Promoting Rasas	Pacifying Rasa
VATA	Pungent, bitter, astringent	Sweet, sour, saline
PITTA	Sour, saline, pungent	Sweet, bitter, astringent
KAPHA	Sweet, sour, saline	Pungent, bitter astringent

Examples of different rasas

Sweet: Wheat, rice, barley, maize, mung beans, masoor beans, honey, sugar, most fruits, milk, butter, ghee, meat of wild animals are some examples of sweet rasa.
Sour: Citrus fruits, other sour tasting fruits like plums, peaches, kiwi etc., tomatoes, rhubarb and so on.
Saline: Various kinds of salt.
Pungent: Ginger, garlic, pepper and many other spices

Bitter: Endives, asparagus, bitter gourd, dandelion, arugula (rocket salad).
Astringent: Spinach, dates, unripe fruits, figs and so on.

Exceptions to the rasa theory:

1. Honey, crystal candy, meat of the wild animals, old rice, barley, wheat and mung beans are not kapha promoting despite having sweet rasa.
2. Amala (a fruit of exceptional energy-promoting qualities from the Northern India) and pomegranate, despite having a sour rasa, are known to bring balance of the three energies.
3. Despite having saline rasa, rock salt does not promote kapha.

Essential Features of Ayurvedic Food Preparation

The essence of the Ayurvedic balanced nutrition lies in balancing the five elements of the body with the five elements of the nutrition we consume. The elements in the food products are present in the form of the rasas and in the body in the form of the energies (vata, pitta and kapha). The fundamental skill of preparing a healthy and rejuvenating food lies in using all the rasas in your meals in a proportionate way so that you have the balance of all the five elements in your body. That in turn will provide you the balance of the three energies—the vata, pitta and kapha. In order to cure an imbalance arising from weather, climate, travelling or any other particular situation, the nutrition would be even more specific to maintain the equilibrium of the three energies. Thus, the concept of balance is very specific and is related to your constitution, space, time and situation.

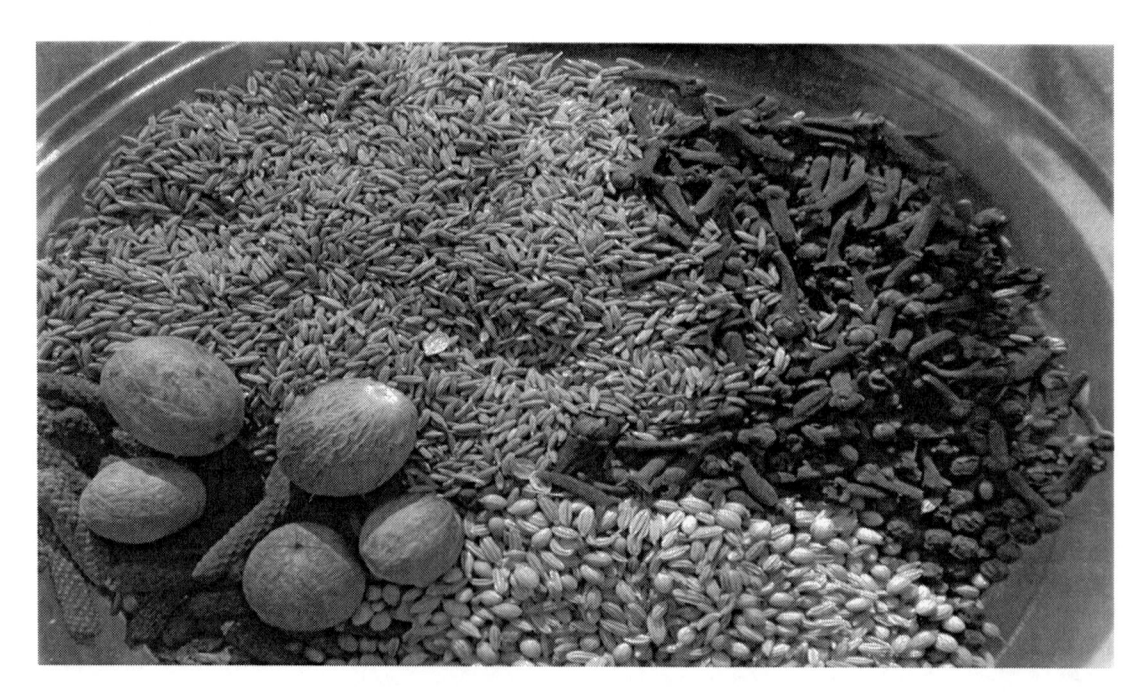

The Five-dimensional learning for Ayurvedic food preparations

Following are five fairly simple and easily comprehensible points you need to pay attention to while preparing or eating your food. They will also help you to understand the rationality of Ayurvedic food preparations in the recipe section of this book.

1. During the food preparation, you should always keep in mind to include all the rasas, and preparations should be extremely dominant in one taste. This is a fairly simple and workable method that requires only a little of your attention. For example, a sour salad sauce made of vinegar can be balanced with some jaggery or a spoon of honey. Onions provide another antidote to the sour rasa of vinegar. Bitter rasa is generally lacking in many menus. You should make an extra effort to include some bitter vegetables and salads or use bitter tasting spices in your meals.

2. Use in your menus a large variety of vegetables, fruits, grains, seeds, herbs, spices and other food substances. Do not repeatedly eat the same things branded as 'healthy'. Do not discard your favourite foods because you are told they are unhealthy. Remember that with Ayurvedic skills you can learn to make a so-called 'unhealthy' food healthy.

3. Try to eat fruits and vegetables nature provides you during the season. If you move from one place to another, try to adapt to the local products and eating habits.

4. A list of heavy to digest foods and the combinations, which are antagonist in nature, is provided in Table 4. Keep in mind that taking foodstuffs antagonistic in nature to each other or to your basic constitution can be very harmful for your health. The negative effect may not be immediate but may accumulate over a period of time. You should also observe carefully if you react negatively to a particular food or some combinations of the foods consumed at a particular time and avoid them.

5. According to Ayurveda, our food should not only provide us the necessary nutrients but also should rejuvenate us and enhance our immunity and vitality. It should also be able to cure our minor disorders arising due to an imbalance of the three energies, which perform all the physical and mental functions of the body. You will learn the use of various herbs and spices to make your food more vitalising and to specifically cure certain minor imbalances in the body. It is fairly easy to do once you have the initial understanding of Ayurvedic principles, the body's inner and outer environments and its relationship to food. Thus, while preparing your meals,

you should try to pay a little extra attention to make your food health promoting and vitality enhancing.

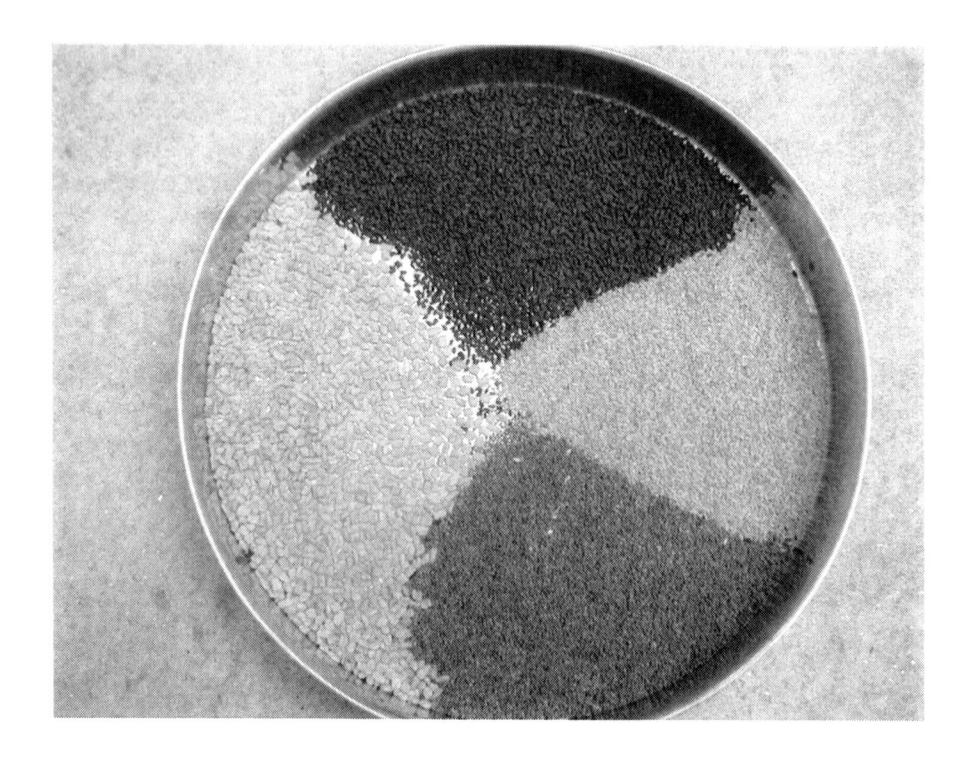

Basic Understanding of the Ayurvedic Food Culture

For understanding the Ayurvedic food culture, I have made the following simple mantra: **WHO EATS WHAT, WHEN AND WHERE, and HOW AND HOW MUCH**. You will get a comprehensive picture of essential factors involved in Ayurvedic nutrition, after understanding each of these key factors.

We will treat one by one the major factors, which should be considered in relation to nutrition. Each time, after the description of a new factor, I will discuss its relationship with our nutrition and then the new aspect will be discussed in the light of the previous ones. For example, first I will explain what is understood by basic constitution in Ayurveda **(Who eats...)**. Then following it, I will relate this to your food and food habits **(Who eats what....)**. Next is the time factor, which relates to your age, time of the year etc. **(When...)**. Following that, I will relate the nutrition to both, time factor and your basic constitution. The third major factor is the place where you reside **(where....)**. The effect of your geographical location on your energies will be discussed and then this effect will be also comprehensively discussed along with the previous major factors—prakriti and time in relation to your food. The fourth and fifth factors are the quality and quantity of food and the manner you consume your food

(How and How much...). Finally, I will discuss different nutritional requirements as they relate to place, time, individual constitution, quality and quantity of food and the way the food is consumed.

WHO ARE YOU?

This part refers to your basic constitution. You have already learnt about prakriti or the fundamental constitution. I will give below some broad outlines as how to determine your fundamental constitution from your way of behaving, reacting or some of your physical features.

Observe yourself carefully and see if you have some of the following tendencies or reactions. You are quick in action, react and decide fast, get up almost with a jump when the telephone or the door bell rings, tend to feel unwell in windy, stormy weather, get easily agitated and emotional, tend to worry rather quickly, have a tendency to get dry skin. All these features show the predominance of the elements ether and air and your **constitution is vata**.

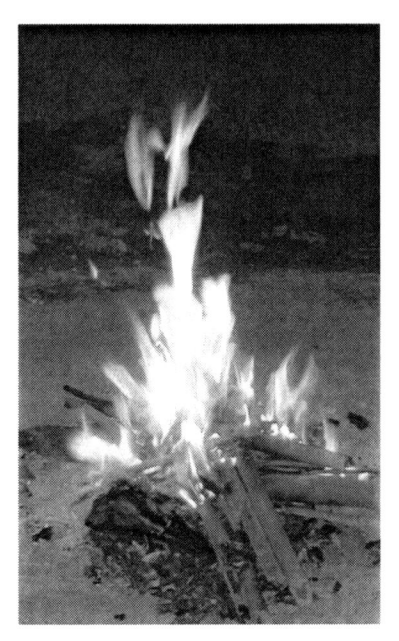

Those of you, who cannot tolerate heat, sweat easily, cannot stand hunger and thirst, have usually a hot face, tend to be intolerant and lack endurance, get easily angry specially shortly before meal times, have certainly the predominance of the element fire and your **constitution is pitta**.

If you are slow to react, have stable movements, you require time to decide, tend to have little hunger and thirst, are tolerant, tend to postpone things, then you are with the predominance of the elements water and earth and thus your **constitution is kapha.**

It is quite possible that after reading the above description, you may feel that you have features from one of the two constitutions—sometimes vata and sometimes kapha and so on. This means that you have a **mixed constitution.** Thus, we have three more types of constitutions in addition to the above three and these are **vata-pitta, vata-kapha, and pitta-kapha**. The seventh type of constitution is **samadosha** which means that all the three energies are in state of equilibrium. Thus, there are **seven principal types of constitutions.**

Introduction to the Ayurvedic Food Culture

> **RELATIONSHIP OF FOOD WITH YOUR CONSTITUTION**
>
> The five elements perform all the physical and mental functions in the form of the three principal energies of the body—the vata, pitta and kapha. These energies are constantly used and the intake of food, water and air replenishes them constantly. The equilibrium of these three energies is fundamental for good health and therefore it should be maintained with nutrition, which is well balanced in all the rasas. Our food should have all the rasas in it to maintain constantly the equilibrium.
>
> In addition to this basic equilibrium in food, we should be careful about our predominant energy. Food and other factors like weather, age etc. can easily affect the sensitive energy that is already predominant and create an imbalance and thus can give rise to a state of non-health or vikriti (minor disorder). For example, if your vata is dominating and you happen to eat dry, cold, preserved food dominating in pungent, bitter and astringent rasa, you may have vata vitiation. Vitiated vata may cause one or more of the following: stiff body, constipation, dry skin, disturbed sleep or sleeplessness, restlessness, dry throat, shivers and so on. Thus, if your vata is dominating then your food should not be predominant in vata. You should try to balance it with some specific herbs and spices. It is the similar logic for the other two energies. The information about specific herbs and spices will be provided in the proceeding Chapters.

WHEN DO YOU EAT WHAT

This refers to the time in terms of your age, time of the day and time of the year.

AGE

During childhood the kapha is enhanced. The water and earth elements predominate. Childhood is the period of growth. Recall that kapha is the energy which is responsible for the formation of the solid structure of the body. As a child grows older, the kapha energy lessens gradually and the pitta energy begins to dominate. According to Ayurveda, the childhood is considered up to 17 years. Pitta dominates during youth and during this time one has more of the fire element. As we grow older, gradually the pitta diminishes and vata begins to dominate. The old age is vata promoting.

TIME OF THE DAY

The early hours of the morning as well as of the evening are predominant in kapha. That means the time around the sunrise and the sunset; let us say from 6 AM to 10 AM and from 6 PM to 10 PM. This period is followed by the dominance of pitta. That means from 10 AM to 2 PM and from 10 PM to 2 AM. Thus the noontime as well as midnight is predominating in pitta. Later part of the night as well as of the afternoon is vata dominating. From 2 PM to 6 PM and from 2 AM to 6 AM are the vata times of the day. The precision of the hours given here is flexible according to summer and winter months and I am giving these timings just to give you an approximate idea.

TIME OF THE YEAR

Since different seasons are during different times of the year in various parts of the world, let me give the specifications of the climate. Dry, cold and windy weather is vata dominating. Cold and rainy weather is kapha dominating whereas hot and dry summer months are pitta dominating. Hot and humid weather is predominantly kapha-pitta.

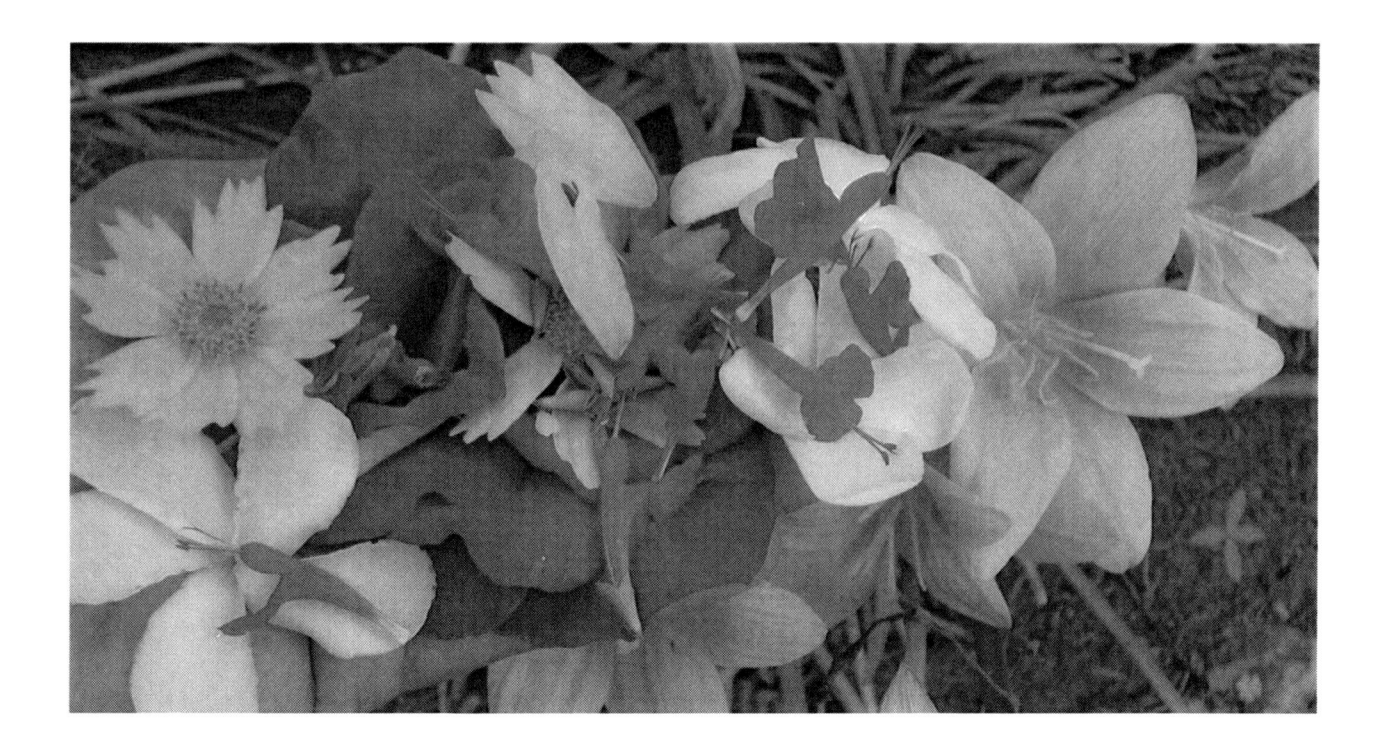

Table 2. Relationship of the time of the day, age and climate to human constitution or prakriti.

ENERGIES	TIME	AGE	CLIMATE
KAPHA	Morning Evening	Childhood	Humid-Cold
PITTA	Noon Midnight	Youth	Dry-Hot
VATA	Afternoon Night	Adulthood	Dry-cold & Windy

Note: The hot and humid climate is pitta-kapha promoting.

RELATIONSHIP OF FOOD TO YOUR CONSTITUTION AND TIME

In the kapha predominant childhood, children with kapha constitution tend to be more sensitive to the vitiation and disorders of kapha. In addition to that, the babies are fed on milk, which is kapha dominating. We all know that babies tend to throw up to varying degrees and are prone to chest congestion. Kapha vitiation in babies leads to suppression of pitta just as the water and earth will suppress the fire. Thus, by adding some fire element through food, we can solve this problem. Simple ingredients like garlic, ginger, pepper, fenugreek and basil in the nursing mother's food or addition of a very small quantity of pepper and basil in baby's milk can solve this problem.

Youth is pitta dominating and persons of pitta constitution may get vitiation of this energy if they do not take appropriate care. They may suffer from rash, acne, tearing of the skin, outbursts of anger, sense of dissatisfaction and so on. The foods with fire element will enhance these problems in this situation whereas the nutrients cold in nature like rice, milk, anise, and substances dominated in bitter rasas will prevent the problem of pitta vitiation.

Old age is predominantly vata and generally people do not alter their food with age. If someone has already a vata dominating constitution and through wrong food and life-style vitiates this energy, its bad effects will come to light particularly at this time of one's life. That is why we see that many people after their fifties suffer from vata ailments like hypertension, insomnia, haemorrhoids, various pains and aches, arthritis and so on. All these ailments are the result of vitiated vata for a long time. With little care, we can save ourselves from this category of ailments, which essentially arise due to self-created imbalance.

Thus, according to age, one should change one's nutrition and the specificity of this change depends upon your constitution.

With respect to time, there are two more factors—the time of the day and the time of the year. According to the predominance of rasas, in a simplified way, the nutrients can be divided in cold, hot and balanced categories (see Table 3 for more details). The logic is that on a winter night, if we eat a meal that is predominantly cold in its Ayurvedic nature, it will have an ill effect on us. The ill effect will be even more pronounced if the prakriti is kapha or vata, and it is childhood or old age. Similarly, consuming things, which are hot in their Ayurvedic nature on a summer noon, may lead to troubles related to pitta vitiation, more so during youth and for pitta prakriti.

WHERE TO EAT WHAT

In the mountains the climate is predominant in vata-kapha whereas on the coastal areas it is kapha-pitta dominating. The forest is vata predominant whereas the desert is vata-pitta dominating. The climate of midlands is dominating in none. Thus where we live is very important to what we eat and all the other factors we have discussed above.

RELATIONSHIP OF FOOD TO YOUR CONSTITUTION, TIME AND PLACE

Now we have an additional dimension to consider along with our fundamental constitution and time factor. Who we are, when it is and where we are, have to be considered in reference to what we eat. For example if you live in the mountains, your diet should have things, which are hot in their Ayurvedic nature to save yourself from vata-kapha vitiation. You have to take even more care in this respect if you are already predominant in vata and you are no more at the prime of your youth. Children have to be equally protected from the vitiation of kapha. In addition to this, during the windy cold air of winter in the mountains, one has to take even more precautions.

> If we move from one geographical location to the other, it is very important to change our food habits accordingly. Otherwise, even if we take care of the other factors like our age, time of the day and our constitution, we can create an imbalance due to the effect of the nature of the place we live in. For example, from midlands, if we go to the mountain area, which has also forest, the change of place may affect us immediately if we do not take care of our nutrition. It does not mean that we have to entirely change our food items, it is just the addition of some herbs and spices can take care of this change. For instance, the use of ginger, garlic, fenugreek and few more grains and herbs alike will take care of this problem. In a similar manner, we have to pay attention to coastal areas with the dominance of kapha-pitta and the desert with the dominance of vata-pitta.

WHAT TO EAT IN SPECIFIC CIRCUMSTANCES

There are prescriptions of foods for the states of weakness, fatigue or when you lead a hectic life style or contrary to that when you have a sedentary lifestyle. The specific circumstances may be there due to sudden untimely change of weather or travelling or the specific nature of your job. Another aspect of this theme is the presence of minor disorders produced either due to internal imbalance of the body (imbalance of vata, pitta, kapha) or due to external attacks of bacteria, viruses or parasites or due to accidental injuries or mental shocks. This is of course a very expansive subject and I will not deal with every topic related to this theme in the present volume. The most important theme will be fatigue that most people suffer from one way or the other. According to Ayurveda, to get over fatigue, we need to enhance ojas in the body. Ojas is the immunity and vitality of the body. When ojas is up, we feel invigorated and energetic. Ojas is increased by the intake of rasayanas in our food. Rasayanas are those products, which have rasas in concentration. A most common example of rasayana in our food is garlic. Garlic is a strong rasayana. Cumin, coriander, Curcuma (turmeric), ginger, basil, cardamom and saffron are other examples. Besides the specific rasayanas, the balanced nutrition will help establish the lost equilibrium and will enhance ojas. In my previous books, I have given several recipes of rasayanas made simply and out of easily available Ayurvedic spices and other kitchen ingredients. In the present book, the food recipes are designed in such a way that you prepare rejuvenating foods, which enhance your ojas.

HOW AND HOW MUCH YOU SHOULD EAT

Inappropriate way of eating, like eating while standing or walking or eating too fast or too slow or in a state of anger and so on, can give rise to several ailments. Eating too frequently and in large quantities also leads to disorders. In fact, these factors are the cause of numerous ailments amongst the wealthy folks on this earth. Even if you cook the balanced Ayurvedic food but eat too much, or too frequently or in an angry or anguished mental state, the food will show its harmful effects. Here are the Eight Golden Principles of the Ayurvedic food culture that you should never forget.

THE EIGHT GOLDEN PRINCIPLES of Ayurvedic Food Culture

1. Food should be warm, unctuous and fluid and should be **served** in a beautiful manner to create the congenial and aesthetic atmosphere for its consumption.
2. Never **consume** food under stressful circumstances or under any emotional restraint. If you happen to be in such a state shortly before your meal, wait for a while, do some breathing exercises, wash your face with cold water and then sit comfortably for taking your meal.
3. **Before beginning your meal**, bring your mind to your food, which is the fundamental basis of body's energy. Look at your food and make a wish that the five elements of the food may provide you with equilibrium, vigour and good health. Say a little prayer or mantra to bring your mind to stillness.
4. The food should be **eaten neither too slow nor too fast.** You should not speak with the food in the mouth.
5. Ayurveda recommends **drinking** either before or one hour after the meal. If required to drink along with food, one may consume liquid in small quantities. Ayurveda recommends drinking only very good quality of wine or beer in a small quantity with food. Juices and milk should not be taken with food. Water is highly recommended. The food should be fluid and should include some soup or something similar.
6. Never eat anything **before the previous meal is completely digested.** According to Ayurveda, it is poisonous for the body if one eats when the body is still in the process of digesting the previous meal. Do not eat anything four hours after having eaten something. For your stomach, a little thing like a piece of chocolate or a fruit is also food to be worked upon and digested. Thus, strictly do not eat anything between meals. Leave a gap of 10 to 12 hours between dinner and breakfast and at least two hours between dinner and going to bed.
7. Many people make themselves sick by eating too much. According to Ayurveda, you should always eat that quantity, which fills the **stomach to two thirds and not totally full**. It means, eat to the limit when you feel comfortably satisfied and not so full that you cannot eat any more. The logic of this is that the three energies also require place in the stomach for the digestion of the food. If the stomach is made full to its utmost capacity, during digestion, the energies are pushed out and give rise to vitiation causing thereby various digestive troubles. This may also give rise to

amadosha. Amadosha is the partial digestion of the food and undigested food remains in the stomach and intestines, ultimately leading to toxicity in the whole body. For the well-being of the body and for avoiding serious ailments related to digestion, it is absolutely essential to have discipline for the quantity of food you consume.

8. Never take a **shower or bath immediately after eating**. Wait at least two hours, preferably three hours. In any case, it is better to have shower or bath before eating. Also avoid any form of vigorous exercise after food. All these vitiate vata. Going for a slow walk after dinner is highly recommended.

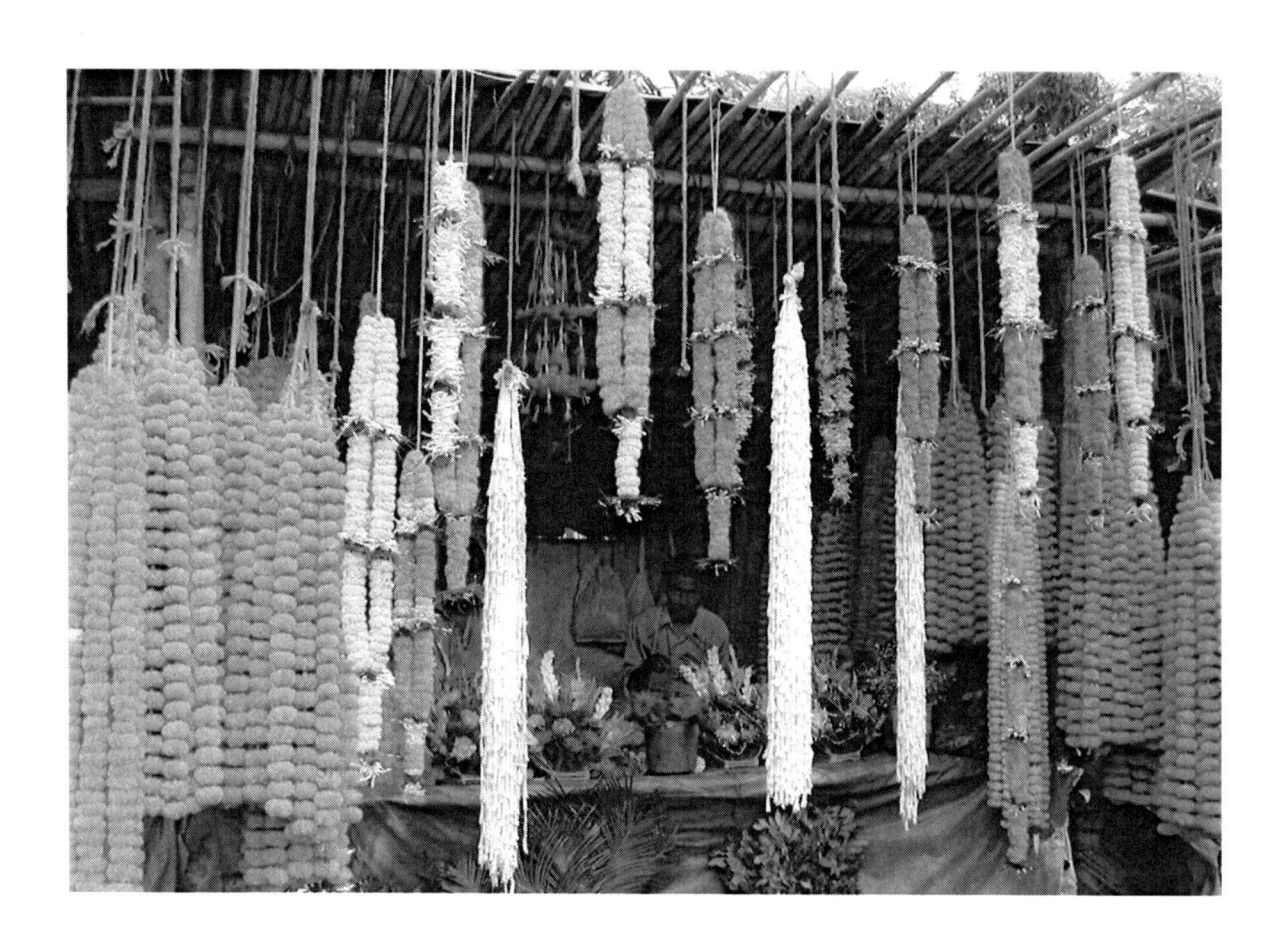

The Practical Aspects of Ayurvedic Food Preparations

When people grow up in a particular culture, they assimilate the wisdom of life related to that culture without searching for how and why. They intuitively follow the wise pattern because it was always done like that. Finding the wise ways for life, which benefit humanity, their rationalisation and analysis is done generally by intellectuals and sages. Ayurvedic cooking has been a part of Indian life for many thousand years and an average home follows this wisdom in a simple and practical way. For practical purpose, foods are either hot or cold. Hot foods promote pitta whereas cold ones promote either vata or kapha or both. There are some foods that have a natural equilibrium of the three energies and these foods are health promoting by establishing an equilibrium of the three energies. Contrary to that, there are nutrients, which do not have natural balance. Hot and cold foods should be balanced with each other to create equilibrium. The balanced foods should be taken often and especially during and after an illness or when one is suffering from weakness and fatigue. The foods that are not balanced in nature should never be consumed without appropriate herbs, spices and other combinations to make them balanced. They should never be consumed in excessive quantity.

Individuals have also hot and cold constitutions. Hot constitution is pitta, cold is kapha or vata. Vata is dry cold whereas pitta is wet cold. Hot and cold state of an individual may also be temporary due to some special situations like fatigue, sickness, and sudden change of place or of weather and climate.

The first and foremost effort should be to prepare a balanced meal. A balanced meal will be good for all types of constitutions and will also gradually cure the imbalance of the body. However if the imbalance is too great or it is to the extent of being a minor disorder, you need some treatment with some of the things from your Ayurvedic cuisine. For example if you are suffering from menstrual pains, half teaspoon of kalonji should be used everyday in your soup or vegetables. For lactating mothers, use of kalonji, dried ginger and fenugreek will help enhance quantity and quality of the milk. For those who have too much heat in their bodies and show signs of pitta dominance or vitiation, fennel, liquorice and coriander should be enhanced in diet. In case of kapha dominance or upon having the signs of its vitiation, hot and spicy food should be taken. Fatty and sweet food should be avoided.

The Practical Aspects of Ayurvedic Food Preparations

I am often asked how one should cope with cooking in a family where people are of varied constitutions. I grew up in an extended family that was equivalent to about six nuclear families. From an Ayurvedic point of view, balanced meals were prepared but those who felt that they required something special for their conditions, heated the specific spices and grains they required in ghee and added these to their food. One of my childhood memories is that my grandfather always wanted to add asafoetida and garlic in his *dal* (a preparation of dried beans or lentils) and my grandmother detested the smell of these both. She being a pitta person needed something sweet and mild to pacify her fire whereas the grandfather wanted to control his vata and to rejuvenate himself. Along with the description of the spices, I will give some suggestions regarding their use for healing.

Ayurvedic nutrition in its theory as well as in practice is not what you will find written in some of the recently published books on the subject. Ayurveda never tells you that according to your different constitutions you should choose to eat certain food items and leave out others. If it were so, then where is the skill of balance? Ayurvedic wisdom tells you with what to balance your favourite food so that it does not harm you. Imagine your little daughter who very often asked you for potatoes but she is pitta in her constitution. First of all, while preparing potatoes, which are hot in their Ayurvedic properties, you should add spices like anise and coriander. Secondly, you should add to the meal the other things, which are cold in their Ayurvedic nature. For example, desserts with cream and sweet fruits, vegetables like pumpkin, carrots or similar kind that help create equilibrium.

Rasas in practice

It is essential to train oneself to feel the total effect of a substance in reference to its taste. Nature provides us with fruits and vegetables, which automatically have a balancing effect on us according to various seasons. For example the presence of many juicy, sweet fruits or bitter vegetables or salads in summer has a cooling effect on our body. Fruits with sour taste in winter provide us with the fire element. The best method to enter into the Ayurvedic food culture is to begin by remembering the foods, which are hot, cold and balanced by nature. There are also heavy to digest and antagonist foods. I give below a list of these four categories. To balance hot vegetables, use spices which are cold in their Ayurvedic nature or else eat the hot foods in combination with the cold foods. Besides that, take care of the individual constitution, time, place or any other specific situation simultaneously.

In Table 3, I have classified the major foods of the world into three categories: hot, cold and balanced. In the sections of cold foods, it is indicated specifically the foods which enhance excessively vata and thus should be carefully cooked with ginger, garlic or fenugreek or other spices which are hot in nature. They should be also avoided when you have already vata imbalance or you have been doing vata actions like travelling, keeping awake at night or a hectic life style. When the weather is windy or stormy (vata promoting), these foods should be avoided or prepared carefully with appropriate spices. They should also not be consumed in large quantities. In case, you do that in certain circumstances, take half a teaspoon of ajwain with some rock salt or normal salt and some drops of lemon on it. Take this mixture after food and swallow it with some warm water. This way, the counter effect of an unbalanced food is taken care of and you save yourself from vikriti.

In Table 4, I have classified foods, which are heavy to digest and should be consumed less frequently and in small quantities. This table also contains the list of antagonist food combinations, which are extremely harmful for health and should be absolutely avoided.

Table 3. Classification of major food products according to their cold, hot or balanced Ayurvedic nature

FOODS COLD IN NATURE

Grains: Wheat, rice, maize (promotes vata), barley (increases vata), common millet and Italian millet (enhances vata), masoor beans (also called red lentils) (promotes vata), young green peas, ripe green peas (strongly vata promoting, chick peas
Vegetables: Spinach, cabbage and Brussels sprouts (vata), okra, green beans, bitter gourd, endives, fennel, aubergine, onion, celery, cucumber, beetroot, sweet paprika (without seeds), dandelion, asparagus
Fruit: Apples (sweet), bananas, pears, apricot, guava, muskmelon, watermelon, figs
Dairy products: Milk, ghee, butter
Meat: Frog, seafood, sea fish, mutton
Herbs and spices: Clove, coriander, fennel, anise, dill leaves (not the seeds), liquorice
Others: Sugar

FOODS HOT IN NATURE

Grains: Urad beans, soya beans
Vegetables: cress salad, potatoes, cauliflower, tomatoes
Fruit: Oranges, grapefruit, lemon, grapes (which are not absolutely sweet), peaches, plumbs, kiwis (specially the black seeds in kiwi), nuts (almonds, peanuts, hazelnuts, walnuts, pine nuts and others), sour apples
Dairy products: Yoghurt, processed cheese

Meat: Pork, horse, beef, freshwater fish
Herbs and spices: Greater cardamom, cumin, cinnamon, black pepper or white pepper, fenugreek, kalonji, garlic, basil, dill seeds, ajwain, mustard seeds, nutmeg, mint
Others: Honey, vegetable oils, eggs (hen, fish)

FOODS WITH NATURAL EQUILIBRIUM

Grains: Finger millet, mung beans, chickpeas at the beginning of germination
Vegetables: Carrots, turnips, small radish (not over-ripped), zucchini, pumpkin (just ripened),
Fruit: Sweet mangoes, papaya, pomegranate, grapes (sweet)
Meat: Deer, goat, chicken
Herbs and spices: Small cardamom, ginger, turmeric or *Curcuma*

Table 4. List of heavy to digest and antagonist foods

HEAVY TO DIGEST FOODS

Vegetarian foods: Urd beans, over-ripe peas, animal or plant fat, nuts or preparation from nuts, any vegetables or fruit or a preparation of food that has an extreme taste like sour, sweet, pungent, bitter, astringent, salty and when consumed in excess, unripe or over-ripe vegetables and fruits, yoghurt when eaten several times a day and specially at night

Non-vegetarian foods: Pork, beef, meat of animals kept under stressful conditions, animal fat or foods containing animal fat in large quantities.

ANTAGONISTIC FOOD COMBINATIONS

1. Milk in combination with sour foods, radish, water melon or fish
2. Honey in any heated form or taking a hot drink immediately after taking honey
3. Fatty food in combination with cold drinks or cold water
4. Use of diet adverse to a person's food habits
5. Combination of too hot and too cold foods
6. Food antagonism to time, place and constitution
7. Foods excessively dominating in one particular rasa like excessively salty, sweet, sour etc.

Methods for Balanced Food Preparations

Besides the above-described groups of food (hot, cold, balanced, heavy to digest and antagonists), there is another dimension that you should be aware of—the preparation method. In a prepared food, its effect is in relation to what we have made out of the ingredients and not the individual effect of all the ingredients. For example, with semolina, butter or ghee and some sugar, you can make biscuits (cookies). According to Ayurveda, it will be a dry and cold food and since this can be kept for a long time, it becomes also *basa**. Thus, this preparation will possibly vitiate vata, and also kapha due to the consumption of cold fat, especially when eaten frequently. With the same ingredients, you can make a warm preparation like a halva, which is easy to digest and is specially given to pacify vata (see the recipe Section).

After having learnt the basic qualities of some most common foods in the world, you can now take into consideration some other aspects we have discussed above. For example, during summer months, you should use cooling products as compared to hot ones. In extremely hot weather, leave out the products, which are hot in their Ayurvedic nature, specially the spices like fenugreek, dill seeds, kalonji, garlic etc. In case you use them, combine them with cooling spices like anise or fennel, coriander, clove etc. Similarly, in winter, the reverse should be kept in mind. Always remember that the food products are not good or bad for you. The same food can have a healing effect on you at one time of the year or in one particular situation, whereas it may prove to be disastrous and may make you sick at another time. Take a simple example of cold sweetened milk. In summer, it is anti-heat and thus is extremely good to counteract the heat. After an over-spiced meal that may give you a burning sensation, the cold sweetened milk is curative. It also cures acidity and is advised to be taken after meals to cure this ailment. But the same cold sweetened milk, taken during winter nights may cause kapha vitiation, and may have an excessively diuretic effect. If taken regularly, you may end up having various kapha-related disorders. In winter, drink hot sweetened milk with a pinch of saffron in it. It will rejuvenate you and will save you from catching cold.

In brief, food products are not good or bad for health and all that brings harmony and balance is good, and all that takes away the equilibrium and pushes you towards a state of vikriti (an unhealthy state) is bad. The nature of the food and your constitution are the basic important factors along with time and place. Some special circumstances may give you a temporary imbalance and that should be taken care with specific menus.

Discovering the Rasas of the Cosmos

Ayurvedic pharmacology is based upon rasa theory. These principles are applied on nutrition as well as on medicines. The remedies, which are generally a combination of several plants and minerals, are balanced by adding specific

---

* *Basa* is that food which is not freshly prepared or kept for several days after preparation. Foods kept in refrigerator or freezer or preserved with other methods to enhance shelf life are also considered basa. These foods cause vata vikriti.

rasas to counter their side effects. Similarly, the food products, which are heavy to digest and are known to have a strong effect on the body, are balanced in their rasas by adding other substances. Now, the question arises, since there are innumerable food items, how can one possibly know the Ayurvedic properties of all of them? In fact it is fairly simple to learn that with rasa theory, do the following in three different steps:

1. Put a small morsel of food on your tongue and concentrate on it. There are dominant rasas and there are subtle rasas, which you may detect after a little while. But you need to concentrate on your tongue and note its reactions to the piece of food.
2. If the food has tiny seeds which are also eaten, then you need to do this rasa experiment in three different steps:
   - with a mixture of those tiny seeds with pulp
   - with the pulp alone
   - with the crushed seeds alone.
3. Eat the food in different quantities and observe carefully its effect on yourself.

Write all the data on a piece of paper. If you detect more than one rasa, write them in a sequence of their domination. First consult the rasa table (Table 1) and find out the properties. In fact, if one rasa is dominating and other is very mild in proportion, it is likely that the substance has the properties of the dominating rasa.

Then eat this particular food in a sizable quantity and see if it has some special effect on your body. For example, if the food is hot in nature, you may feel excessive heat inside you, your urine may turn yellow or it may have some other effect like enhancing the hunger and so on. It may be possible that you may get constipation or dryness from your food under test and obviously, it is vata in qualities. Suppression of hunger or sense of saturation after consuming a particular food denotes its kapha characteristics.

Alcohol and Tobacco

Ayurveda recommends a modest quantity of good wine (madira) or beer (sura). In ancient India, they made a large variety of wines from various health promoting and rejuvenating plant products. For the consumption of alcoholic beverages, I have the following suggestions.

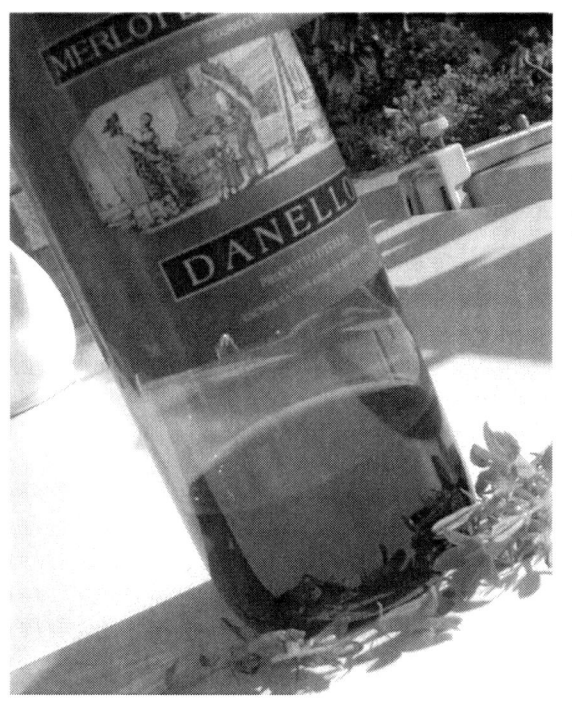

1. You may drink a good quality alcoholic beverage regularly but only in small quantities. A maximum of two drinks are suggested. Never compromise with cheaper wines or other beverages. They may harm you if consumed frequently. The bad effect may be on your stomach and nerves. Replace low quality alcoholic beverages with pure water.

2. Observe carefully the effect of a particular beverage on yourself. Sometimes, artificial colours or flavours are used, which may give rise to allergies or other side effects. Some beverages may give you headache even when they are consumed in a small quantity.

3. Never drink any alcoholic beverage on an empty stomach. In Ayurveda, it is recommended that you drink with your meals. If you wish to drink something before a meal, than make sure that you take a little something with or before the alcohol. French do well to drink wine with their meals. Intake of alcoholic beverage on an empty stomach may harm the epithelial cell lining of the stomach, thus causing ulcers or other stomach disorders.

4. Alcoholic beverages are pitta promoting. Persons with a pitta constitution should be especially careful with the side-effects of alcohol.

5. Beverages with bitter substances like Wormwood (Vermouth or absinthe) or orange peels have a counter-effect on alcohol and thus are better than the others.

6. Avoid wines which are sour in taste. Always remember that any rasa taken in extreme is harmful.

7. Do not continue drinking alcoholic beverages after meals. In some countries, people drink hard liquor after dinner under the pretext of having to digest the meal. Brandies can be helpful in case of low blood pressure or extreme cold or during trekking in the high mountains. In normal circumstances, you may use some fruit alcohols for flavouring the fruit salads or other desserts.

Tobacco is not considered as food. But according to Ayurveda, all that is taken inside the body through any mode is considered as nourishment. Generally people smoke tobacco but in many parts of the world, they chew it. Tobacco came from the New World but in Ayurveda, several other plants are recommended for smoking. It is suggested to smoke very ceremoniously for relaxation. As in case of alcohol, very moderate quantities of smoking herbs are recommended. Smoking is recommended in some cases as a remedy. In case of sickness or indigestion, it is sometimes helpful to smoke.

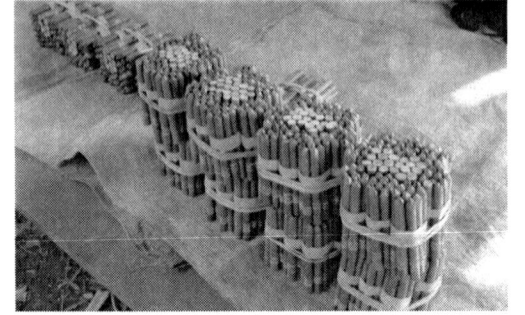

Food as Nectar or Poison

The equilibrium of food is essential for good health and harmony, because an unbalanced diet can lead to vikriti. I cite some case studies to show how through ignorance, people can gradually harm themselves and impair their vigour and looks.

1. A young deliveryman once sought my medical help to stop his hair from falling. He told me that he was not married and if he became bald, no woman would marry him! He was quite desperate and started buying from me a hair oil for treatment. I told him that external treatment alone would not help and I needed to know about his diet and life-style. One day I casually asked him what he ate for breakfast. He told me that he was taking 4 or 5 eggs and bread, among other things. The reason for his loss of hair was quite evident; eggs are hot, and in a hot place like Delhi, he built too much heat in his body. Pitta vitiation causes hair fall, wrinkles in the skin and skin eruptions. You may have several or one of these problems.
2. A young lady who despite being attractive looked listless and drab came to me for consultation in Germany. Her trouble was dry skin, nervousness and disturbed sleep that she has been having for the past few months. These are all vata vitiation symptoms. It turned out that she has been following an American diet prescription to lose weight that allows you all except animal fat. It is well known in Ayurveda as well as in modern biology that our body needs both animal and plant fat. Animal fat is taken in the form of meat, butter, ghee, milk, cheese, yoghurt and other milk products. Lack of animal fat in the body disturbs vata and you will get various symptoms of vata vikriti.
3. There are many cases that have a contrary situation than the above. People eat excessive fat, or some antagonist nutrients or drink a lot and bad quality wine and alcohol, it tells upon their liver besides their weight. Liver malfunction can give rise to white or brown spots of the skin.

Many stomach problems are caused due to amadosha. Ama is the presence of partially digested food inside the stomach. Ama hinders the stomach to perform its full functions and also brings impurities in the blood. This later can cause skin problems. Ama builds up in the stomach either by eating too much or too frequently or taking antagonistic foods. If this happens, take boiled food with little ghee for few days and then follow the eight principles of Ayurvedic food culture. If you are suffering from amadosha for a long time, you will need special treatment. Nutrition therapy alone may not be sufficient.

Your Menu in Case of Vikriti

Persons of any prakriti may suffer from any vikriti but generally the dominant energy is more liable to get vitiated. For example, if you have vata prakriti and generally you get this energy vitiated due to windy weather, exposure to cold or eating dry, cold and preserved food or due to some other reason that is vata promoting. However, it is also possible that you get kapha vitiation due to eating too many fatty things, rice, and chocolates during wet and cold weather. You may get sweet taste in your mouth, feel drowsy or get other symptoms of kapha vitiation. Similarly, eating too spicy food or too much garlic or too much sour food, you may get pitta vikriti. It is important that you learn to diagnose yourself and alter your nutrition to get back to prakriti. I give below some suggestions of food you should take in case of each vikriti.

Vata vikriti makes you yawn, you may get dry throat, body ache, constipation or just fatigue. First measure to cure is to drink hot cardamom water or just any hot drink. Avoid all that is cold. Warm and liquid food like a nice carrot soup or in the morning semolina breakfast (see recipes) are highly recommended. To cure vata vitiation, it is essential to eat unctuous food. Ghee alleviates vata vitiation. Do not eat any preparation of lentils and avoid grains except wheat. Use Mixture B, D and F in your cooking (see the details of the spice mixtures on page 79-82).

Pitta vitiation is cured with cold water and with cold drinks made of syrups or sharbats. Brahmi, almond and khas sharbats are recommended. Eat fruits like papaya, sweat grapes, bananas, pears, sweet apples and apricots. Cold milk is recommended. Avoid spices like pepper, garlic and dill seeds and use fennel, coriander, cardamom, fresh ginger and clove to spice your food. Use spice Mixture C to reduce excess heat in your body.

The Practical Aspects of Ayurvedic Food Preparations

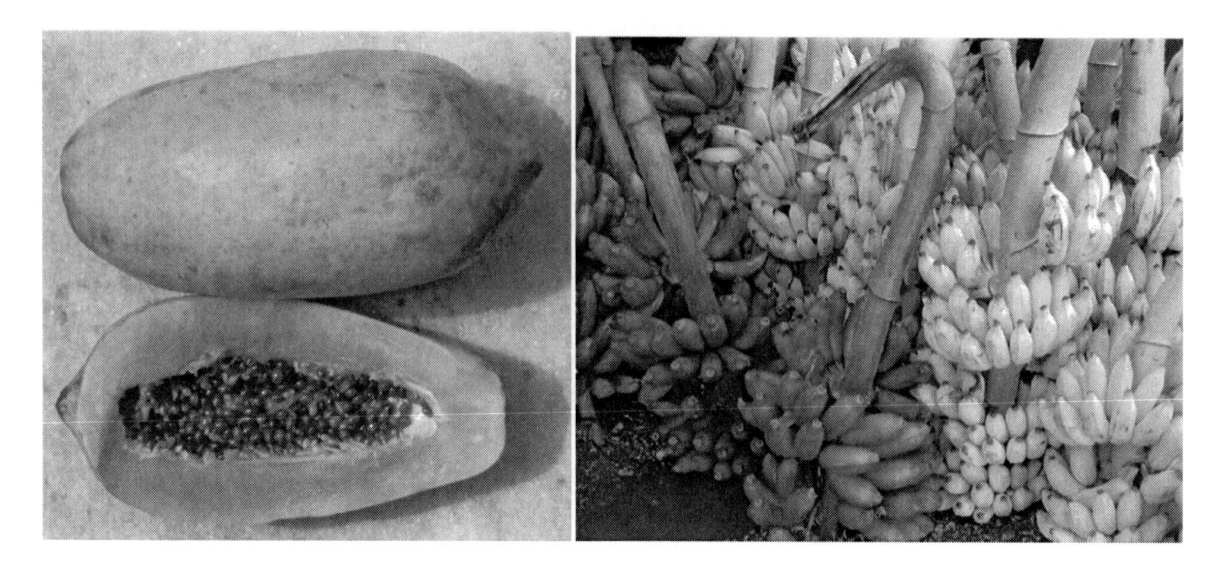

Kapha prakriti cases suffer from vikriti after consuming fatty and sweet food. This kind of food will affect them more than vata and pitta dominant persons. They may suffer from heaviness in the body and may lose initiative. Balance can be restored with the use of ginger, garlic, saffron and other spices that promote heat. Eat vegetables like bitter gourd, spinach and potatoes and fruits like peaches, plumbs, oranges and grapes. Avoid milk and milk products. Do not use ghee but oil for cooking.

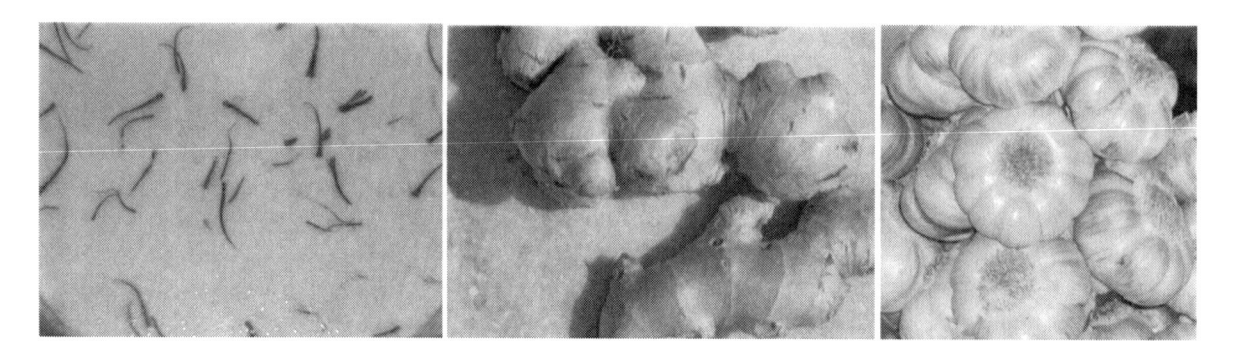

The use of different kinds of tea for treating vitiation of energies is given in Section II (see Beverages). If you are still confused and unsure about what kind of food to have when you feel unwell, eat very simple food with balanced ingredients (see Table 3). Spice it moderately and eat small portions. Give your body time to recover.

Prana in your Food

Prana means life itself or consciousness. The cause of consciousness is the soul in the body but the factor that holds the body and the soul together and is responsible for continuous vivacity is Prana. Through breathing or intake of the cosmic energy, which we call Prana, our link with the dynamic cosmos is maintained. When Prana stops, the body and the soul separate and death occurs. Breathing is not just a mechanical phenomenon that gives fuel in the form of oxygen for making the body machine work, as is thought by those who compare the living body with a machine. I have explained in one of my previous books* that the air we inhale does not constitute only the element air but all the five constituent elements of this universe.

Our food comes next to breathing for the continuity of our existence. The five fundamental elements, which are constantly supplied to our body through food, constitute the three principal energies (vata, pitta, and kapha), which perform all the physical and mental functions of the body. From the holistic point of view, nutrition does not merely fulfil the energy needs of the body, as I have pointed out above in the context of breathing. Our food contains prana energy in the form of rasas, colours, flavour, forms etc. We not only consume food in terms of its value in calories, but we also consume a subtle energy in it in the form of the 'living element' or prana. It is important that we relate to this living aspect of our food in the sense of its past and present and we consume foods which still have prana in them. The past of our food is that it was living before it was cut, chopped and prepared for our consumption. When it was living, it had an independent system of its own. In its entire form of plant or animal, it had a distinct character, form, appearance, colour, flavour etc. There are a variety of seeds we consume as food. All these are capable of giving rise to living plants. However, if they are too old, this potential of propagation is terminated in them.

---

* *Patanjali and Ayurvedic Yoga*

Prana in your Food

The seed which is consumed by most of us in large quantities, is wheat. Before you have a piece of bread on your table, it was in the form of flour. Before that there were grains and even before that, these grains were hanging on the little golden plants of wheat. Imagine all that effort which goes on to sow the seeds, care for them until the crop is ready and obtain grains. Each piece of fresh bread we consume, not only provides us energy in the form of calories to perform our bodily functions but also brings the living element or prana to us. The prana shakti or the living power in the grain depends upon the conditions and circumstances under which it is grown. If there is vitiation of Prana in that atmosphere, obviously, the food grown in the area will also be vitiated or will lack Prana. Pollution may prevent the sunrays to reach the growing plants; earth may not be appropriate in its quality or may be polluted with chemical waste and so on. Vitiation is not only caused with man-created pollution, it may be caused with natural disasters like too much or too little rain, wind or sun, and abnormal heat or cold.

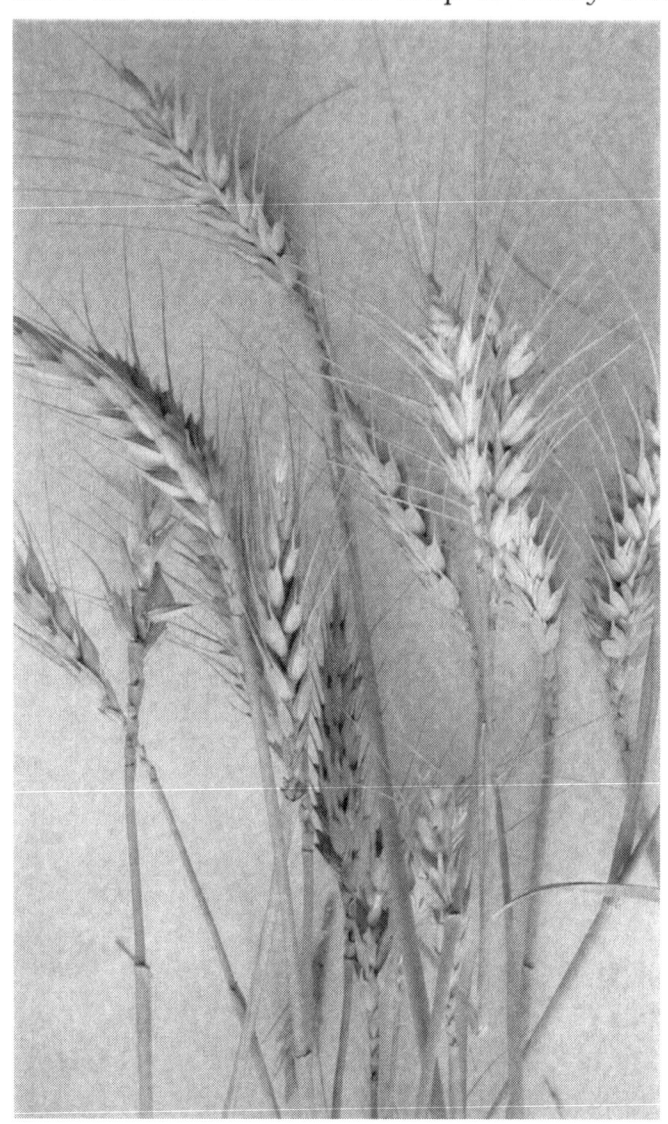

In the tradition in which Ayurveda was developed, it is believed that the manner in which the food is grown or the animals are kept has a direct effect on the physical and mental state of the person who consumes this food. Similarly, the mental state and the feelings of the person who prepares food have an effect on the taste of the food as well as on the mental state of those who consume it. It is recommended that the food should be prepared with a peaceful mental state and with love and care.

Thus, we see that there are some subtle aspects of Ayurvedic food culture, which are extremely relevant for the actual preparation of the food. Without this understanding, you will not be able to see the holistic aspects of Ayurvedic food culture, but merely look at the Ayurvedic cosmic principles in a very narrow and mechanistic way.

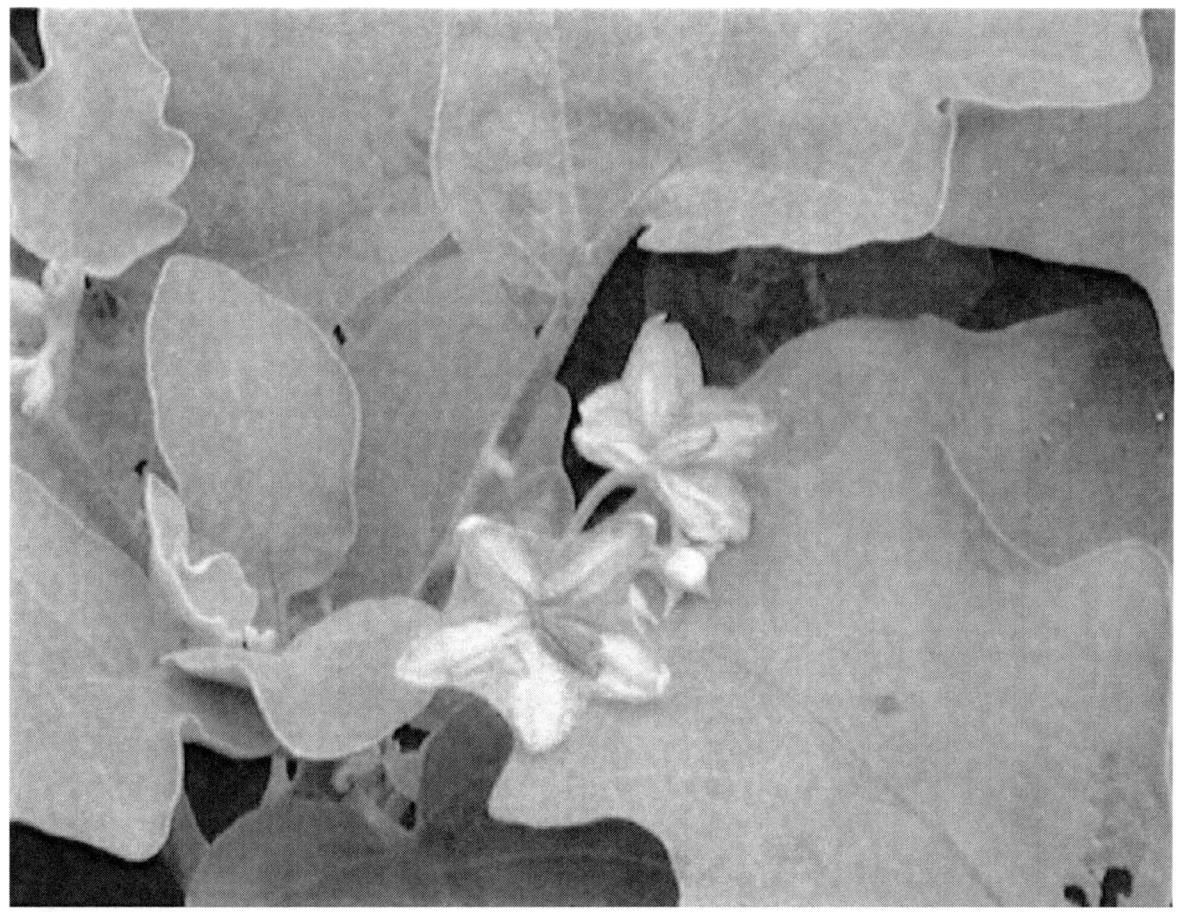

Aubergine flowers

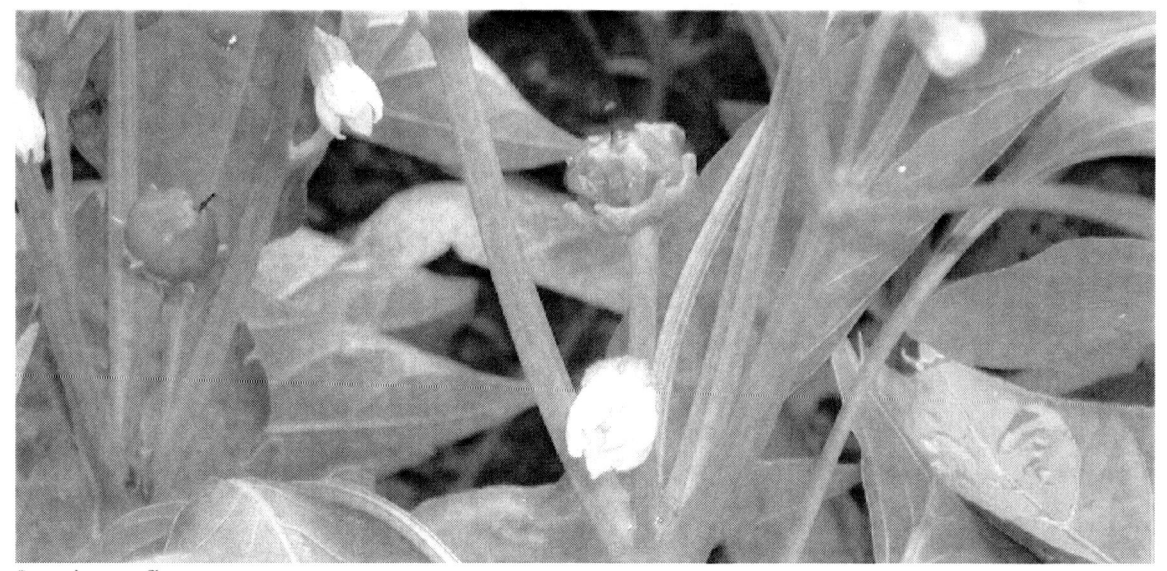

Capsicum flowers

Six Dimensions of Food

In Ayurveda, the food is not only qualified in terms of vata, pitta and kapha, but also in relation to the three qualities of the Prakriti—sattva, rajas and tamas. An over-cooked and over-spiced meal is tamasic and will give rise to tamasic qualities. Similarly, the food prepared in an angry and irritated state of mind (the tamasic qualities of the mind) will induce tamasic qualities when consumed. Simple and rightly proportioned health promoting food will promote sattva and is called sattvic. Those nutrients which promote activity and energy and cater to sensuous fulfilment have rajas qualities and are rajasic. Rajasic food will have a variety of spices, herbs and other ingredients to make it rich and delicious. There is not a hard line between foods of these three categories. The qualities may be mixed and in various proportions and it also depends upon the mode of preparation and processing. For example, over-cooked, over-spiced or preserved food and over-ripe foods will have tamasic effect on the body. Whatever the quality of the food, if over-eaten, it will have tamasic effect.

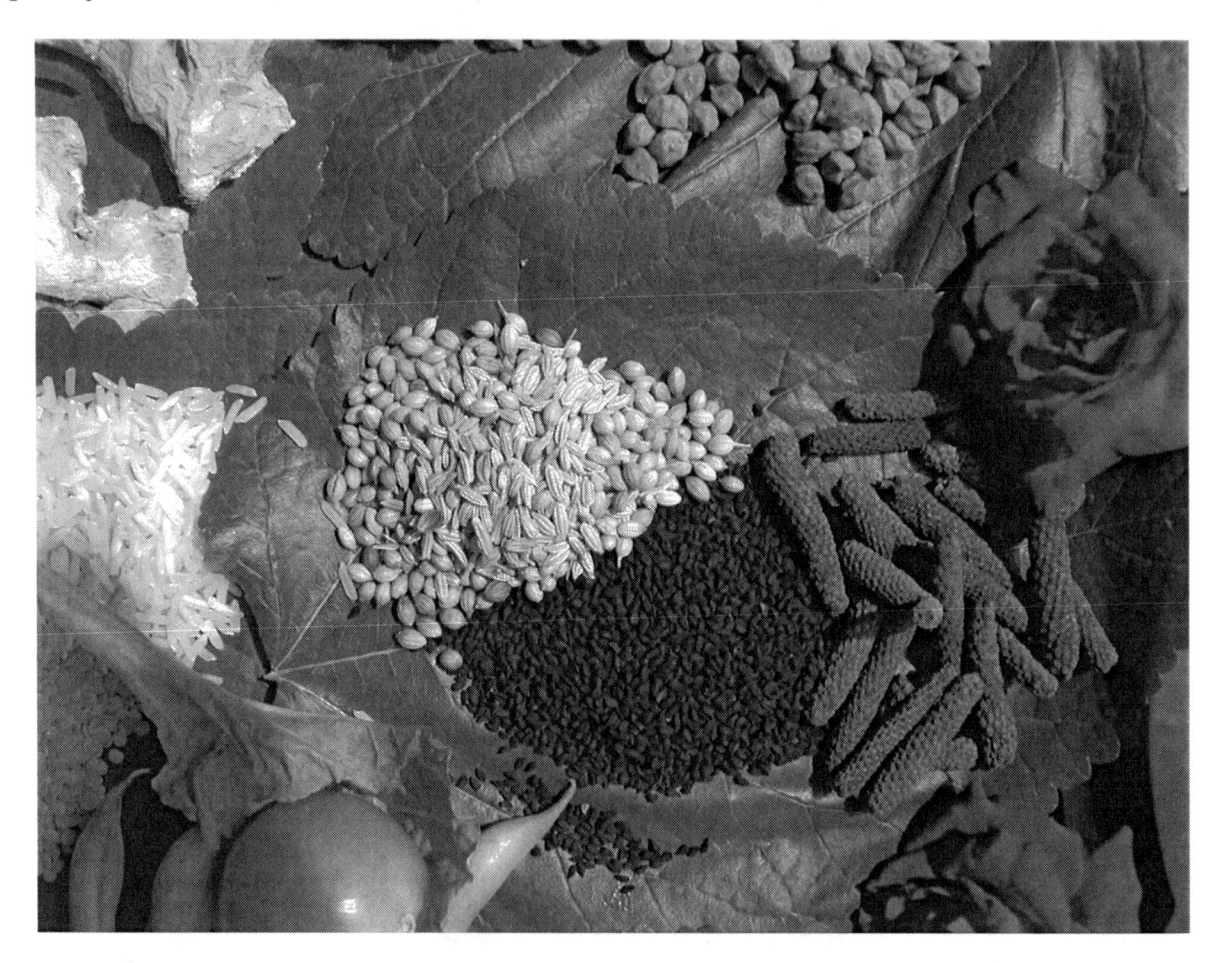

Predominantly sattvic substances are milk, rice, curd (yoghurt), ghee, vegetables of the zucchini variety, pumpkin, sweet tasting fruits, coconut, fennel, cardamom etc. A good variety of meat, wine, most spices, a large variety of fruit are predominantly rajasic in qualities. Strong smelling and sleep inducing foods and substances with narcotic effect are tamasic. Onions, oily or fatty foods, bad quality alcohol, drugs, coffee, tobacco, and so on are the substances which are tamasic in nature.

All kinds of preserved foods, drinks made with various chemical substances, fruit juices which are not freshly pressed), frozen and canned foods etc. are tamasic in their qualities. Similarly, the foods grown with chemical fertilisers and sprayed with insecticides are tamasic in nature. In developed countries, most available foods are transformed into tamasic foods. Consumption of these foods evokes tamasic thoughts in you and they also make you sluggish. Such foods lack Prana in them and are unable to provide you with appropriate vigour, energy and immune response called ojas in Ayurveda. That is why people are constantly tired and even young people look pale without any radiating and youthful energy. Fortunately, a new consciousness has arisen and people are getting aware of the harm caused by inappropriate food technology. All over the world, there are too many industrially processed foods and fast food joints that offer us anti-health products. The consumption of such products is strongly reinforced by heavy advertising tempting ordinary and poor people to consume such anti-health foods.

Our Relationship with Food

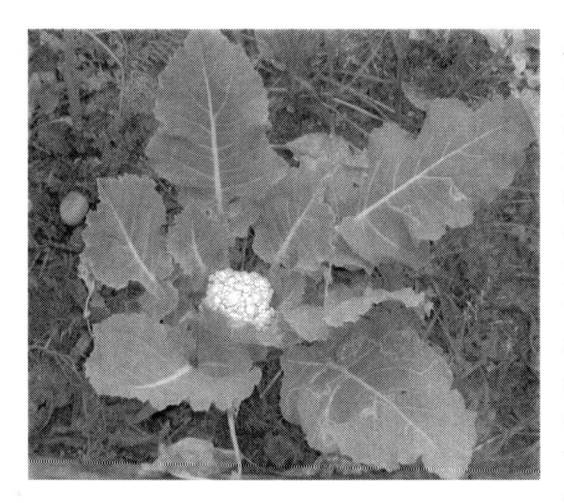

According to the Ayurvedic food culture, we should recognise the living element or Prana in our food and build a relationship with our food. We should make an effort to know about our food before it is on the table to be consumed. We should learn more about plants and animals which nourish us. If these living beings are not kept in good conditions, they cannot provide us the appropriate *shakti* or power to live. The ill effect of meat from the stressed animals is well known. Plants grown in artificial conditions and noisy and polluted environments are bound to carry their prana vikriti into us. This vikriti may not be immediately evident in our body but gradually over a long period of time, it begins to show its accumulative effect. Similarly, the food grown in a healthy environment gives us prana shakti and enhances our ojas. We look radiating, become more resistant to ailments and our work efficiency enhances. We should not forget that air and food are our life, and that the quality of our life is dependent upon them. I have a living experience of this when I am in our Himalayan centre where the food is grown with organic farming and most cooking is done in a solar cooker. After two or three days of being there, I feel the difference in my looks, energy and way of thinking. I feel that I develop more patience and tolerance and am able to work more.

The six dimensions of our food directly affect the six dimensions of our being. Besides promoting our immunity and vitality through the food we eat, we can also alter our thought process and beautify our appearance. For example, if you feel very restless and are unable to concentrate, eat sweet and unctuous things. Feeling restless and to have a wandering mind are due to vata vitiation. Vata is constituted from ether and air, which signify movement and vastness. The thought process is rapid and not bound by space. The elements ether and air are light. Balance in them is brought by heavy elements like water and earth. Thus, when you eat food with more of these elements, the mind acquires stability. At another level, we can say that the rajas state of mind stabilises with the sattvic food.

Enriching the Food

We all know that when we visit an open market with fresh farm vegetables and fruits, it looks quite different than the vegetable and fruit corner of a super market. Packed in plastics and ripened with artificial means, the fresh products look less fresh with rather a dead expression on them. When the vegetables and fruits are growing, they have all kinds of interactions with various insects, butterflies, frogs, earthworms, birds, wind, dew, sun, day and night. Thus, a ripe cucumber or okra, a mango, a guava, an orange or a banana brings us that living part of the dynamic cosmos with them. If we kill all the insects and frogs with sprays or grow products in controlled climate in the green houses, the cosmic energy does not come to us with the food. We should make our best efforts to enliven our food preparations with various herbs and spices. We can grow some fresh herbs even in pots in order to enrich our food with some cosmic energy. Simple things like basil, coriander, fenugreek, dill etc. are very easy to grow.

You will see that in the Chapter on recipes, each recipe contains a variety of ingredients. If you look at it from the point of view of the modern science, all these ingredients bring us various vitamins, minerals and other essential elements for our body. From the Ayurvedic point of view, the variety of ingredients brings us the five elements of the cosmos and in addition they bring us the prana, which is the dynamism of the cosmos. Always make sure that the food you consume is not dead and has prana in it. Besides the cosmic interaction of the ingredients, the energy and feelings of the person who prepares the food is also very important. Canteens and restaurants not only use foods with less pranic energy but their mechanical preparation also often renders the food lifeless. It is because of the prana through the love of your mother or grandmother that you never forget certain good items prepared during your childhood. Therefore, when you cook, bring your concentration on it and always stir the food gently and tenderly. Your bhavana or devoted emotions bring in food a seventh rasa which is subtle and more intense than the six rasas you integrate in your food.

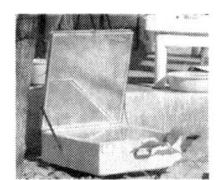

Solar cooking makes the food delicious. The food cooked in solar cooker acquires a different colour. I suggest that you cook the food on low fire also when you cook on the stove. I do not recommend the use of pressure cooker. Slow cookers are excellent. In the recipe section, I have given you many preparation methods on very low fire with the lid on. In brief, always think and make best of your efforts to preserve and add the 'living element' in your food.

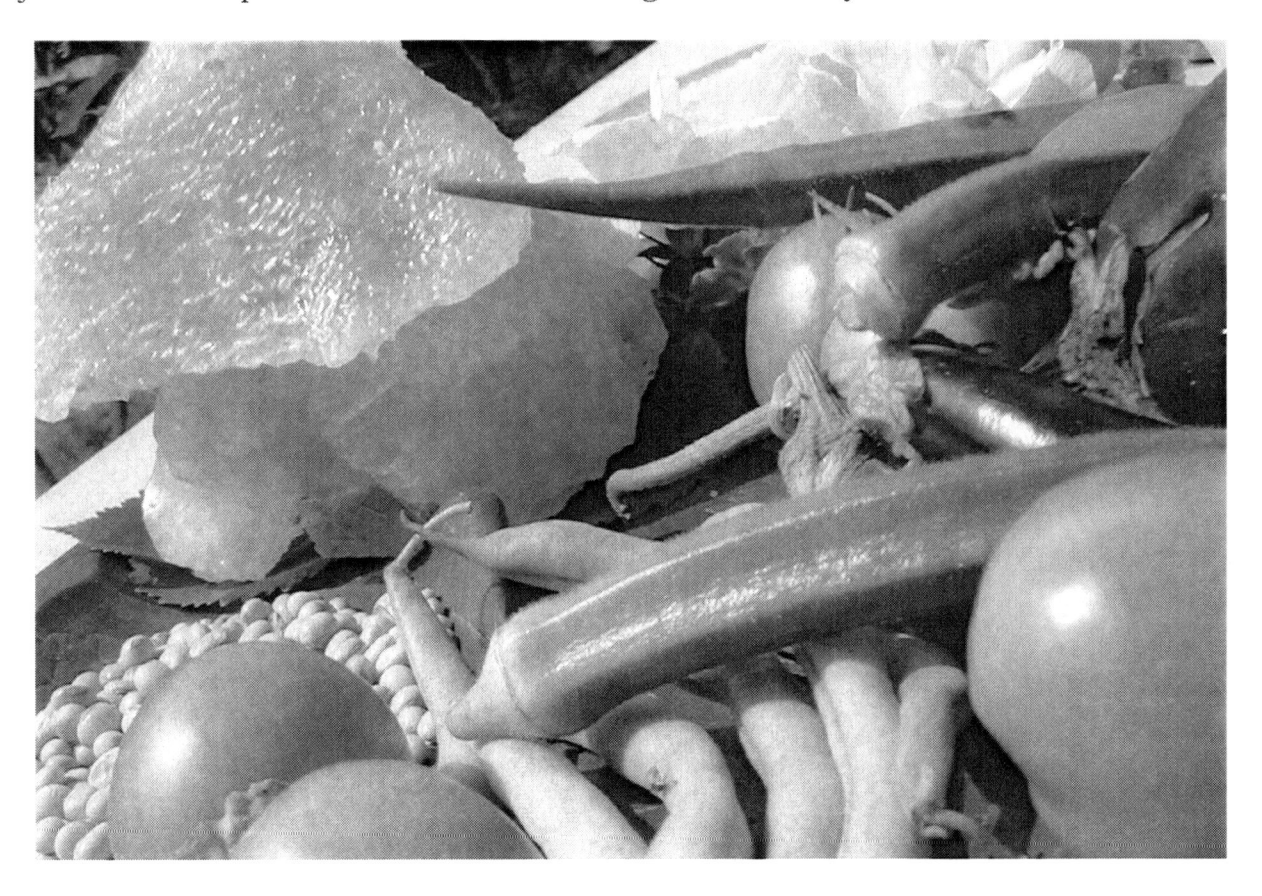

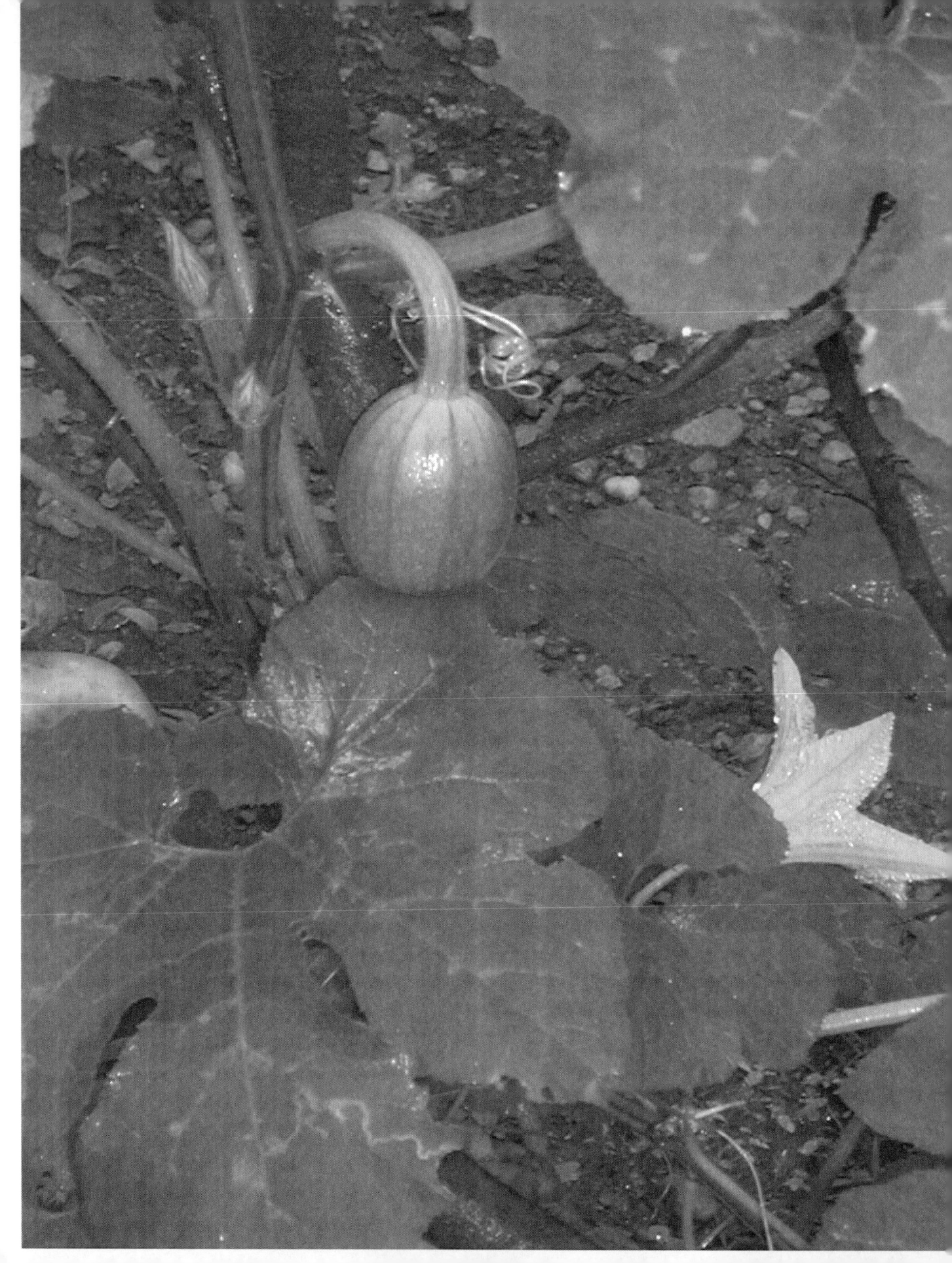

Preparation of the Basic Ayurvedic Cuisine

This chapter gives a list of some fundamental ingredients essential for Ayurvedic cooking, and explains how to prepare some basic things like ghee, curd (yoghurt), sprouts, etc.

For Ayurvedic cooking, you need to stock up your kitchen with a collection of about 25 herbs and spices, and some other fundamental products like different kinds of flours, grains, rice, ghee, etc. This will not only help you to prepare healthy and delicious meals but also provide you a small apothecary of healing herbs.

Later in the chapter, I will describe some basic equipment to set up a modern kitchen for Ayurvedic cooking. I have also described certain key preparations for Ayurvedic cooking like spice mixtures, ghee, yoghurt etc. and some simple ways to germinate seeds and grow some herbs.

Herbs and Spices

I will start with the most simple and common things which many of you may already know and then with the other ingredients that some of you may not be familiar with. For each product, I will explain the Ayurvedic nature of the products and their pharmacological importance.

Salts

Most people in the world are familiar with the sea salt, which is widely used. From Ayurvedic point of view, there are four kinds of salts. For the purpose of cooking, there are two kinds of rock salts which are important besides the generally available sea salt.

Sendhav or *Sendha* salt is transparent or white rock salt, which has shades of other colours in it as it is enriched with other minerals. The name of Sendha salt is from the great river Indus, which is called Sindhu in our language. These days, it is marketed as Himalayan Salt in the West but it is not truly Himalayan. Most of the river Sindhu is in present day Pakistan and this salt is imported from there.

Krishan lavan or *kala namak* or black salt is generally dark brown because it contains iron and sulphur.

Sea salt is kapha and pitta promoting but vata reducing. However, rock salts are exceptions for not promoting kapha. They are good for digestion and are a remedy for loss of appetite. It is suggested to use a mixture of these three salts. You can make a concentrated solution of these three salts in water and can use the fluid salt.

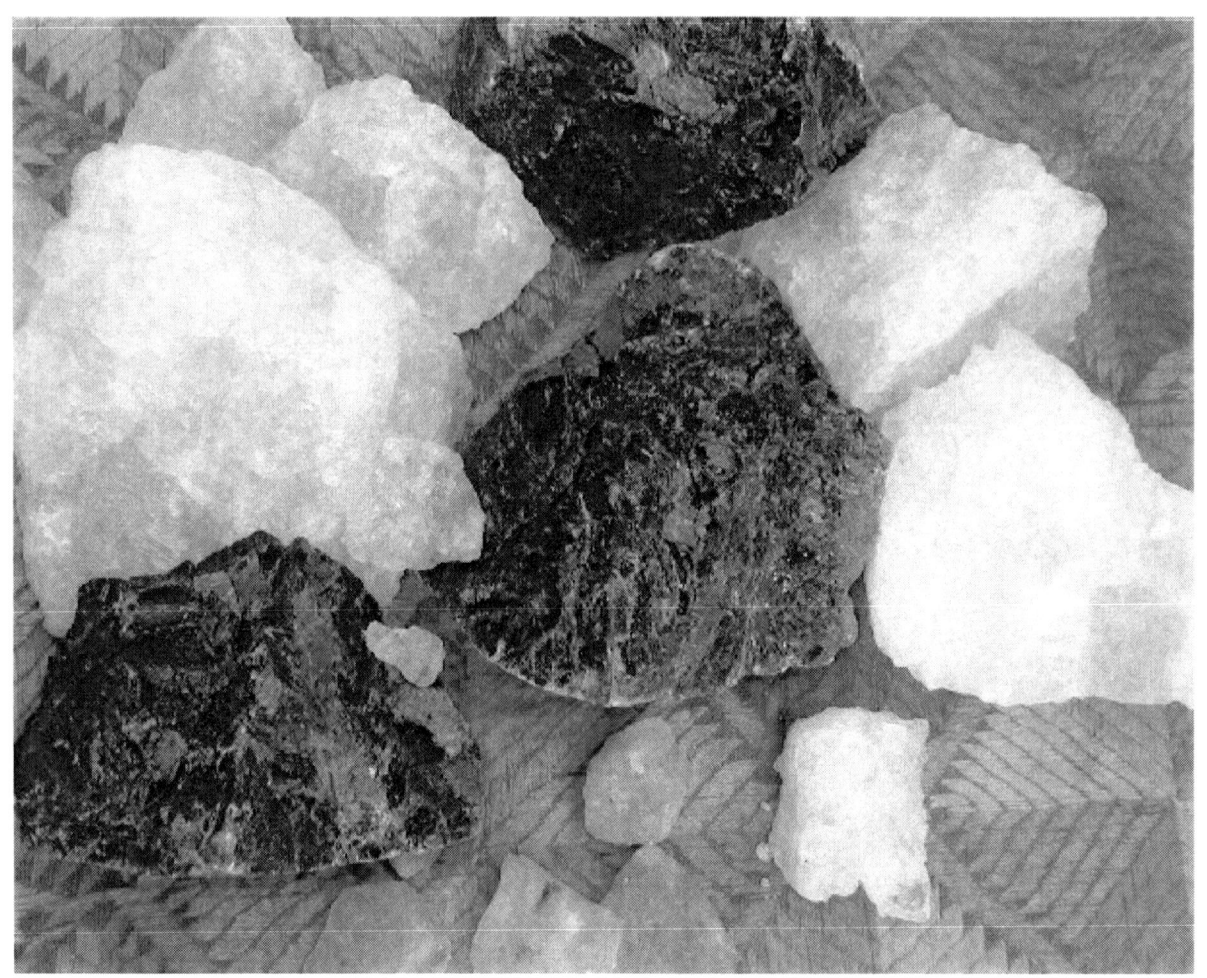

Various kinds of rock salts

Note: In areas with iodine depletion, it is essential to mix normal sea salt sold in the market with rock salt, as the former is enriched with iodine.

Pepper

Most common spice in the world is black pepper. Besides India, it is grown in Malaysia, Indonesia and Sri Lanka. It is a creeper with big leaves about 15 cm (6 inches) long and about 8 cm (3 inches) wide. The leaves have tentacles, which help the creeper to stick to trees. The flowers and fruits are in bunches. The fruits are green when unripe and later they turn red. On drying, they turn black and that is what we call black pepper. **White pepper** is prepared from the ripe fruits of black pepper. Black pepper is soaked in water and the husk is removed. The seeds are then dried to get white pepper. After removing the husk, the pepper becomes less sharp than the black pepper.

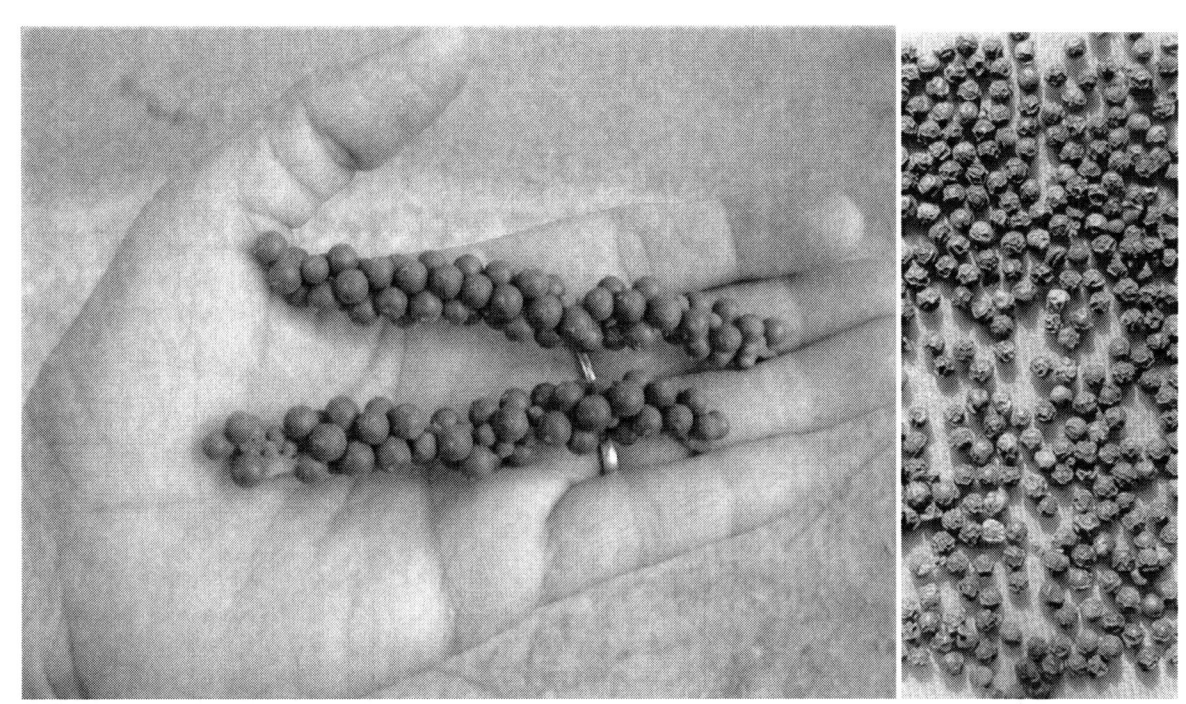

Pepper: Fresh and dried

Pepper is hot in its Ayurvedic nature. White pepper is milder than black pepper. Pepper is recommended to cure aggravated vata and kapha but it enhances pitta.

Long pepper or *Piper longum* in Latin (Peepal or Peepali in Hindi)

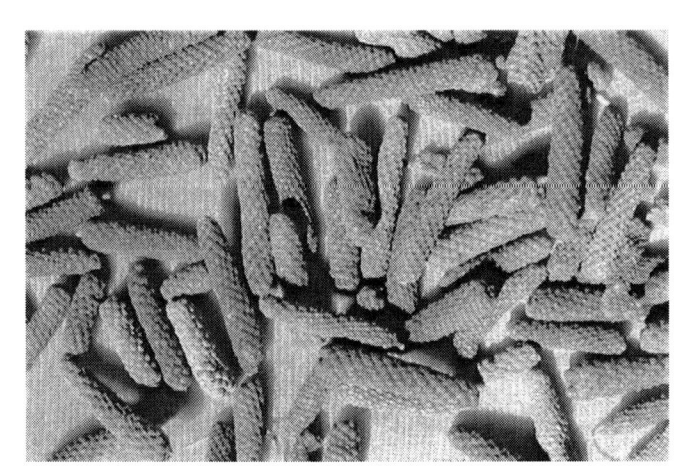

There are two varieties of it available. One is small and thin, about 1-2 centimetres (0.4 to 0.8 inch) long and ½ cm (0.2 inch) in diameter. The second variety is double the size than this. Long pepper has a granular surface. From the surface, both the varieties are alike.

This plant is also a creeper but has heart-shaped leaves, which are about 8 cm (3 inches) long. The ripe fruit is red but dried is dull brownish black.

Long pepper is less hot than the normal black pepper. It is recommended to use it in spice mixtures and some teas. It is very good for the nerves.

Cinnamon (*Dalchini in Hindi*)

The cinnamon tree is 7 to 10 meters high (22 to 33 feet) and its bark is used as spice. Normally, there are two different kinds of cinnamon available. One is thick and dark brown and the other is reddish brown and thin, and the bark is rolled down. The dark and thicker one is stronger in taste and flavour than the thinner one.

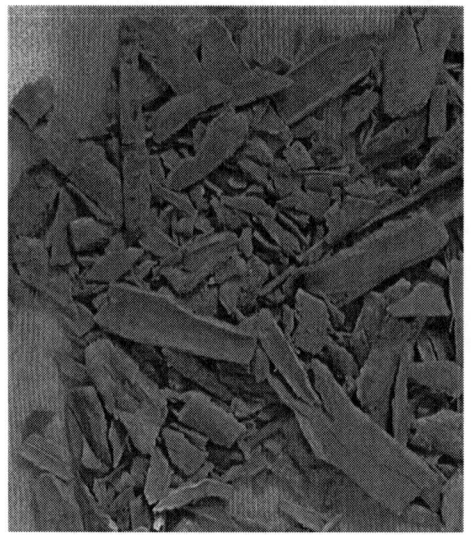

It grows in abundance in Northwest Himalayas until the height of 1200 meters, Southwest India and Srilanka. The southern variety is thinner and milder.

Cinnamon is hot in its Ayurvedic properties.

Cinnamon leaves are called Tejpatra and are also used as spice. They are particularly used to perfume rice. In fact, cinnamon leaves help to recognise the tree as they have specific profound lines running all along their length. The tree has very thick foliage.

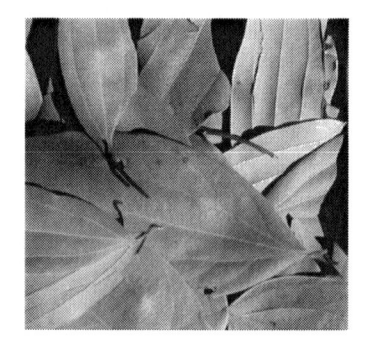

Clove (*Lavang or Long in Hindi*)

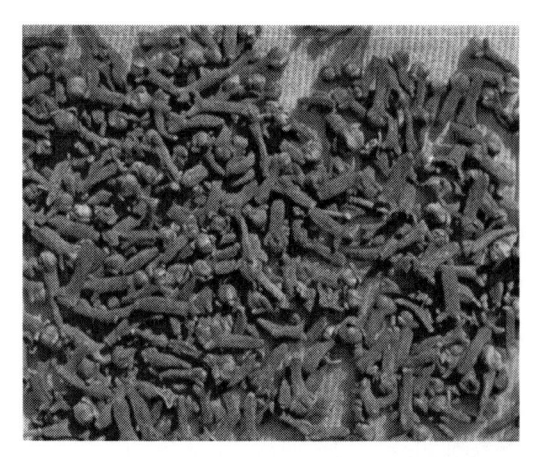

Most people in the world know this spice. Even those who have not seen these little dried flower buds may have smelled it at a dentist, as clove oil is used to relieve toothache and to prepare fillings with different polymerising substance.

Clove tree is big and can grow up to 12 meter (40 feet). This tree has a very long life; it could live up to 100 years. At the age of 7-8 years, the first buds appear. The maximum yield is when the tree is between 30 and 60 year old. The buds are plucked at a very specific time when they are just beginning to turn from green to pink

Clove is cold in its Ayurvedic nature.

Both clove and cinnamon have antibiotic qualities and cure minor digestive disorders. Most spices are rasayanas (promote immunity and vitality) but these two in particular are very important.

Cardamoms (small and big) (*choti* and *Badi ilayachi* in *Hindi*)

The cardamom most of you know is also known as lesser cardamom or choti ilyachi in Hindi. This name is in comparison with bigger cardamom, which is very different in its Ayurvedic properties as compared to the lesser or small cardamom but belongs to the same family of plants called *Zingiberaceae*. Both the plants are bushy with long leaves emerging from the root. The buds appear at the lower end of the leaves near the ground. Smaller cardamom is grown in Southern India and Sri Lanka whereas the bigger cardamom grows in the lower Himalayas. It requires sloppy land with plenty of water but the water should not stay.

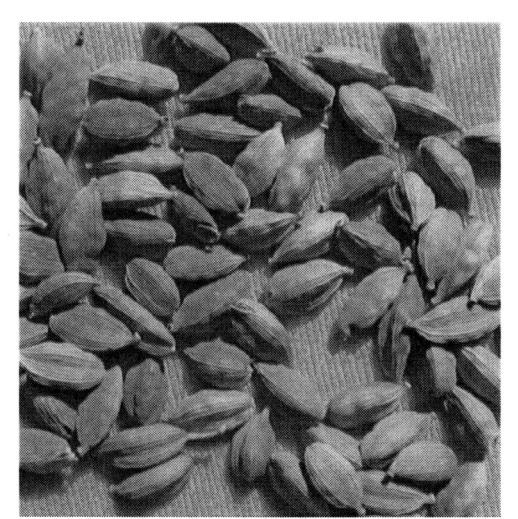

Small cardamom has light green flowers and fruits are light green or yellow, about 1 cm (0.4 inch) in length. Inside the fruits, there are 15-20 brown or black seeds. For the spice, the seeds are used.

Small cardamom is used in many sweet as well as salty dishes and various tea mixtures. It creates equilibrium of energies and is good for throat and heart. It promotes digestion and is good for teeth. Eating it after meals is very beneficial as it cleans and perfumes the mouth and promotes digestion.

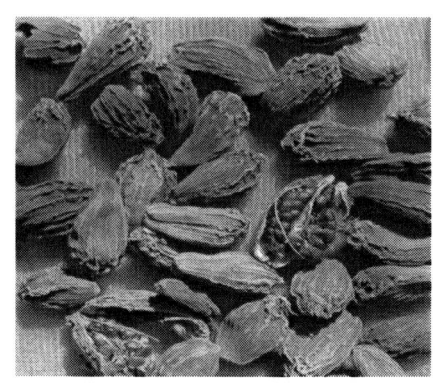

Greater or big cardamom has yellow or white flowers and fruits are dark brown and are about three times the size of the smaller cardamom. It has small seeds inside. The seeds are used as a spice and for medicinal purpose.

Ayurvedic nature of big cardamom is hot. It is a wonderful medicine for curing low blood pressure. Therefore, the persons with hypertension should avoid it. It is used in cough medicines and is useful for fever, and mouth and throat ailments.

Big cardamom has very strong flavour as compared to the delicate flavour of the small cardamom. It is generally used in spice mixtures.

Cumin (*jeera* in Hindi)

The cumin plant is about 30 cm (1 Foot) high with very fine leaves. The tiny flowers are white or pink in colour and are in bunches. Fruits are elongated, brown and about ½ cm (0.2 inch) long. It is cultivated all over India.

Cumin is hot in its Ayurvedic nature. It has a delicious taste and a great flavour. It promotes digestion and therefore it should be particularly used when preparing something, which is hard to digest or is rich.

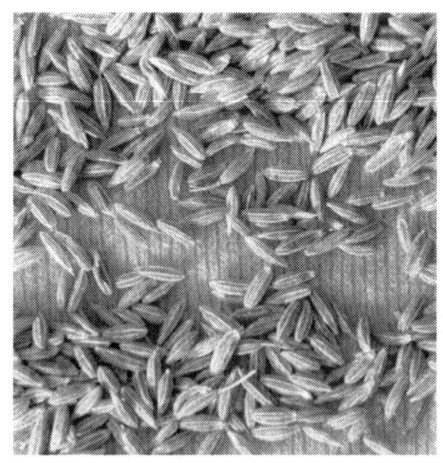

Cumin has a number of medicinal usages and some prominent ones are, it is strength promoting and anti-fatigue, it is used in many women's ailments especially after childbirth to promote milk. It is very beneficial in loss of appetite.

Fennel (Saunf in Hindi)

It looks a little like cumin but bigger in size and is green. The plant is about one meter (3-4 feet) high. It has tiny leaves and the flowers are yellow and are in bunches. The fruits are elongated, light green and have five clear lines in them. If the leaves are repeatedly trimmed, the root becomes bigger and is eaten as vegetable.

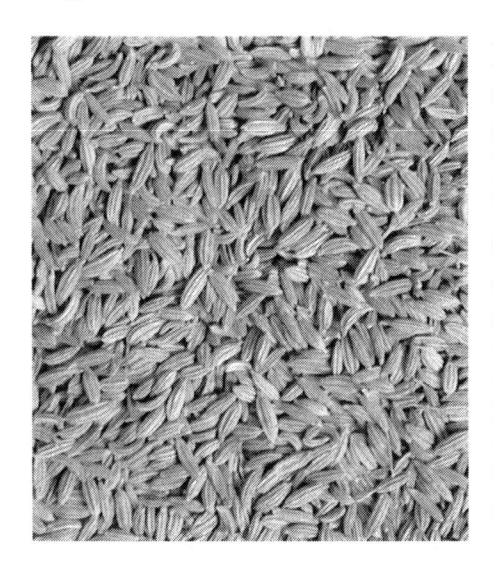

Fennel is cold in its Ayurvedic nature. It has a delicate flavour and sweet taste. It promotes digestion and perfumes the mouth. That is why, like small cardamom, it is also recommended to be eaten after meals. It is used in desserts as well as in spices. It is used to pacify the hot effect of other spices. Entire grains used in different dishes render them a soft taste and help create a balance with strong smelling onions or garlic. Fennel cures vitiated vata and pitta. It is used in herbal teas also. Too much of it may cause constipation. One of its medicinal uses is to cure diarrhoea.

Anise has small round grains and is similar in qualities to fennel. Its taste and flavour are also nearly the same accept that it has slightly bitter rasa.

Coriander (dhaniya in Hindi)

The coriander plant is about 60 cm (2 feet) high. Its leaves are used to perfume various salads and hot dishes. Its seeds are used as spice. The leaves are rounded with various indentations. Flowers are purple and white and are in bunches. Fruits are yellow and round, and upon being pressed, they split into two. These are two seeds of the plant. Therefore, they should be split before plantation. Coriander is cultivated all over India. You may plant it in your garden or even in pots.

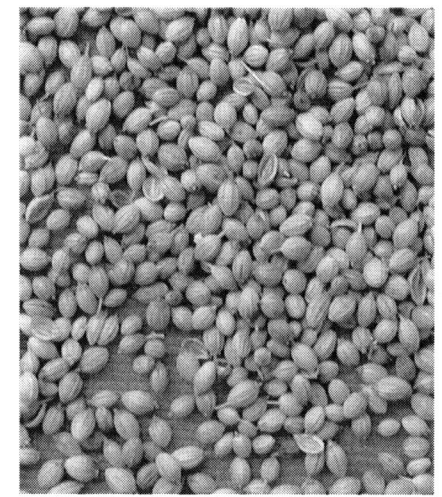

Coriander is cold in its Ayurvedic nature. In spice mixtures, it is used to have equilibrium of the sharp and hot spices. Amongst its many medicinal qualities, it strengthens the nerves.

Kalonji

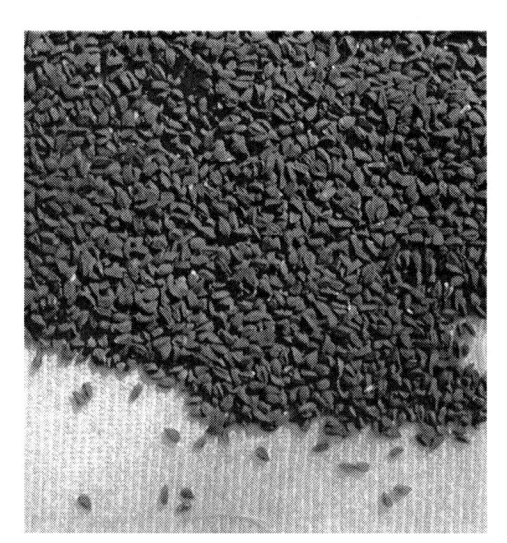

Kalonji is a Hindi word and has no equivalent in English. Like coriander, it is also a small plant but leaves are bigger. The flowers are light blue and fruits are round. Each fruit has several seeds. Seeds are dark black and heart shaped. Kalonji is called by several erroneous names like black cumin or small fennel or onion seeds etc. outside India. One should be very careful buying it and make sure that the word 'kalonji' is written on the packet. Its Latin name is *Nigella sativa*. It is originally from southern Europe but now a very important Indian spice, which is cultivated all over India.

Kalonji is hot in its Ayurvedic nature. It has a strong taste and flavour and therefore it should not be used in very delicately flavoured dishes. Amongst the many medicinal qualities of kalonji, it is used to cure painful menstruation.

Preparation of the Basic Ayurvedic Cuisine

Fenugreek (*Methi* in Hindi)

This is also a small plant of about 60 cm (2 feet) in height. The rounded leaves are in the groups of three. Flowers are white and yellowish and fruits are in tiny beans with each containing 10-20 seeds. The seeds are round with uneven surface and dark yellow in colour.

Fenugreek seeds are used as spice and for medicinal purposes and leaves are eaten as a vegetable. Fenugreek is hot in its Ayurvedic nature and seeds have very strong taste. This spice is not used in delicately flavoured dishes. It is very good for curing vitiated vata. It is given to women after childbirth to enhance milk. It strengthens the nerves.

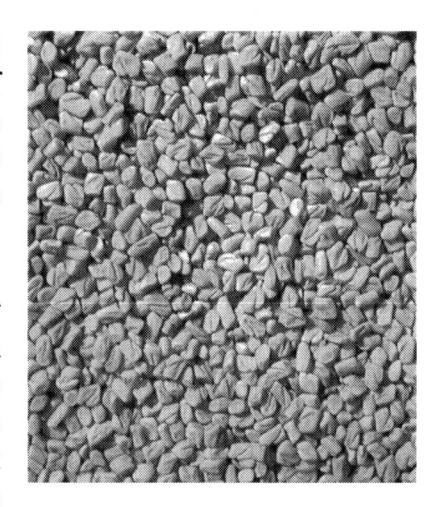

Mustard

This is a well-known plant all over the world. It is a small plant of nearly a meter high (3 feet) and has bright yellow flowers. The fruits are in small bean pods with several seeds in each pod. Seeds are tiny and round and reddish brown in colour. There are several varieties of mustard with a slight difference in colour and size. A variety called the Indian mustard is used as a spice. It is called *rai* in Hindi. It has smaller seeds as compared to the normal mustard, which is planted for obtaining oil. Mustard leaves are eaten as vegetable in some parts of India but they are extremely astringent and therefore need special preparation. Mustard seed oil is used for cooking as well as for medicinal purpose because it is pain relieving and has antibiotic qualities. It is used for curing skin infections.

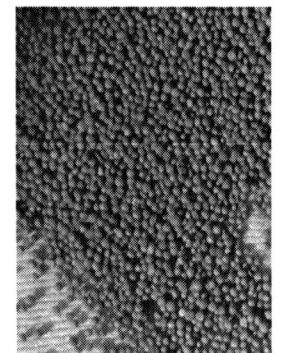

Mustard seeds are hot in their Ayurvedic qualities. These are used in the spice mixtures with other spices.

Ajwain

Ajwain is a Hindi word with no equivalent in English. It is a small bushy plant with tiny and split leaves. The plants are maximum 1 meter (3 feet) high. White flowers in groups are umbrella shaped. Fruits are egg shaped, brown and about 4mm (1/12 of an inch) in length. Each fruit has a single brown coloured seed, which is very tiny, dull brown and has lines on the surface.

Ajwain is too kinds—big and small. Small is 1-2 mm (about 1/20 of an inch) and the big one is double its size. In India, big one is generally given to house animals for various remedies and small one is used as spice and in medicines.

Ajwain is similar to thyme but in thyme leaves are used whereas in ajwain seeds are used. Ajwain is profusely used in food and medicine in India and is cultivated almost everywhere. It is hot in its Ayurvedic nature.

It cures aggravated vata and kapha and enhances pitta. It promotes digestion and is extremely effective to cure several digestive disorders. It gives delicious taste and flavour to various food preparations. It is specially suggested to use it in fried foods, dishes with dough or other fatty foods. Ajwain promotes the liver function and hence helps digest heavy and rich foods. In case of discomfort and heaviness in stomach, you may take half a teaspoon of ajwain with some salt and lemon juice in it.

Dill (*Soye* in Hindi)

Dill plant is 50-60 cm (about 2 feet) high. Leaves are divided into several tiny parts and fruits are yellow and in umbrella shaped groups. The fruits are tiny brown and seeds are even smaller, dull brown in colour, slightly flat and with lines on their surface. Dill is also grown everywhere in India and in some northern states the leaves are used as vegetable.

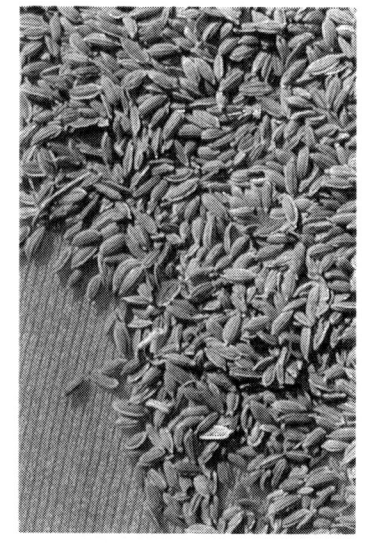

Dill leaves are cold in their Ayurvedic nature whereas seeds are extremely hot. Dill leaves are eaten as herb or vegetable and fruits are used as spice and medicine. Dill seeds are important for women and are used in many remedies to cure menstrual troubles and for the management of post-delivery period.

Dill Seeds render delicious taste and flavour to food. Since they are highly pitta promoting, they should not be used excessively or with foods, which are hot in their nature, and also when the climate is very hot. To neutralise the hot effect of dill, you may use it in combination with fennel and coriander seeds (see Mixture C later in this chapter).

Preparation of the Basic Ayurvedic Cuisine

Turmeric or curcuma (*Haldi* in Hindi)

Everybody knows this spice as bright yellow coloured powder but they are very few in the West who have seen the original spice. Mostly, turmeric powder is sold abroad. The spice is a root and looks like ginger but on removing the skin, unlike ginger, it is bright yellow from inside.

The plant is 70-90 cm (2-3 feet) high with very big leaves. The leaves are 50-60 cm (about 2 feet) and about 15 cm (6 inches) in width.

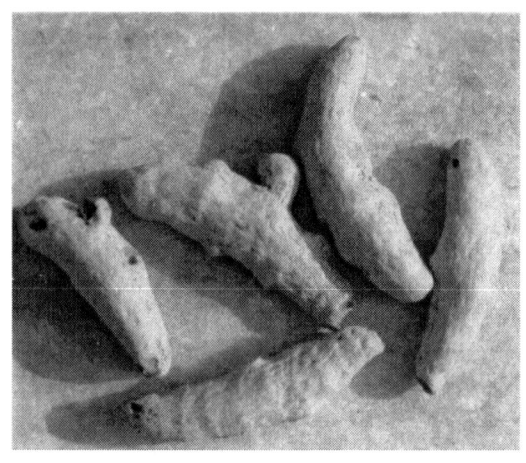

Turmeric makes the food colourful and has also tremendous medicinal value. It is anti-inflammatory, anti-allergic, has antibiotic qualities and is a rasayana. Turmeric brings equilibrium of the three energies but is slightly hot in nature.

Note: Many people abroad confuse turmeric with so called '**curry**'. There is nothing as curry either in India or in Ayurveda. Curry is a British creation from colonial times. The British, who found our spices too complicated, tried a make a mixture of turmeric with all the other spices added to it. From an Ayurvedic and Indian point of view, it is rather silly, because spices are used very specifically according to the nature of the food, climate, season etc. The concept of curry can be equated to mixing all different kinds of French wines in one bottle, and call the mixture as, 'The Great French Wine'.

Ginger (*Shunthi* or *saunth* or *adarak* in Hindi)

The ginger plant resembles that of turmeric with big leaves coming out of the ground. It is similar in size to turmeric

Fresh ginger establishes the equilibrium of three energies and is highly recommended to use in food and in teas. It is a rasayana. Dried ginger is hot in its Ayurvedic nature. Ginger rejuvenates the liver functions and promotes appetite.

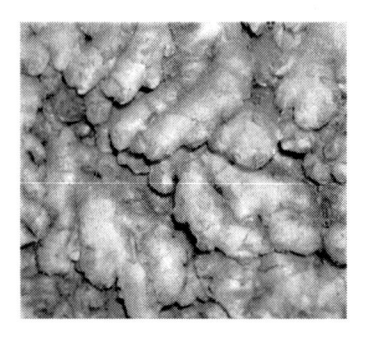

Garlic

The garlic plant is 50-60 cm (about 2 feet) high and has thin and long leaves. There is a big bulb of flowers with numerous white flowers. The white or pinkish bulbous root, which we know as garlic spice is divided into about 12 to 18 parts. Each part is called the garlic clove. The garlic leaves are used in the salad or on the top of the soup or other warm preparations.

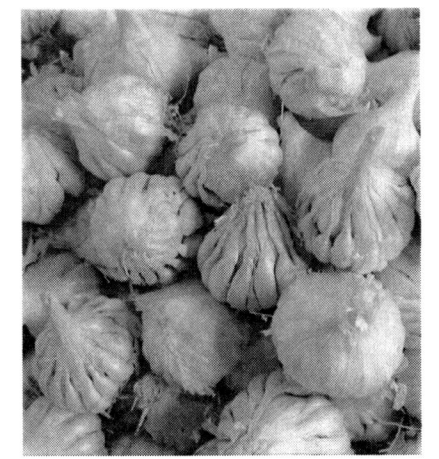

Garlic is hot in its Ayurvedic nature. It is the most important rasayana out of all the spices. It has five out of six rasas. Except sour, it has all the other five rasas. The strong smelling garlic is a highly rejuvenating product. Besides that, it has antibiotic qualities, promotes vision and is an aphrodisiac. For more qualities and medicinal uses of garlic, refer to my other books on Ayurveda.

Despite all the wonderful qualities of garlic, you should be careful with its use. It is very hot and should be used according to the constitution. Even in food, there are people who cannot digest it well and suffer from its side effects like dried throat, excessive thirst, rash on the skin and restlessness. To get over these effects, one should drink a coriander seed decoction. Garlic should be eaten in moderate quantity everyday. To get over its strong smell, small cardamom is highly effective.

Cress (*Chansur* or *Halim* in Hindi)

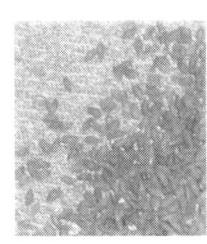

Cress plant is very tiny. It is about 30 cm (1 foot) high. The rounded leaves are around 1 cm (0.25 inch) in diameter and are in groups of three. Flowers are tiny white and are in bunches. Fruits are in tiny spindle shaped pods, each containing one seed. Seeds are elongated and are brown in colour. They are very strong in taste and they are used in several remedies. They are blood purifiers, used in several women's ailments, are strength promoting and enhance sexual secretions.

As you all know, the small, rounded leaves of cress are delicious as salad. In India, the leaves are principally used as fodder for horses, camels and other house animals. There is a similar wild plant in the Gharwal Himalayas, which is used as green vegetable. Because of their tremendous medicinal value, I suggest that cress seeds should be used to garnish various salads or they can be put directly in different dough preparations or in sandwiches and so on.

Cress is hot in its Ayurvedic nature. Leaves are mild hot because of the bitter rasa in them but seeds are extremely hot. Germination makes them milder.

Nutmeg and mace (*Jaiphal* and *Javitri* in Hindi)

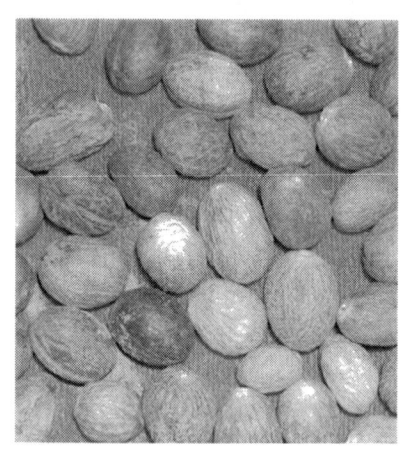

The nutmeg tree grows up to more than 10 meter (33 feet) in height. Leaves are about 8 cm (3 inches) long and are oval in shape. The flowers are yellow and are in bunches and they smell nice. Fruits are oval in shape and are around 5 cm (2 inches) long. They are yellow with a thick and smooth shell. When the fruits ripe, the shell splits into two and inside there is a bright yellowish red aril around a hard light brown coloured seed. When the fruit is dried, the aril separates and is called **mace**. This is used as a spice too. The seed is called nutmeg and is used as a spice the world over.

Both, nutmeg and mace are hot in their Ayurvedic nature. They provide a delicate taste and flavour to food. Mace is milder hot as compared to the nut. Both are used to cure vata and kapha imbalances.

Nutmeg should not be taken in excessive quantity, as it is intoxicating for the nerves. It slows down the thinking process and calms down the nerves. About ¼ of a nut is the maximum daily dose per person. It is good for hyper-excited persons. Nutmeg also slows down the activity of the smooth muscles and is therefore given in diarrhoea and to promote assimilation of the food. Besides these, nutmeg is used to cure menstrual problems as well as several sexual disorders, as I have described in my other books.

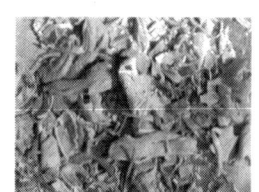

Saffron (*Kesar* in Hindi)

Saffron is like tiny fibres of bright red and orange coloured. These fibres are stamina of the delicate flowers of *Crocus sattivum*. The plant is less than 30 cm (1feet) high with thin long leaves. Flowers are purple in colour and the female flowers have bright red coloured stamina, which are three in number and about 2½ cm (1 inch) long. These are delicately taken out and dried. Plantation and preparation of saffron needs extremely delicate work and care. This is why saffron is very expensive. On the other hand, the quantity required for food and medicine is also very minute.

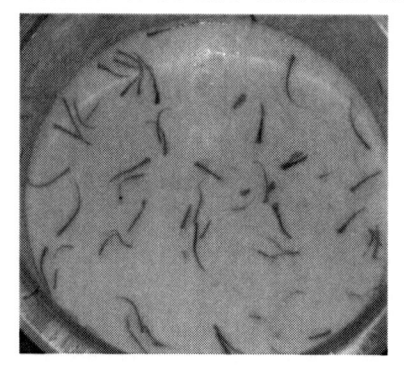

The saffron plant is originally from southern Europe. It is cultivated in Spain, Italy, Greece and France and exported from there in many parts of the world. In India, it is cultivated in Jammu and Kashmir and is also imported from France and Spain.

When taken in small quantities and regularly, saffron helps bring the equilibrium of the three energies. Basically, its Ayurvedic nature is hot and more than 250 milligrams should not be taken daily as medicine and 100 mg daily as food. It is an aphrodisiac and a rasayana. It is also used in many other remedies, especially for women's ailments.

Holy Basil (*Tulsi* in Hindi)

Basil is a holy plant in India and is also called Holy basil or *Oscimum sanctum* in Latin because it is worshipped in every Hindu home. Because of its tremendous medicinal qualities, perhaps the sages made all these rituals for the care and protection of this plant and ensured its ready availability in every home.

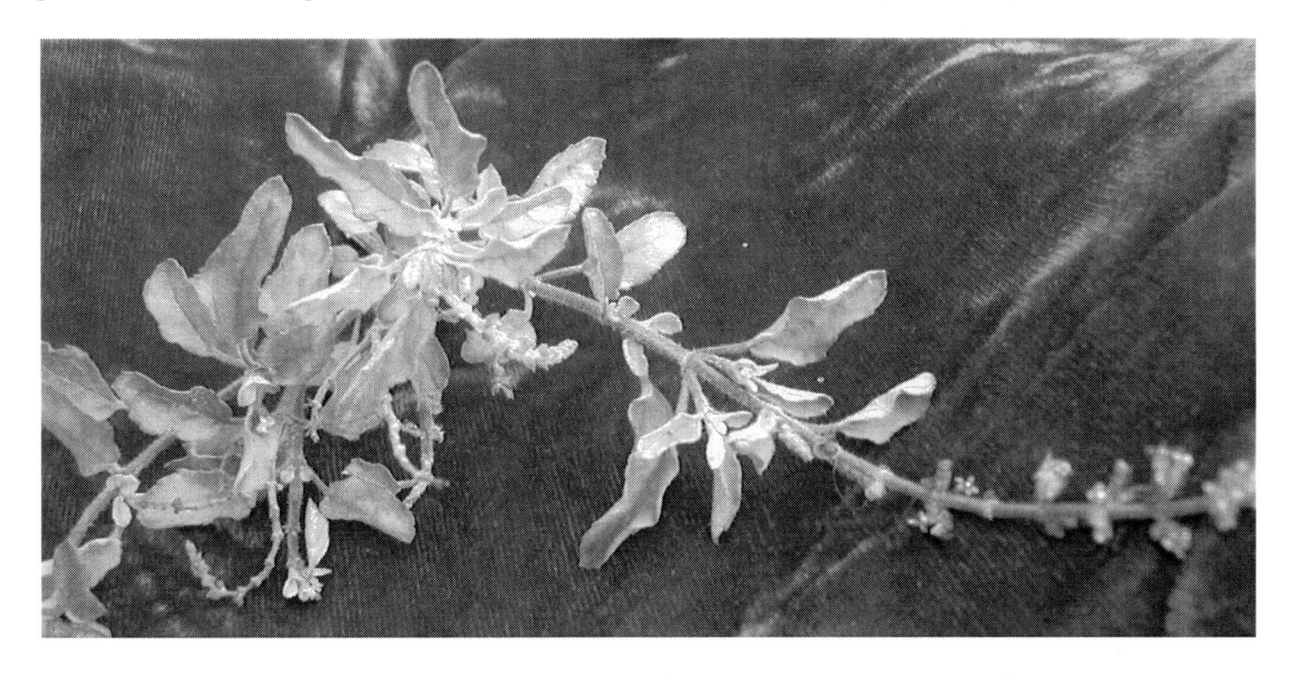

Basil plant is less than 1 meter (3 feet) high. Leaves are generally 2 to 5 cm (1-2 inch) long. The tiny flowers are purple and are arranged in elongated groups. The length of the flower bunch is 10-15 cm (4-6 inches). The seeds are brown and are small and round.

Basil leaves make the food rejuvenating. One should regularly use basil in the form of tea or to flavour the salads. It is a rasayana and strengthens the immune system. It is hot in its Ayurvedic nature and therefore should not be used in excess. Four to five leaves a day are recommended. The European variety of Basil with big leaves is milder and may be taken double this quantity.

Peppermint (*Pudina* in Hindi)

This herb does not need much explanation as the strong flavour of peppermint every body knows through all kinds of sweets and chewing gums and so on. The small plant of peppermint is around 30 cm (1 foot) high. The leaves are thick and slightly round. The flowers are tiny purple. But the leaves of the young plants before flowering are tender and they are used as herb. There are many varieties of peppermint like garden mint, wild mint, Himalayan mint and so on.

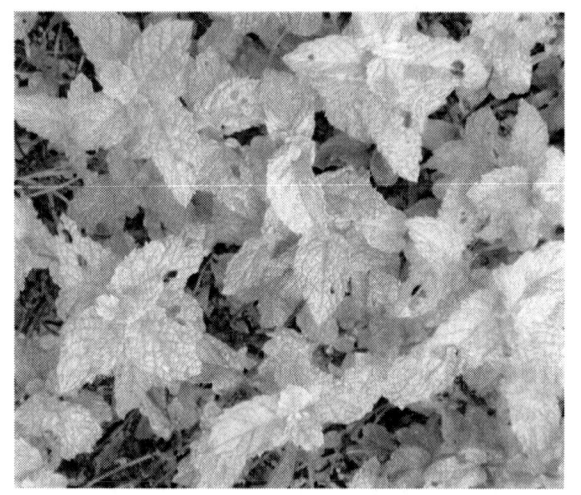

Peppermint is hot in its Ayurvedic nature. It promotes appetite. A delicious chutney can be made from peppermint (see the recipe Section).

Asafoetida (*Heeng* in Hindi)

It is an oily resin from a small tree of about 2 meter (6-7 feet) high. The tree is found in the high Himalayan Mountains. The resin has extremely strong smell because of the presence of some sulphur salts in it. It is difficult to obtain the pure spice as its synthetic imitation is made in large quantities. The pure product is expensive and rare. Sometimes, a resin from another tree is mixed with a synthetic substance and is sold.

Asafoetida is very hot in its Ayurvedic nature and cures vitiated vata and kapha but enhances pitta. It is generally used in heavy to digest lentils and beans, which tend to cause vata vitiation. Asafoetida is used to cure the ailments of old age which are generally vata ailments like joint pains, fatigue, gout etc.

It is very difficult to use asafoetida in modern kitchens because of its extremely strong odour.

Chilli

This spice comes from the New World but now widely and rather too much used in India along with the other spices. The small plant of chilli is less than a meter high (3 feet). Small and long leaves are pointed in front. The flowers are white. The green fruits are long and contain many seeds. There are many varieties of chillies with varying sizes of fruits. The green fruits turn red after they are ripened and dried.

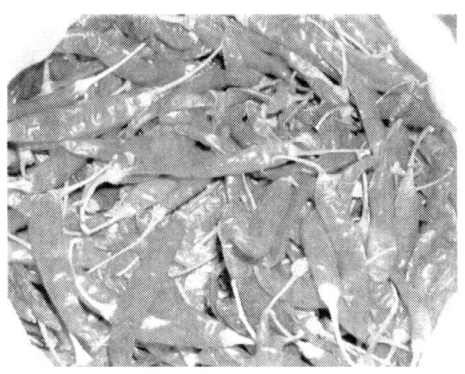

Chillies are hot in their Ayurvedic qualities. They are good to cure vitiated vata and kapha. In excess amount, they give heartburn. If you are not used to chillies or you have pitta constitution, they are not recommended. Their use is optional in the recipes given in this book. Many people think that hot taste can be only due to chilli. In fact, many of the spices give pungent and sharp taste. Since different chillies have varying degrees of pungent taste, be very careful with the amount you use.

Cleaning and Storage of Spices

Before storing the spices, they should be cleaned properly. Mostly the spices sold in the industrial packing are clean but still it is essential to check them once more. For cleaning, put the spice in a plate and go through it with your fingers to get rid of any straw, stones etc.

For storage of the spices, I suggest glass jars, which can be closed tightly. They should be absolutely dry before you put spices in them. Sundry them briefly or dry them in the oven at low heat. Drying is especially necessary in humid places.

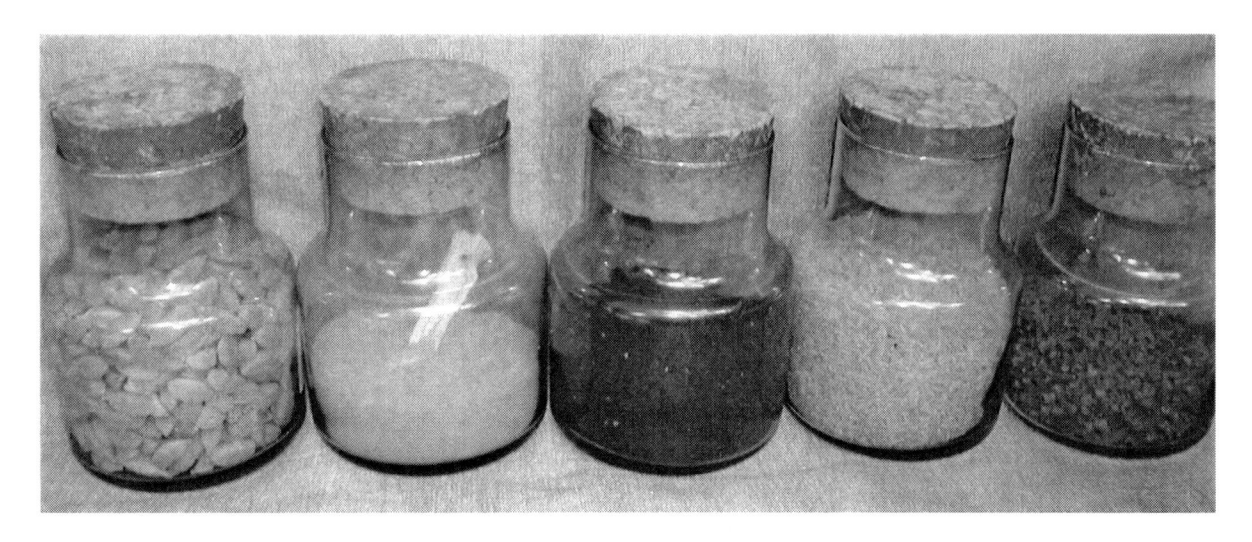

Collection of Ingredients

Grains and flours: For preparing a basic Ayurvedic kitchen, you need to have different kinds of flours like wheat, chickpeas, maize, millet and so on. You also need good quality wheat for germination. There are different varieties of beans and lentils recommended in Ayurveda. These are particularly important as a source of protein for vegetarians. I have given below the description of some of these you may include in your diet.

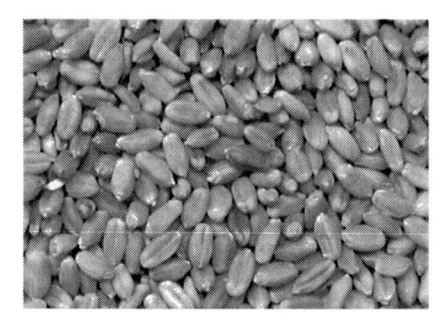

Wheat: Clean and dried wheat can be made into fresh flour with a little grinder. You also need to have wheat grains for certain recipes. In Indian shops abroad, they sell the wheat flour as *Chapati* flour.

There are many qualities of wheat and they seem to have different Ayurvedic properties. The best is the smaller grains with darker colour. The big grain wheat is more kapha promoting and bulk promoting than the small grain wheat.

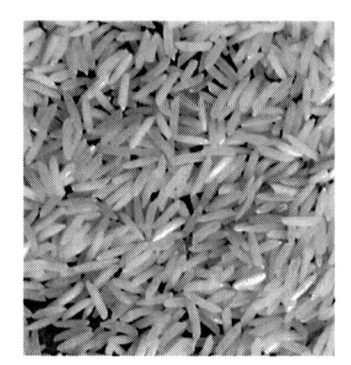

Rice: Rice is the most eaten food in the world. I recommend buying basmati rice, as it is easier to cook. It is recommended for wheat and rice both that they should be one year old and should not be more than two years old. However, in the modern way of living, it is impossible to find such details about the food we eat. You also need to get some round variety of rice, which are more starchy than basamati and is used in some recipes given in this book.

Maize: Americans call it corn. I have given recipes with its flour. Maize flour cannot be kept for a long time as it turns sour. That is why, in India, it is only used during the season when fresh flour is available. I experienced buying sour flour from the stores in Europe. Be very careful and check the packing date.

Chickpeas: You are required to buy chickpeas, as well as chickpea flour, which is called *Besan* and is available in Indian stores. Chickpeas are two kinds, the bigger white one and the smaller dark brown called also the black gram.

Finger millet: Finger millet is a health promoting diet. I have given recipes with its flour.

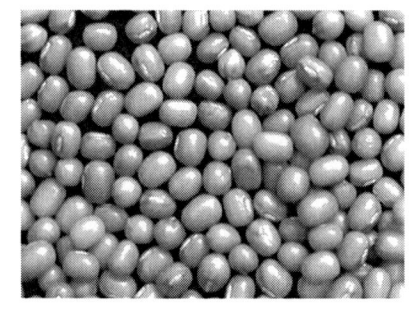

Mung beans: You require mung beans as well as mung dal (crushed beans without husk). Both are health promoting and are easy to digest and therefore are highly recommended food.

Urd beans: Urd beans are very heavy to digest and long to cook. Therefore, I have written recipes for urd dal. Like it is said above, dal is without husk and crushed.

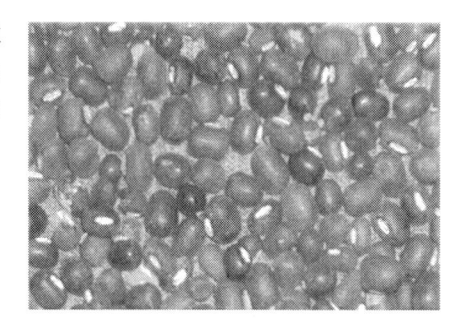

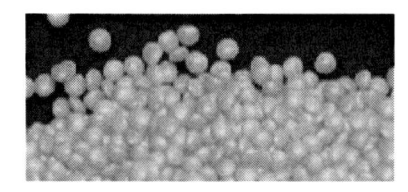

Masoor dal: They are also called red lentils abroad as after removing husk and crushing, they are dark pink in colour. They make very delicious soup and are very good to heal vitiated pitta.

Semolina: Semolina is made from wheat starch. It is a very light food. It is particularly good when one is unwell. Besides that, it is very quick to prepare breakfast or a small meal from semolina.

Ghee and different kinds of oils: It is important to have both, animal as well as plant fat. Amongst the animal fat, in Ayurveda, it is suggested to use ghee, which is butter fat. Butter is normally 85% fat and the rest is protein and water. Ghee is also called clarified butter. It can be preserved like any other oil without refrigeration. One can buy it readymade or can make it easily at home from unsalted, good quality butter. The method is described on the following pages.

Amongst the plant fat, Ayurveda highly recommends the use of sesame oil.

Sesame seeds: Sesame seeds can be used directly in some salad sauce or to make a winter dessert.

Tamarind Fruit (*Imali* in Hindi): If you eat beans and other things like lentils, etc., keep some tamarind fruit in the kitchen. It promotes digestion and is recommended to put in bean preparations.

Mango powder (*Amchoor* in Hindi): A variety of mangoes, which is called pickle-mango because it is used to make pickles and chutneys is cut into pieces and dried. It is powdered and is used to give the sour taste to many dishes. Mango powder is sold as a spice. It can be also used to replace tamarind in bean preparations.

Some other products: Always keep fresh milk, fresh ginger, garlic, some onions (if you like them), lemon, some green herbs and some fresh vegetables.

Preparation of the Basic Ayurvedic Cuisine

Equipment

For Ayurvedic cooking, it is essential to have different kinds of mortars and grinders.

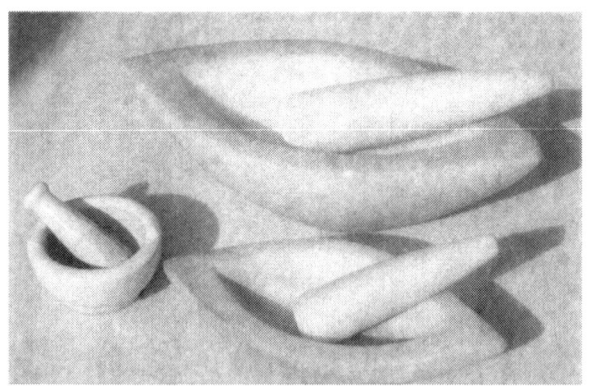

Porcelain mortar: A porcelain mortar is required for pounding some delicate herbs and spices and for those cases where you need to pulverise some substances in small quantities. For example when you wish to powder a half teaspoon of roasted cumin or crush some basil leaves for a tea and so on, you need porcelain mortar with pestle. Porcelain mortar is delicate and therefore do not beat or pound strongly with it. Crush the substances by rubbing repeatedly with the pestle.

Stone mortar: Small stone mortars are generally made of marble but they could be of some other stones too. These are stronger than the porcelain mortars and can be used to crush slightly more hard substances. If you want to make powder of a hard substance, first crush in stone mortar and then pulverise it in porcelain mortar. Because of the shape, it is easier to make fine powders in porcelain mortar.

The big stone mortars are made of a hard variety of stones and pounding is done by a rounded wooden rod. They are meant for hard substances and also for making chutneys. These are generally too big for modern kitchen and also too noisy for apartments. They can be replaced with some modern equipment, which is mentioned later.

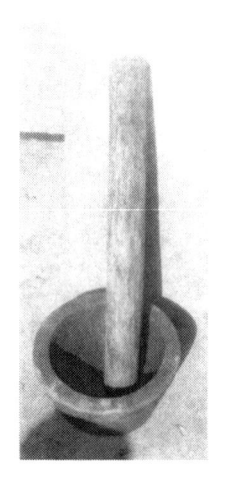

Metal mortar: Metal mortars are made of copper or wrought iron. I suggest that you buy a small one for crushing hard things. They are made deeper as compared to the above-described mortars so that the substances do not fly out when you pound them. This mortar will be useful for taking off the cardamom shells by pounding them.

Flat stone with rounded stone pestle: This is used to crush ginger, garlic or some green herbs. It consists of a flat stone with slightly rough surface and a smaller pestle which is rounded from below. (See picture on page 16).

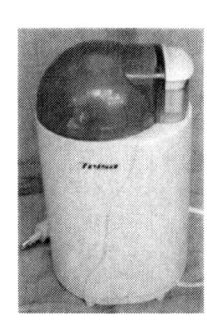

Coffee grinder: For making spices in bulk, I suggest that you buy a small electric coffee grinder. In India, this is generally called a dry grinder for spices. This grinder is very useful and practical for making various spice mixtures. Its motor does not get hot, as it has to be run in small fractions of time. Therefore, the flavour of the spices remains intact.

Hand mixer: A small electrical hand mixer for making soups or mashing tomatoes is a very practical and time saving equipment you may have in your kitchen. It saves you from washing big equipment as it can be used directly in the pot or in any other container.

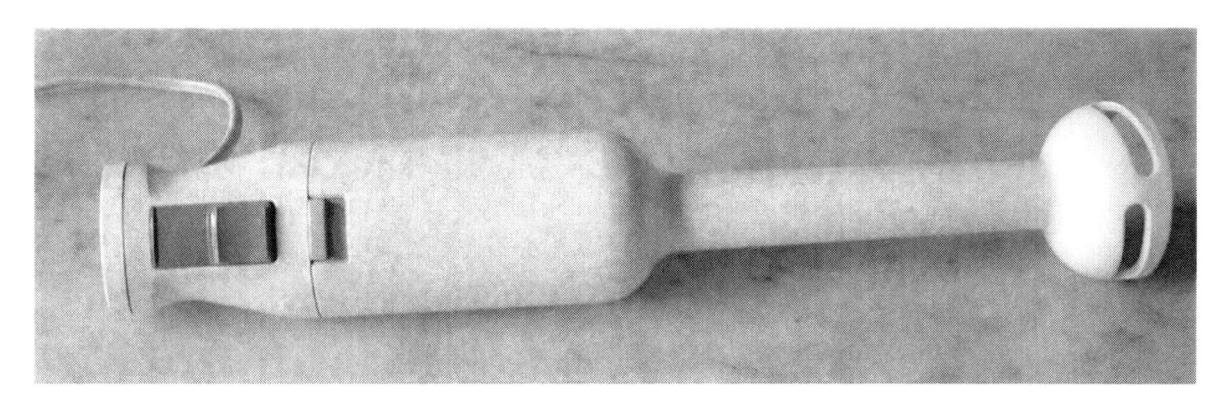

Wet grinder: It is also called meat grinder in the West. It is essential equipment for some recipes I have described. It is also used to make chutneys and some wet spice mixtures. It is essential for making germinated wheat breads.

Grating equipment: Generally, in each home, there is some kind of grater, whether it is a hand grater or electric. For some recipes, you need grated vegetables.

SOME FUNDAMENTAL PREPARATIONS

For Ayurvedic cooking, you require to learn fundamental preparations of some Ayurvedic spice mixtures and other basic ingredients like making ghee, yoghurt (curd), paneer (Fresh cheese).

Spice Mixtures

It is convenient to make various spice mixtures as it saves time and makes cooking easier. However, you need to have most spices also in individual containers, as in some preparations the individual grains are required. The

Preparation of the Basic Ayurvedic Cuisine

recipes for spice mixtures given below are according to my own classification and I have also described mixtures A and B in one of my previous books. The mixture A in this book is an improved version.

Mixture A (a rejuvenating mixture): Mixture A is an intensive ojas (immunity and vitality) enhancing combination of the following 9 spices.

1. Coriander   100 gm (½ cup)
2. Cumin   100 gm (½ cup)
3. Big cardamom   50 gm (¼ cup)
4. Black pepper   25 gm (1/8 cup)
5. Long pepper   25 gm (1/8 cup)
6. Clove   50 gm (¼ cup)
7. Cinnamon   50 gm (¼ cup)
8. Nutmeg   25 gm (6-7 nuts)
9. Mace   10 gm (2 tablespoons)

Clean the spices individually after weighing them. Remove the shells of the big cardamom. The best way to do this is to put few of them in the mortar and strike a little with the pestle. The shells will loosen and it will be easy to remove them by hand. Break the nutmegs into smaller pieces in the mortar. Put everything in a big plate or tray and dry them in the sun for half an hour or in a mildly heated oven for about 15 minutes. If you have none of these available, heat a wok and put the spices for a minute in it while stirring. It is important that the spices should be absolutely dried before grinding. Now put the spices in the coffee grinder, which should be kept exclusively for the spices. Fill the grinder only two thirds each time and grind. Do not grind too fine. Keep the sand like consistency of the powdered spices. After you have ground all the contents, pass them through a sieve. Make sure that the sieve does not have very fine holes. Generally metal sieves are good for this purpose. Ingredients which do not go through the sieve, grind them again and pass through the sieve once more. If still something is left in the strainer, you may discard it. Store the mixture in a dry, tightly closed jar and keep it in a cool place. Keep a small quantity of the mixture in a bottle for everyday use.

Mixture B (an enriching mixture): Mixture B is one of the classical mixtures used in India. It is very simple to prepare, as there is no grinding involved and spices are mixed as such in their entire form. It contains the following spices in equal quantity:

1. Coriander   50 gm (¼ cup)
2. Cumin   50 gm (¼ cup)
3. Fennel   50 gm (¼ cup)
4. Fenugreek   50 gm (¼ cup)
5. Mustard seeds   50 gm (¼ cup)

6. Kalonji   50 gm (¼ cup)
7. Ajwain   50 gm (¼ cup)

Clean spices and then mix them together. Shake the spice mixture each time you use it so that they are mixed well and are used in right proportion.

Mixture C (a cooling mixture): This mixture contains fennel and coriander in equal proportions. Since both of them are cool in their Ayurvedic nature, it is a recommended for those who have excessive pitta. Since mixture A tends to be hot, in summer or if you are a pitta person, you may use this mixture along with it. It should be also used to spice foods, which are hot in their Ayurvedic nature.

1. Coriander   50 gm (¼ cup)
2. Fennel   50 gm (¼ cup)

Clean the above two spices, dry them and grind them as is explained for the mixture A. Store it in a clean and dry jar.

Mixture D (a hot mixture to heal vitiated vata and kapha): This mixture is contrary to the above and is hot in nature. It is especially for cold weather or for those who have vata-kapha vitiation.

1. Dried ginger   50 gm (¼ cup)
2. Ajwain   50 gm (¼ cup)
3. Cumin   50 gm (¼ cup)
4. Black pepper   25 gm (1/8 cup)
5. Long pepper   25 gm (1/8 cup)
6. Fennel   25 gm (1/8 cup)
7. Clove   10 gm (2 tablespoons)
8. Dill seeds   15 gm (3 tablespoons)

Dry and grind all these spices together. Break dried ginger pieces into smaller bits in a mortar before grinding. Store the spice mixture in a clean and dry jar.

Mixture E (a spicy mixture for pickles and for rapid preparations): This mixture is generally used to make pickles from vegetables. This spice mixture is also handy when you are rushed for time while preparing vegetables or other food items. It gives a nice and spicy taste to the food.

1. Ajwain   50 gm (¼ cup)
2. Dried ginger   50 gm (¼ cup)
3. Cumin   50 gm (¼ cup)
4. Black pepper   25 gm (1/8 cup)
5. Long pepper   25 gm (1/8 cup)
6. Clove   10 gm (2 tablespoons)

Preparation of the Basic Ayurvedic Cuisine

7.	Cinnamon	10 gm (2 tablespoons)
8.	Small cardamom	10 gm (2 tablespoons)

Grind everything together accept ajwain which should be left as it is. Remember to take off the pods of small cardamom and make smaller pieces of the dried ginger before grinding everything in the electric grinder.

Mixture F (a spicy and sour mixtures): The Mixture F is essentially for making spicy vegetables and fruit salads. Since it contains rock salt, do not use salt whenever you use this mixture.

1.	Ajwain	50 gm (¼ cup)
2.	Dried ginger	50 gm (¼ cup)
3.	Cumin	50 gm (¼ cup)
4.	Black pepper	25 gm (1/8 cup)
5.	Long pepper	25 gm (1/8 cup)
6.	Clove	20 gm (2 tablespoons)
7.	Cinnamon	20 gm (2 tablespoons)
8.	Small cardamom	20 gm (2 tablespoons)
9.	Rock salt	100 gm (¼ cup)
10.	Mango powder	50 gm (¼ cup)
11.	Dill seeds	25 gm (1/8 cup)
12.	Dried peppermint leaves	50 gm (¼ cup)

Grind everything together as explained earlier.

Mixture G (A Green Mixture for Soups): This mixture is made with dried herbs like parsley, coriander, mint, basil, celery, dill, oregano, laurel leaves and other kitchen herbs one uses. If you have a garden, collect each of the herbs during the season, wash them and dry them. Otherwise, buy them during the season and dry them. Herbs should not be dried in sun for too long. Spread them on a napkin in a warm place. In the hot climate they dry very rapidly even in shade. Collect as many as possible but make sure that you have them all in almost similar quantity. When they are all dry, crush them with your hands and mix them together. Then grind them with the electric grinder. You will realise that a large quantity will reduce to a very small amount after grinding.

This green mixture is used for garnishing soups. Use about ¼ of a teaspoon for each serving of the soup.

Mixture H (A Mixture for Rayata and Salads): Rayata is a salty preparation made with curd (yoghurt). Curd is kapha promoting and therefore heavy to digest. Mixture H promotes agni or the body's digestive fire. Similarly, green salads and other raw vegetables require strong digestive power. This mixture promotes digestion.

1. Cumin (slightly roasted on a pan)   50 gm
2. Dill seeds   30 gm
3. Ajwain   50 gm
4. Black pepper   25 gm
5. Long pepper   25 gm
6. Peppermint leaves (dried)   50 gm

Grind all the ingredients and mix them well.

Preparations with Milk Products

Making ghee from butter: Normally, ghee is available in Indian grocery stores abroad. In some countries, something similar to ghee is sold but unfortunately, they add preservatives and its use is not recommended. To make ghee from butter is fairly simple and you may make in larger quantities for several months.

Take good quality unsalted butter. Put it in a pot and place on medium heat. After all the butter has melted, reduce heat and let it cook for about 15 minutes. Stir from time to time and wait until all the water evaporates. The ghee is ready when you see the transparent fat in the pan. Test to make sure that no traces of water remain in the ghee. Otherwise the ghee will get fungus. To test, take a metal lid and put on the top of your pot for half a minute. Pick it up and touch it to see if there is any trace of water left on the lid. Cook until there is no dampness on the lid. As soon as there is no moisture, take off the pot from the stove. If you continue to cook after all the water has evaporated, the fat will burn and the ghee will turn brown.

The last part of this process is to strain the preparation. Wait until it is not too hot and strain it through a piece of thin cotton cloth in order to separate the burnt out proteins. Do not let it cool down as it solidifies and you will not be able to filter it. Preserve the ghee in clean and dry jars. When the ghee cools down, it becomes semi-solid. If kept in refrigerator, it becomes hard. The ghee is between light yellow and white depending upon the quality of the milk.

Making yoghurt from milk: It is very simple to transform milk into yoghurt (curd). You need not have a special gadget for this purpose. There are two different kinds of bacteria called lactobacillus or streptococcus, which convert milk into yoghurt when their culture is put in milk at an appropriate temperature.

Take fresh milk and boil it. Put the milk in an earthen vessel. Let it cool down until it is as hot as a real hot bath water. Add half a teaspoon of good quality plain yoghurt with living bacteria into this hot milk and stir so that it mixes up properly. Put the lid on and cover the yoghurt pot with a small blanket or use an old pullover. Leave it for 7-8 hours. It is best to put it at night and then pick up in the morning. The best temperature for the bacterial culture to grow is about 37⁰ C (99⁰ F). The reason to cover the pot is to maintain this temperature for a while. In hot climatic conditions, the room temperature is generally high enough for the bacteria to grow and one may not require covering the pot. Once the milk is coagulated and the yoghurt is made, either consume it within few hours or put it in the refrigerator. If it is left too long at room temperature, the bacteria will grow further and the yoghurt will become sour.

Fresh yoghurt promotes pitta and kapha and cures vitiated vata. It is strength promoting. Yoghurt should not be consumed too much and never at night. Those who have any kind of inflammation in the body or any muscular or joint pain should not eat it. In the West, many people are used to eating sweet yoghurts. Commercial sweet yoghurts are generally prepared with some fruit jams and added starch to thicken them. In homemade yoghurt, you may add some fresh fruits and honey or some home made fruit jam.

Creamy yoghurt: It is easy to prepare delicious creamy yoghurt from the homemade one. Hang the fresh yoghurt you have prepared in a thin muslin cloth as shown in the picture on the next page. Leave it for about fifteen minutes. The excess water will come down from the cloth and you will be left with thick, creamy yoghurt.

Note: Some people think that if they eat something creamy, they will put on weight. It is always the excessive quantity of food, which makes you put on weight. For example, in present case, if you are eating one cup of yoghurt or draining out the water from it and eating slightly lesser quantity, it does not make any difference at all.

Cheese from yoghurt: For making cheese from yoghurt, you have to do the same as above (hanging the yoghurt in a muslin cloth) but for about two hours or a little more. You will be left with semi-solid contents of the yoghurt. Add different spices and herbs into it.

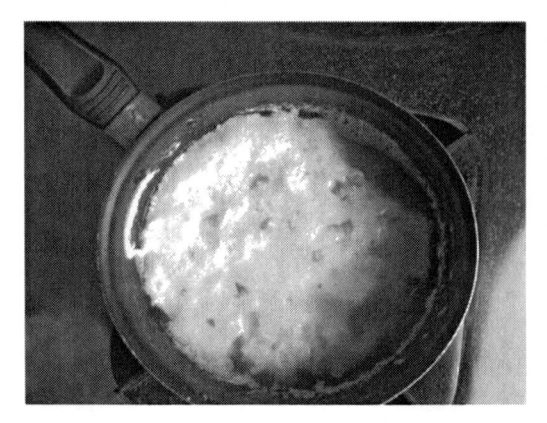

Paneer from milk: Paneer can be compared to fresh cheese. Solids of the milk are separated by adding some sour substance into the boiling milk. Take a litre of full cream fresh milk, put it in a pot and heat it. Wait until it comes to a boil. Add immediately a tablespoon of lemon juice. The solids of the milk will begin to float in the semi-transparent liquid. In case it does not happen, add a little more lemon juice. Once the solids of the milk form lumps in the watery substance, the paneer is ready. Normally one tablespoon full of lemon juice is enough to make paneer from 1 litre (5 cups) of fresh milk but due to the pasteurisation and homogenisation of the milk in many places in the world, you may require a little more lemon juice than that. Depending on the recipes, you may need to separate the solids from the liquid. For that, pass the contents through a thin muslin cloth as you have done above in case of yoghurt and hang it to drain out the rest of the water. For making cubes, put the whole thing (paneer inside the cloth) on a flat surface like a wooden board and place some weight on it. The idea is to squeeze out the rest of the fluid and obtain a solid round piece, which holds together and can be cut into small cubes.

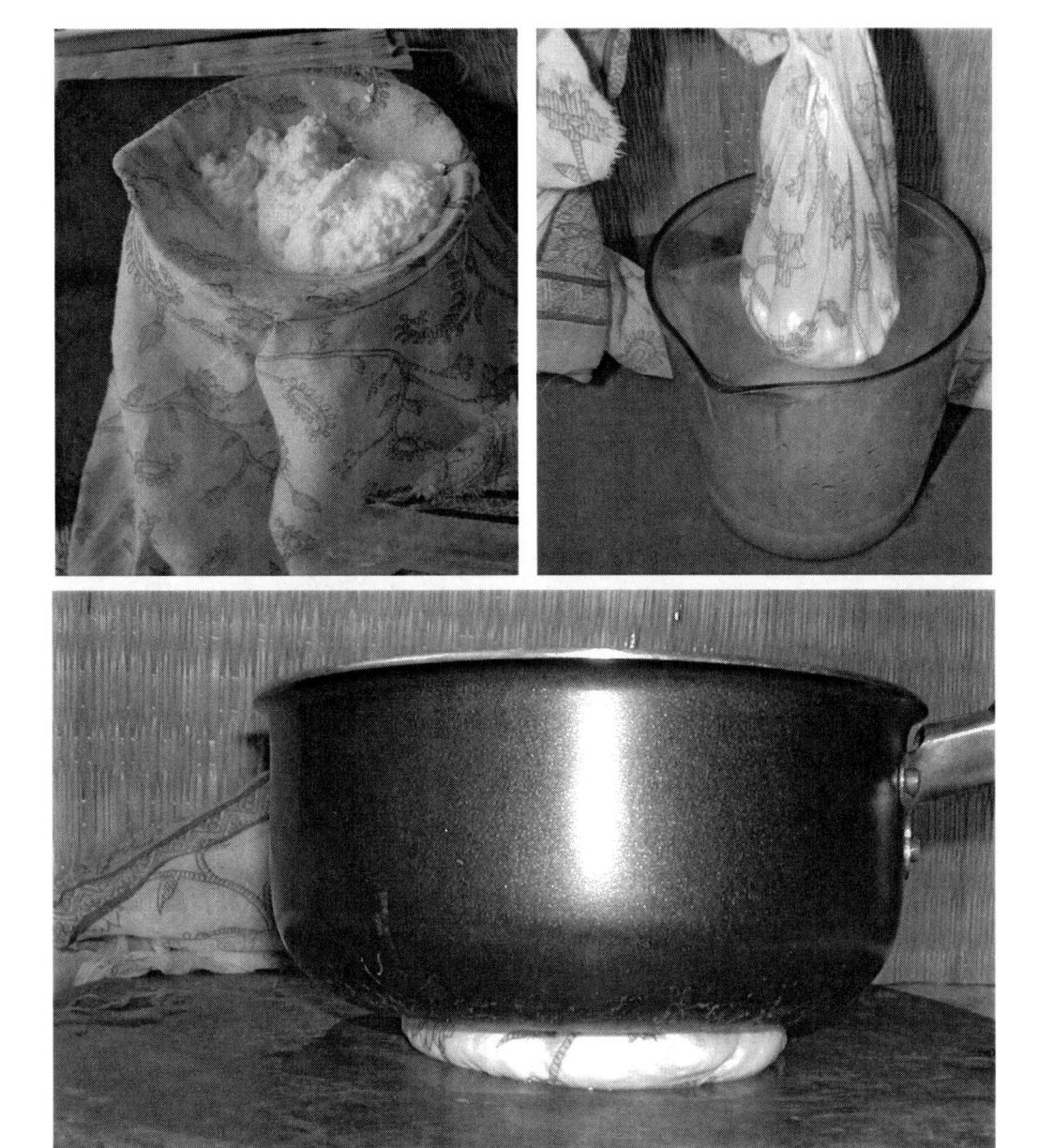

Various stages of obtaining solid paneer pieces

Germination of seeds and growing herbs: According to Ayurveda, for promoting health, the best period of germination is when this process just begins. This means that you observe a tiny sprout at a stage when it is just beginning to emerge. For this kind of sprouting, you do not need any special apparatus. Soak the grains for about 24 hours in water. If it is hot, you may even need lesser time. If the temperature in your kitchen is around 18 ^{0} C (about 63º F), you may require a little longer time until the seeds reach a state when they just begin to germinate.

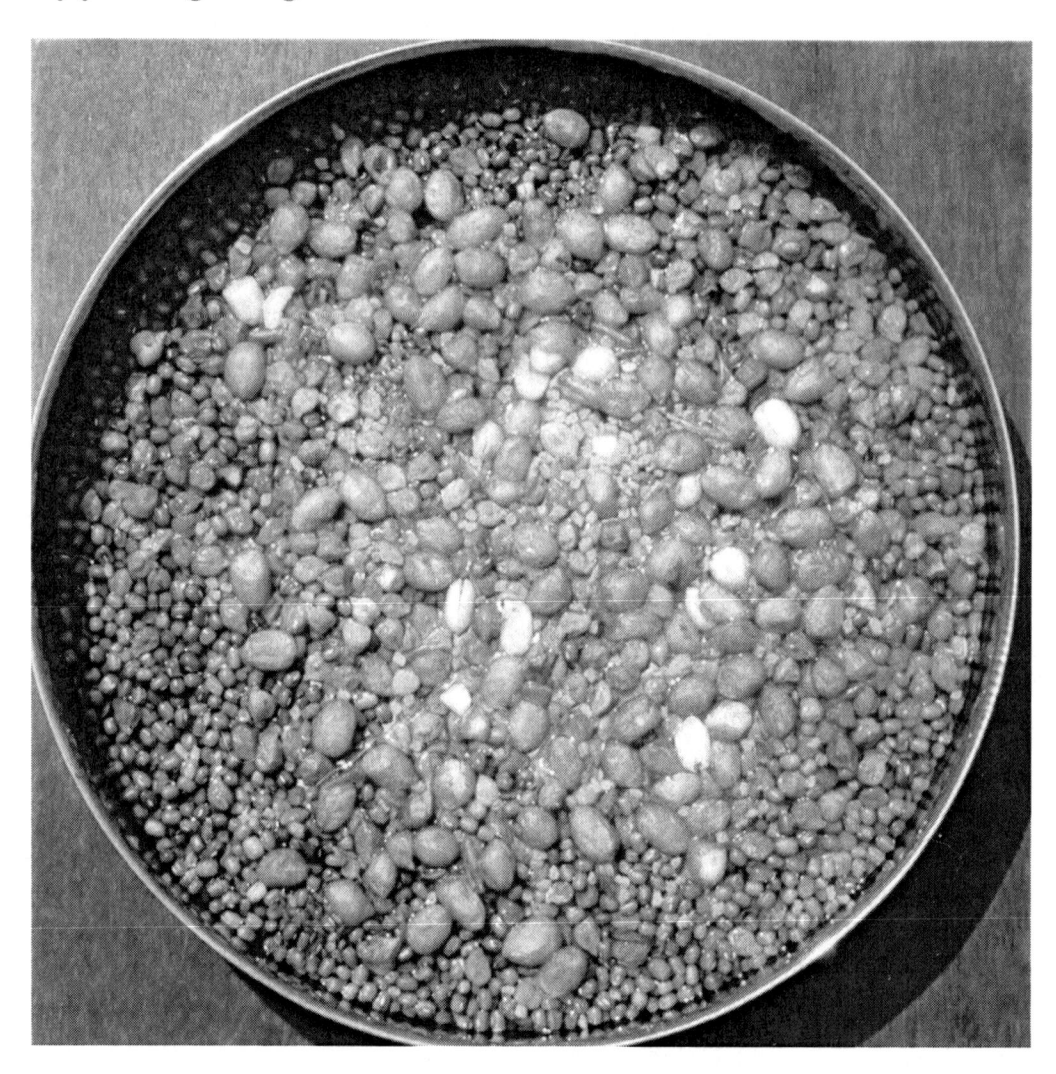

In the recipe Section, there are various dishes with germinated seeds. In particular, the wheat bread made out of these slightly germinated grains is highly strength promoting and alleviates fatigue.

There are certain things, which you may grow even in the apartment in pots. It is important to have some fresh herbs like basil, peppermint, coriander, dill etc. and they are fairly easy to grow in pots. Take good soil with a lot of manure in it and plant the seeds. Sprinkle a little water on it everyday. Keep near the window or outside. Fresh herbs add beauty and prana to your dishes when mixed with salads or used to garnish cooked food.

Fenugreek and cress may be grown to get fresh winter salads. They are winter plants. They grow very rapidly. Since they are hot in their Ayurvedic nature and alleviate vata, their use is highly recommended during winters.

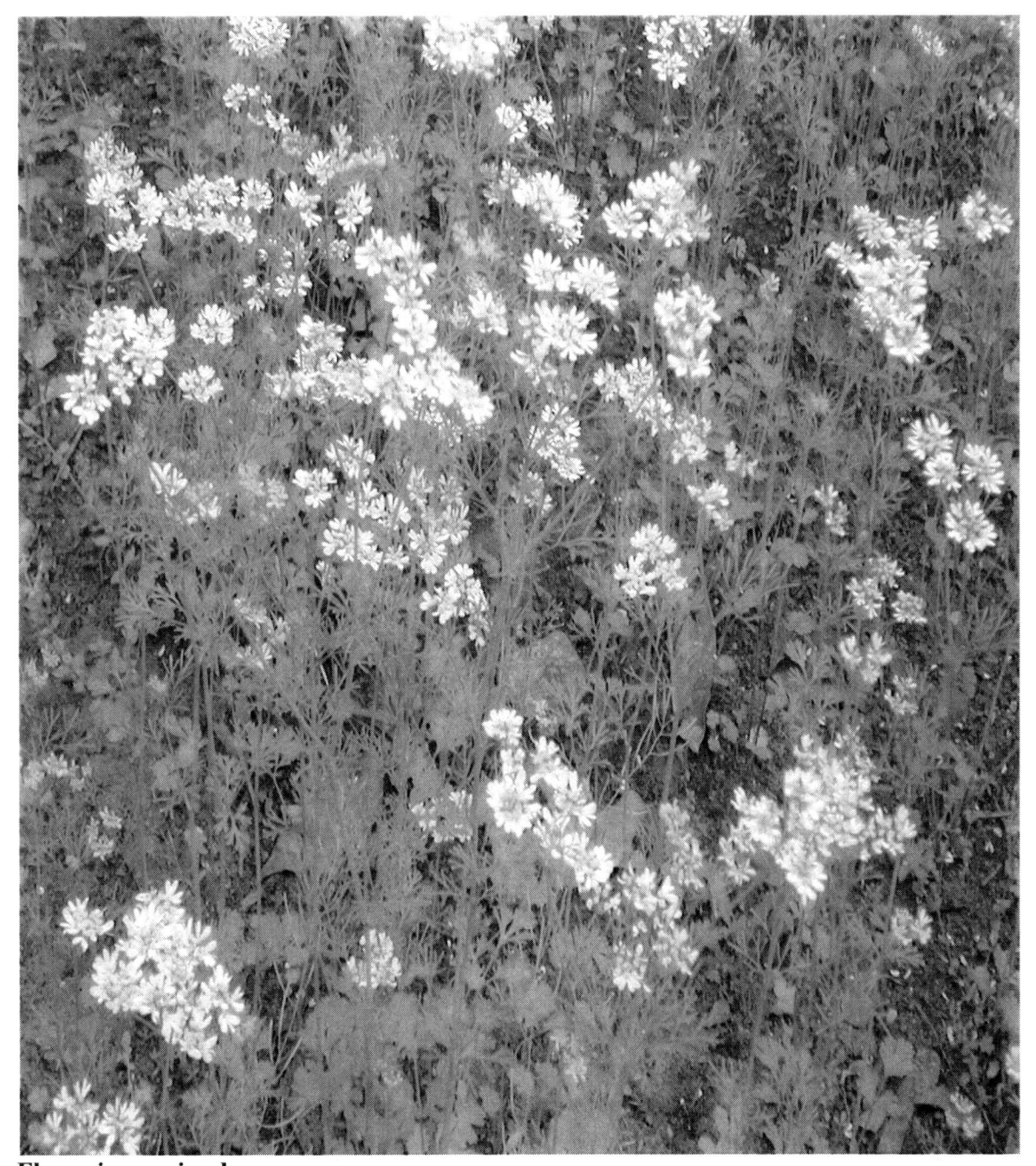

Flowering coriander

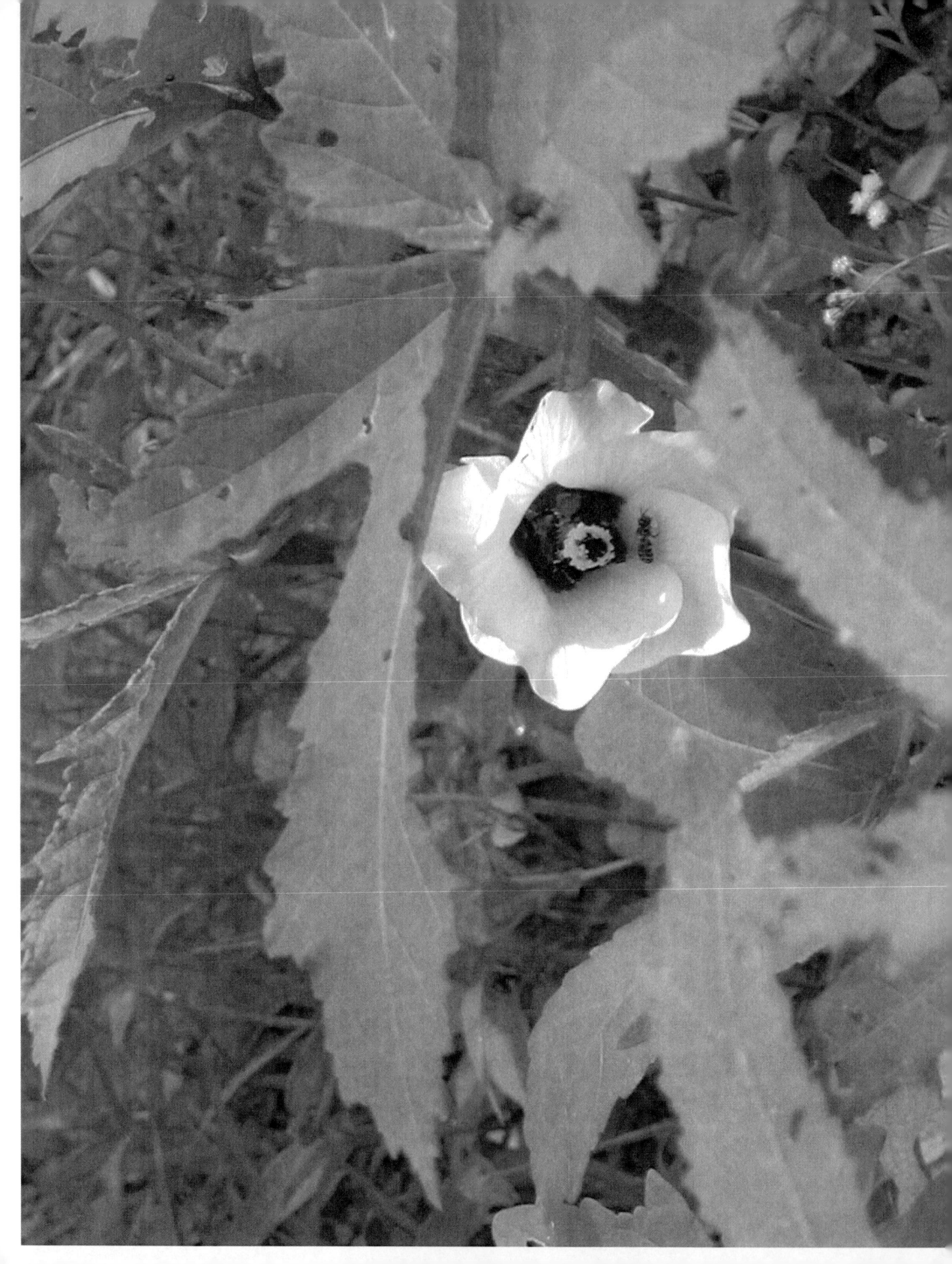

SECTION II

THE AYURVEDIC FOOD RECIPES

The body is the product of food, whether eaten, drunk, licked or devoured. ...Wholesome and unwholesome food produce good and bad effects on the body respectively.

One desirous of happiness should follow the regimen prescribed for the prevention of unborn and alleviation of born disorders. Although activities of all creatures are directed intuitively towards happiness, the good and bad course they adopt depend upon the knowledge and ignorance respectively.

Charaka Samhita
Sixth Century BC

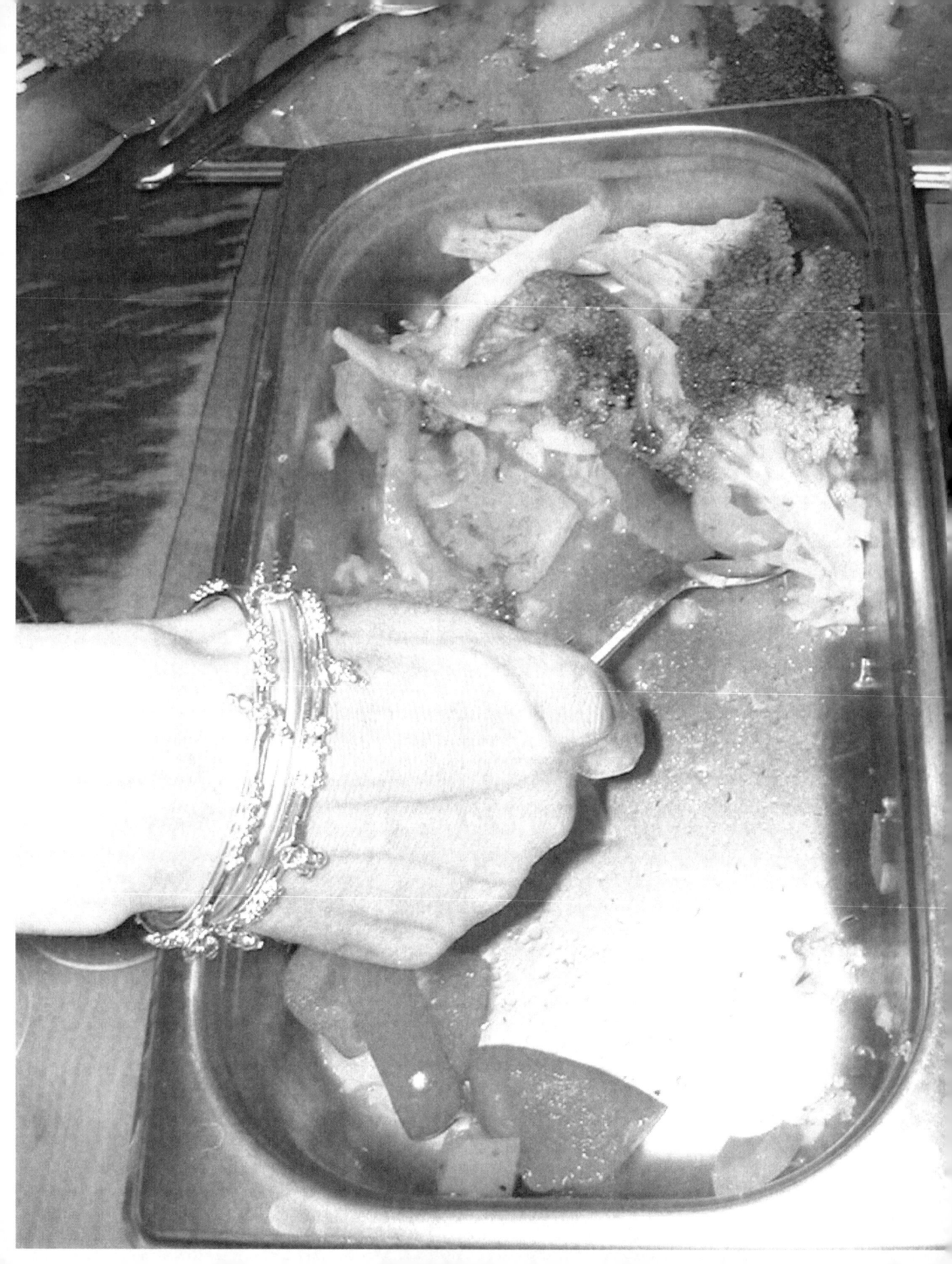

INTRODUCTION TO THE RECIPES

Ayurveda recommends eating warm, well-prepared and well-cooked food. The cold preparations include side dishes like salads, chutneys, *rayatas* (yoghurt preparations) and some drinks and desserts. Warm, well-cooked food assimilates better in the body and helps keep vata equilibrium. Thus, you will find that recipes for all the meals including breakfast are warm. Meals should be always freshly prepared. Pre-cooked meals or any kind of food preparation done many hours or a day in advance are called *basa* and they cause vata imbalance.

I have specially taken care that the recipes are easy and quick to prepare. The recipes given here are international and I got the inspiration from many different countries in the world. In fact, when I say 'Ayurvedic recipes', it means the food preparations which will help maintain an equilibrium of the three energies of the body with the help of some herbs and spices or by adding some other specific ingredients. It is thus possible to convert practically any of your favourite dishes into Ayurvedic ones. Therefore, the following recipes should also inspire you to use the Ayurvedic methods and ingredients in your routine cooking in order to have easily digestible, tasty and health promoting food.

In the West, many of the food products are partially pre-prepared, and people generally do not know what all they are eating. Many times, I have encountered such persons who claimed that they do not eat any salt or sugar because they are supposed to be bad for health. They did not have these two ingredients in their kitchens. They were quite unaware that the bread and the cheese they are generally eating are full of salt. Most chocolates have 50% sugar and several cakes and other desserts contain significantly more than 25% sugar. Long ago in the United States, in the canteen at the NIH (National Institutes of Health), Bethesda, I took a fruit yoghurt, which was supposed to be without sugar. When I tasted it, I realised that it had much more sugar than normally fruits would have. I started to read what it said on the container. The contents of this yoghurt were 'Full cream yoghurt with blueberry jam'. With many food products, people are often misled like that. People hardly ever realise how much salt and sugar they are eating, leave aside all chemicals such as preservatives and colours etc. That is why several students in my cooking classes in Europe, as well as when they come in India to our centres show their amazement at the amount of salt, sugar, spices and other ingredients we utilise. When we prepare

Introduction to the Recipes

our food from basic ingredients, at least we know what we are eating, to what we are reacting and therefore, we can control the ingredients in our food.

It is important to eat homemade food in order to enhance the quality of life and to rejuvenate oneself constantly. It is equally important to observe the reactions of various foodstuffs on your body and to modify the food according to your well-being. Warm and unctuous food with an appropriate quantity of rejuvenating spices and herbs, taken in a moderate quantity can cure your minor ailments and enhance your vitality.

Earlier, I pointed out that not all Indian food preparations are Ayurvedic and that Ayurvedic food does not necessarily have to be Indian. I will explain this by giving some examples so that you understand the concept of Ayurvedic cooking better. In some Indian homes and largely in restaurants, when they make the basic sauce for some vegetable or meat dishes with onions, ginger, garlic, curd is added to it. Although the sauce is delicious, it is very heavy to digest and Ayurveda does not recommend this. According to the Ayurvedic principles, the sauce is too sour. The curd (yoghurt) becomes sour when it is heated. In some places they add cream to this sauce. Milk and cream are antagonist to the sour of the tomatoes, and therefore it is not recommended. Similarly, tomato cream soup, a European recipe, tastes very good but due to antagonism of sour and cream, it is not healthy. One can alter it by not adding fresh cream and using something to sweeten it or to add extra herbs and spices to lessen the extreme sour. Addition of a potato or an extract from corn flour or cornstarch and so on are some of the ways to do this.

Garlic is a rasayana and should be used in small quantities, almost everyday. Garlic has many volatile oils which are sensitive to heat. Thus, to safeguard the medicinal values of garlic, it should be added in the end of the cooked preparation, as you will notice in all the recipes given below. However, in many Indian homes and restaurants, garlic is added with onions and ginger in the beginning of the preparation and thus it loses most of its health promoting qualities.

In some recipes I have given the reasons for a specific way of preparation so that you can use those ideas in other recipes you know. It is also important to vary preparations according to your constitution, weather and climate. For example, if you have a pitta constitution and feel that one of my recipes is giving you too much heat in the body, you may leave out hot things from it like mixture A or garlic. You can use mixture C instead to beat the heat. You can do the same in excessively hot climate. You can also enhance the use of bitter salads and vegetables in hot climate. In winter, you can use more dill seeds, fenugreek, kalonji and saffron.

Ayurvedic Food Culture and Recipes

The recipes given in this book are not only to give important examples of how to prepare good and balanced food, but also to teach you the essential wisdom of Ayurvedic cooking.

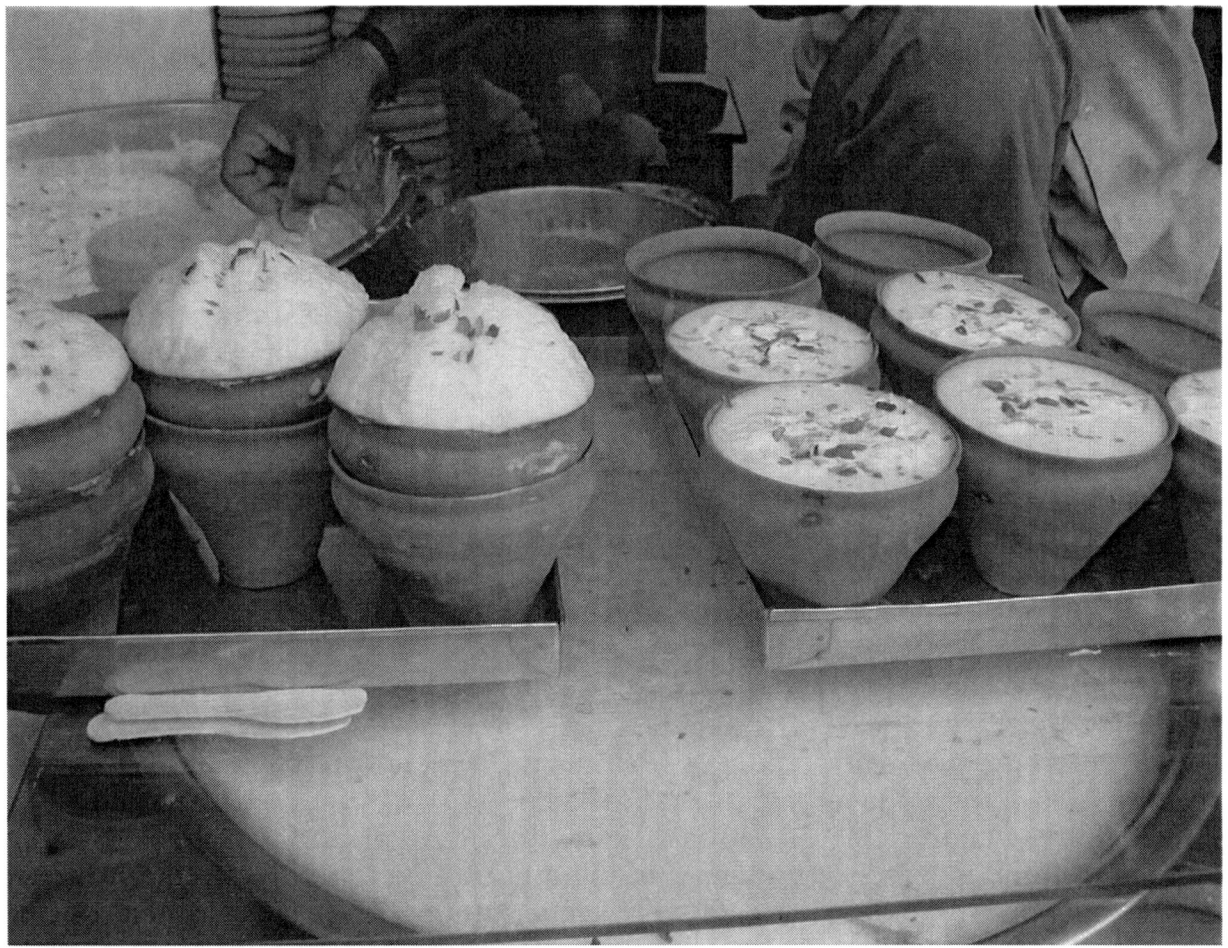

Various Curd (Yoghurt) dishes in Varanasi

A Note for the Indian Reader

The order in which recipes are presented varies according to the food habits of different countries and cultures. In modern day India, we have also a concept of 'small meals' for breakfast. It is because many people eat their lunches very late and the school timings also generally extend up to the middle of the afternoon. Besides that, many Indians are used to eating rice dishes and freshly made breads like chapatis and paranthas and so on for breakfast. We have tremendous variety of foods in India in different states. Though most of our cooking is still based upon Ayurvedic principles, there are also numerous things which are not made by keeping in mind the balance and harmony of the body. For example, in north India, we have Mouglai food which can be good for the pallet but injurious to your health. If eaten frequently, the stomach will revolt. Southern Indian food is balanced and less fat but they do an over-dose of green chilli or red chilli. Mixture of Urd dal and rice that is used for numerous recipes in Southern India is very health and energy promoting. Urd dal is used in Ayurveda in many rasayanas (health promoting substances) and aphrodisiac preparations. However, anything from Urd dal has to be prepared with great caution as it has extreme pitta and kapha energies and can lead to an imbalance in the body. Its combination with rice is ideal and promotes ojas (immunity and vitality).

There are certain ways of preparing some foods, which are not light and healthy according to Ayurveda, and you should keep that in mind. Yoghurt (curd) in cooked form, whether in the Mouglai sauce or Punjabi and Sindhi kadi or in Gujarati dhaukala is heavy to digest and should not be taken too frequently and should be avoided at night. Foods with fermentation (yeast) should also not be taken too often. Bread, rolls and bhaturas have lot of yeast. Excess of yeast leads to vata and pitta imbalance and causes acidity and pain in the joints. The batter for idaly, dosas etc. have also little yeast but that is at the beginning of fermentation.

Yoghurt and dishes made of yoghurt should be strictly avoided at night. Dals should also not be eaten with dinner as they are heavy to digest. One should always have light things for dinner as the shrotas or energy channels of the body are partially closed at night. Body follows the rhythm of the day and as the sunsets, gradually the activities of energy channels also slow down. During sleep, they are in a state of relaxation. Our sages said all this thousands of years ago. Now this rhythm of biological clock is also recognised in modern biology and medical sciences.

BEVERAGES

It is very important to maintain fluidity in our system and therefore beverages are described in the beginning of the other recipes. We lose lot of water during sleep and therefore it is essential to drink something in the morning. For the purification purpose, one should drink one to two glasses of hot water in the morning. Drinking hot water empty stomach cleans the digestive tract well, insures proper evacuation and purifies the kidneys and the bladder.

In traditional Ayurvedic cuisine, there are a number of beverages which are taken in order to create equilibrium in the body under varying weather conditions. For example, in hot summers, various sharbats* (Syrups) are recommended to lessen the side effects of heat. There are a variety of spices and herbs, which are used as teas in winter to maintain body balance. I have also given a recipe for a rejuvenating breakfast tea.

Some drinks are health promoting as well as aphrodisiac. But the most important drink is water. Water varies from place to place and differs in taste as well as in its mineral contents. For example, water containing sulphur is pitta promoting, whereas water containing more calcium is kapha enhancing. Saline water is pitta-kapha dominating. If the water has a slightly astringent taste, it will be vata dominating. With Ayurvedic methods, we can bring equilibrium to water to some extent.

CARDAMOM-WATER

It is better to boil drinking water with cardamom not only to improve the taste and flavour, but also to create equilibrium. Take 2-3 cardamoms, remove the pods, crush them and add them in two litres (4 pints) of water and bring it to boil. In case the water you are using has any biological contamination, boil it for 15 minutes. After cooling down, store your water in clean bottles. For Ayurvedic lifestyle, it is suggested drinking two glasses of warm cardamom water in the morning upon getting up. It cleans up the toxins from the body, purifies intestines and kidneys.

---

* The word sharbat is taken into English language and is spelt as Sherbet. I have used spellings which are more phonetic.

Beverages

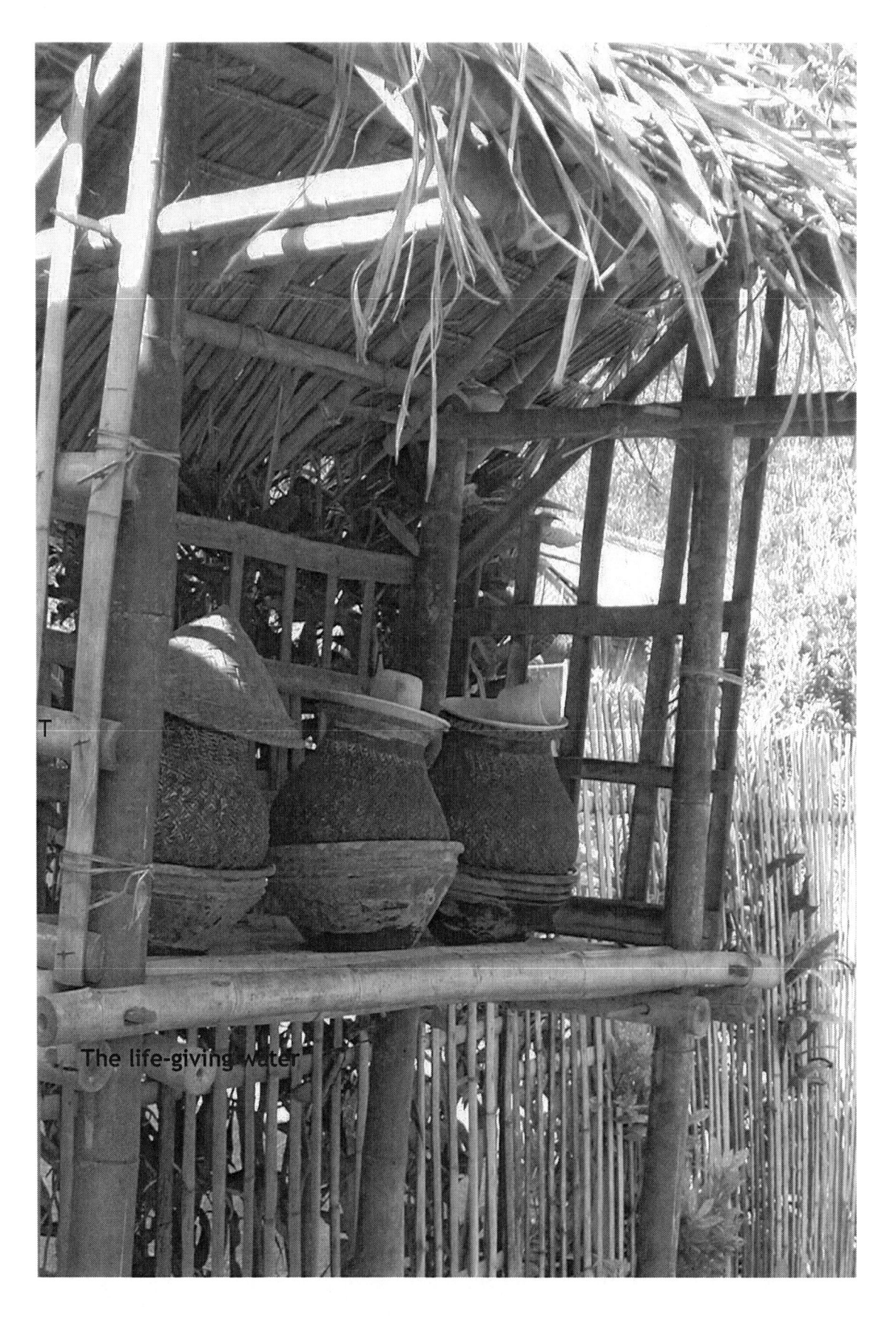

The life-giving water

TEAS

In former times people had not much choice but to use locally produced things. This was true for food as well. In India, various herbal teas were taken in different parts of the country, and black tea was used only in the areas where it was grown.

When the British commercialised tea in India as well as in other parts of the world, gradually the local teas were pushed back and black tea became a predominant drink in North India. Coffee took this place in southern India as over there the commercial coffee plantation was introduced. The usual herbal mixtures came to be known as 'desi chai' (country tea) or Ayurvedic teas. Some important herbal teas were lost forever; others are still alive amongst the tribal communities in different parts of the country. It is noteworthy that the Indian mind which is moulded with Ayurvedic wisdom, did not accept the black tea as such. Indians found it a good drink because it stimulated but thought it was not balanced because it was too sour and too hot in its Ayurvedic nature. Black tea is still regarded by some people as 'that drink which burns your insides'. However, milk and sugar tone down its negative effect. To get rid of the negative effects of the black tea, Indians added various things according to the season and particular circumstances. Ginger, cardamom, clove, cinnamon, pepper etc. can be added in various proportions.

In Ayurvedic food culture, various spices in different combinations are used for healing and rejuvenation. Crush the spices and boil them in water for about 5 minutes with the lid on and on low heat. Afterwards, leave the tea for another five minutes. It is not a decoction in the technical sense of Ayurveda. It is what we call the Ayurvedic tea. You may add into it a little candy sugar. Recall that honey is antagonist to heat. However, if you take the tea warm and not hot, you may add honey. Some teas with liquorice are sweet and one does not require anything else to sweeten them.

I will describe below various combinations of spices and herbs, each for half litre water (2½ cup). I will also indicate the effect of each tea in terms of energies. Remember always that the aim in Ayurveda is to have equilibrium. If we make a tea with a substance that is hot in its Ayurvedic nature, we add something to create equilibrium so that we do not have side-effects. However, in the present context, we are dealing with food and not medicine. There are many things from Ayurvedic cuisine which are also used as medicine. The difference between the two is that medicine is taken in bigger doses and regularly for the purpose of healing. These are not teas but decoctions and there is a prescription for their intake. For example, the combination of ginger, basil, cardamom and pepper as tea may be taken as pleasure after dinner or on a winter evening. But the same

Beverages

tea, made stronger and taken every four hours is a remedy for bad throat, cough and fever etc.

Ajwain tea

Add ½ teaspoon of Ajwain in ½ litre (2 ½ cup) of water and bring it to boil. Keep covered and reduce the heat. Let it simmer for 5 minutes. Put off the heat and allow it to stand for another 5 minutes. Strain and add some candy sugar (mishri) to sweeten it (optional).

Ajwain tea is very good for digestion. It cures the loss of appetite, alcohol hangover, heaviness in the stomach and indigestion. It should normally be taken after meals. Since ajwain is hot in its Ayurvedic nature, pitta-dominated persons should add a pinch of fennel in it.

Ajwain and ginger tea

Along with the ajwain in the above recipe, add ¼ teaspoon of powdered ginger or a 1½ cm (about ½ inch) cube of crushed fresh ginger. This tea helps revive sluggish liver functions.

Ginger-cardamom tea

Add 1 teaspoon of chopped ginger and 2 crushed cardamom in ½ litre (2 ½ cup) water and bring to boil. If you do not have fresh ginger, you can add ¼ teaspoon of dried and powdered ginger. If you find the tea too strong, lessen the quantity of ginger or else add a pinch of fennel or anise. Alternatively, lessen ginger and add one cardamom more.

Ginger-cardamom-basil tea

It is the same as above but add a few leaves of basil into it.

Ginger-cardamom-basil-pepper tea

A pinch of pepper is added to the above recipe.

The last three teas are highly recommended for person of vata and kapha prakriti. The last recipe is good to cure cold, cough and fever; as a remedy, it should be taken every 3-4 hours.

Fennel or anise tea

This tea is made by simply pouring hot water (½ litre or 2 ½ cups) on ½ teaspoon of fennel or anise and letting it rest for about 15 minutes.

This tea is recommended for pitta prakriti persons and specially to those who have frequent bowel movements. Fennel and anise are heat sensitive and lose their medicinal qualities when heated. Therefore, as a remedy, soak 1 teaspoon of anise or fennel in same amount of water as above and keep it over night to make a cold decoction.

Basil-liquorice tea

Few leaves of basil with ½ teaspoon of powdered liquorice should be added to ½ litre (2 ½ cups) of water and boiled for about 5 minutes and then made to rest another 5 minutes. Many people find the taste of liquorice 'medicinal'.

This tea is specifically recommended for persons with pitta prakriti and for those who have weak nerves.

Big cardamom-clove-cinnamon tea

Grains of one big cardamom, 4 cloves and a little piece of cinnamon are added in half litre (2 ½ cup) of water. Boil for five minutes and let it rest for another five minutes.

Big cardamom and cinnamon are hot in their Ayurvedic nature whereas clove is cold. Nevertheless, this tea is hot in its Ayurvedic nature and pitta-dominated persons should avoid it. It should be also avoided in very hot weather.

This is a rejuvenating and anti-fatigue tea but people with hypertension (high blood pressure) should be careful as big cardamom enhances blood pressure. In fact, big cardamom is a very good remedy to cure low blood pressure.

Beverages

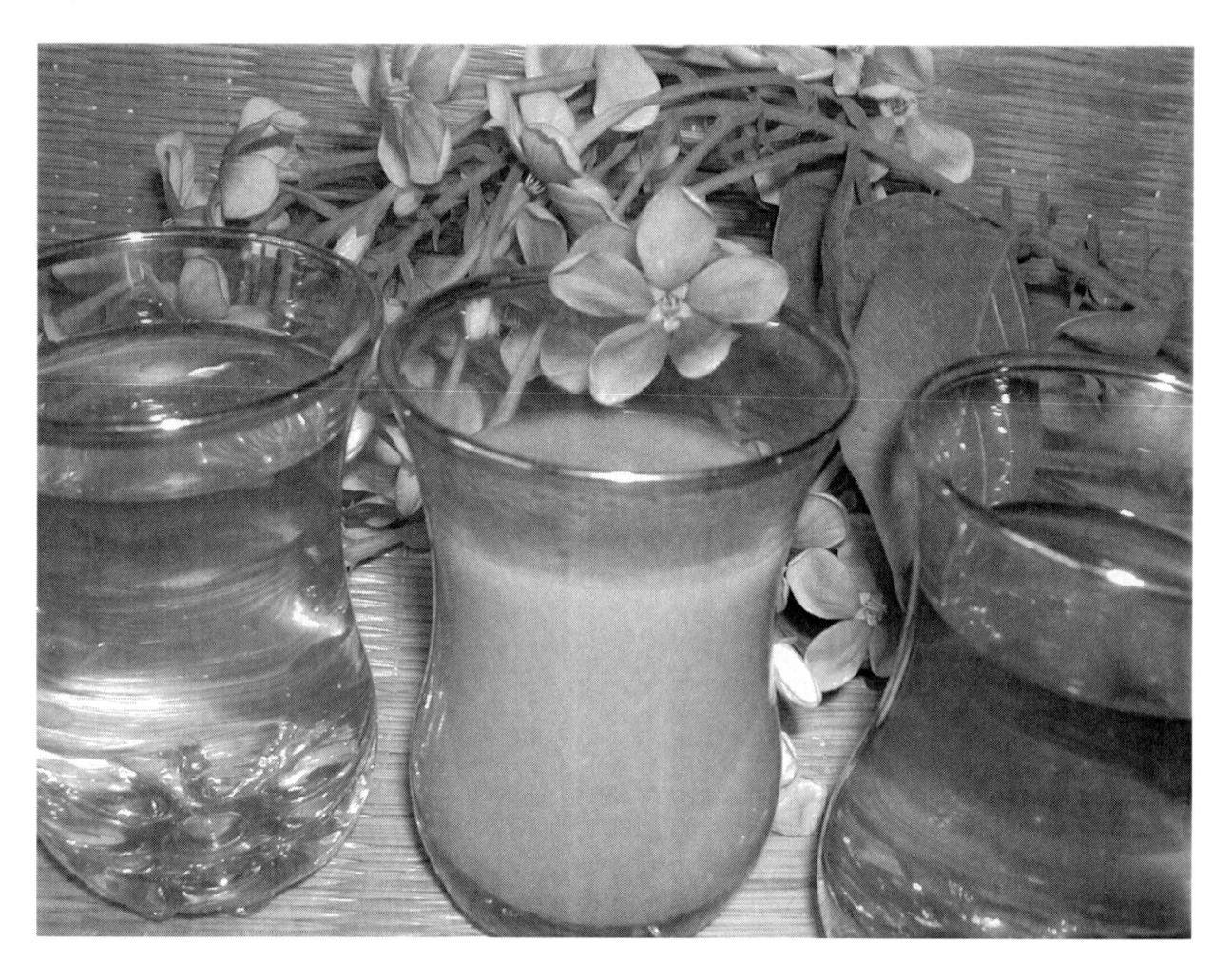

Eleven-spice anti-fatigue and rejuvenating tea

I suggest that you should make this tea mixture in bulk for everyday use.

Ingredients:

Coriander seeds	50 gm	(2 ounce)
Dried ginger	50 gm	(2 ounce)
Liquorice	50 gm	(2 ounce)
Fennel	50 gm	(2 ounce)
Cardamom seeds	25 gm	(1 ounce)
Big cardamom seeds	25 gm	(1 ounce)
Dried basil leaves (*Tulsi*)	25 gm	(1 ounce)
Long pepper*	25 gm	(1 ounce)
Black pepper	25 gm	(1 ounce)
Clove	25 gm	(1 ounce)
Cinnamon	25 gm	(1 ounce)

Clean and powder all these ingredients with the electric grinder. Mix the powder well and sieve it to make sure that there are no big pieces left. Grind once again the contents you obtain on the sieve. Make sure to mix well the final powder you have obtained. Store this powder in a tightly closed dried jar. Take out a small amount for everyday use.

Make the tea by using ½ teaspoon of this powder in ½ litre (2½ cup) of water. Boil the water on low heat for about five minutes with a lid on. Let the tea rest as such for five more minutes before serving.

Note: Those of you who are used to taking black tea or coffee can try the following recipe. Add a teaspoon of black tea (powdered black tea like the English Breakfast Tea) in the above preparation after having boiled the rejuvenation mixture for three minutes. Let the black tea boil with the rest for about thirty seconds. Add about 150 ml (3/4 cup) of milk and some candy sugar (optional). Boil everything together for another minute. Your stimulating and rejuvenating tea is ready. This drink is a very effective substitute to replace coffee.

Black tea

Black tea is hot in its Ayurvedic nature. It is anti-fatigue and anti-sleep. It is good to cure vitiated vata and kapha.

There are hundreds of varieties of black teas. The one that is used to make the above-described spice tea should not be leafy but small and granular tea and in technical language it is called 'tea dust'. The British call it 'The English Breakfast Tea'. There are several varieties of this tea. My preferred brand is Brooke Bond Red Label.

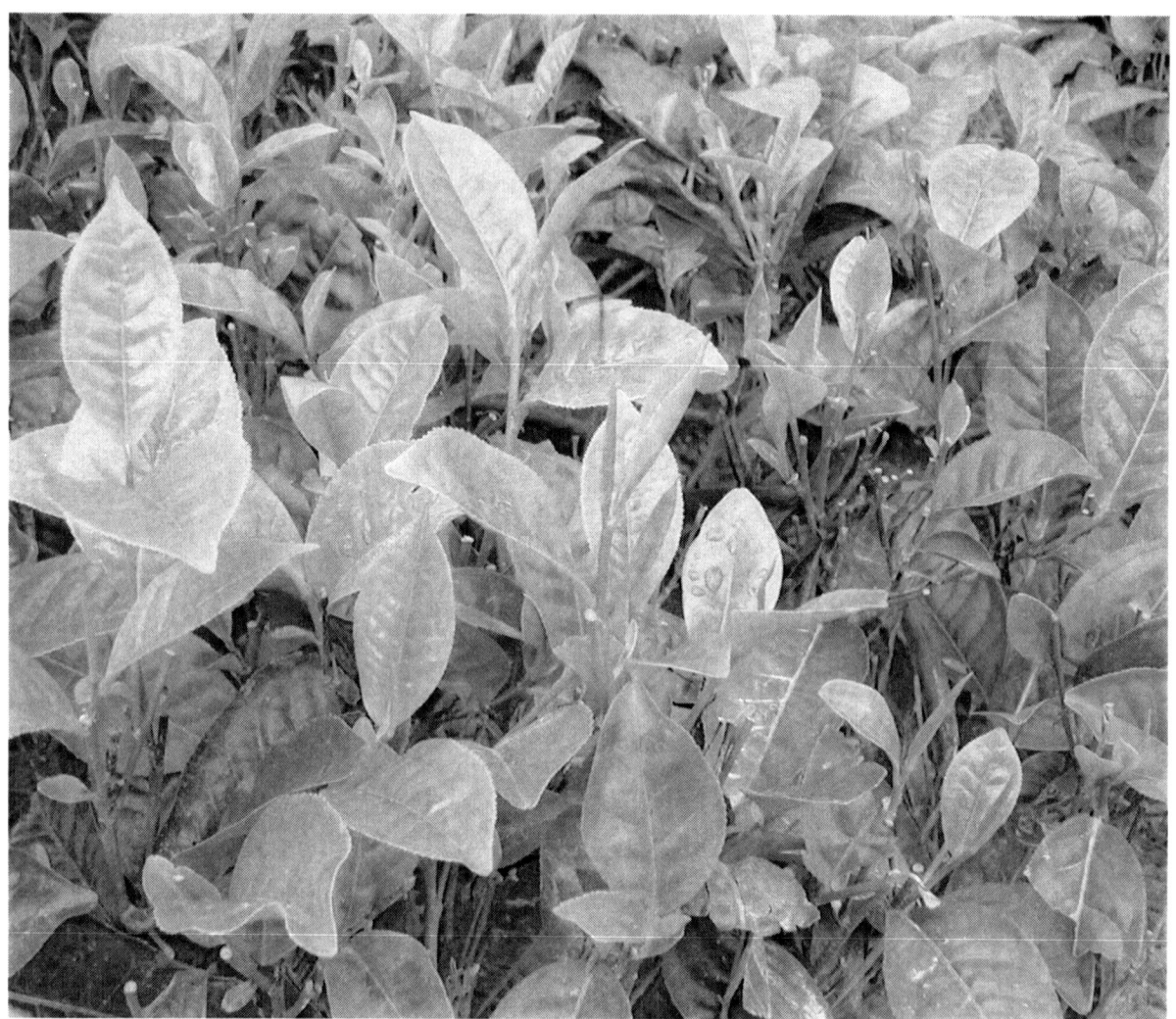

Tea plantation in Assam

Ayurvedic tradition suggests making black tea with some spices, especially with ginger and cardamom. In my experience, the most beneficial and health promoting preparation is with the eleven-spice rejuvenating tea.

For making **black tea with spices,** use the same amount of water and spices described above and boil for 2-3 minutes. Add 1 teaspoon of black tea, boil for another minute and add about 100 ml (½ cup) milk and 1½ teaspoons of candy sugar. Adjust the quantity of sugar according to your taste. Boil for another minute and the tea (called chai in India) is ready.

Black tea with spices has an anti-fatigue effect but since black tea is anti-sleep, avoid taking it after 5 or 6 o'clock in the evening. Too much black tea makes the digestion sluggish and causes stomach acidity.

COFFEE

Coffee is like black tea in its properties but stronger in its effect. It is hot in its Ayurvedic nature, alleviates fatigue and is anti-sleep. Since coffee is hot, adding milk and sugar will make it more an equilibrium drink than black coffee. In any case, black coffee should not be taken on an empty stomach. People with weak nerves or those who get easily worried should avoid taking this drink. Excess of coffee can give rise to arrhythmic heartbeat.

Note: Black tea and coffee, like tobacco, are mild drugs and are addictive. Do not take them in excess.

FRESH FRUIT OR VEGETABLE JUICES

According to Ayurveda, the juice of vegetables and fruits should be consumed fresh, within half an hour of preparation. Juice kept long after pressing the fruits or vegetables vitiates vata.

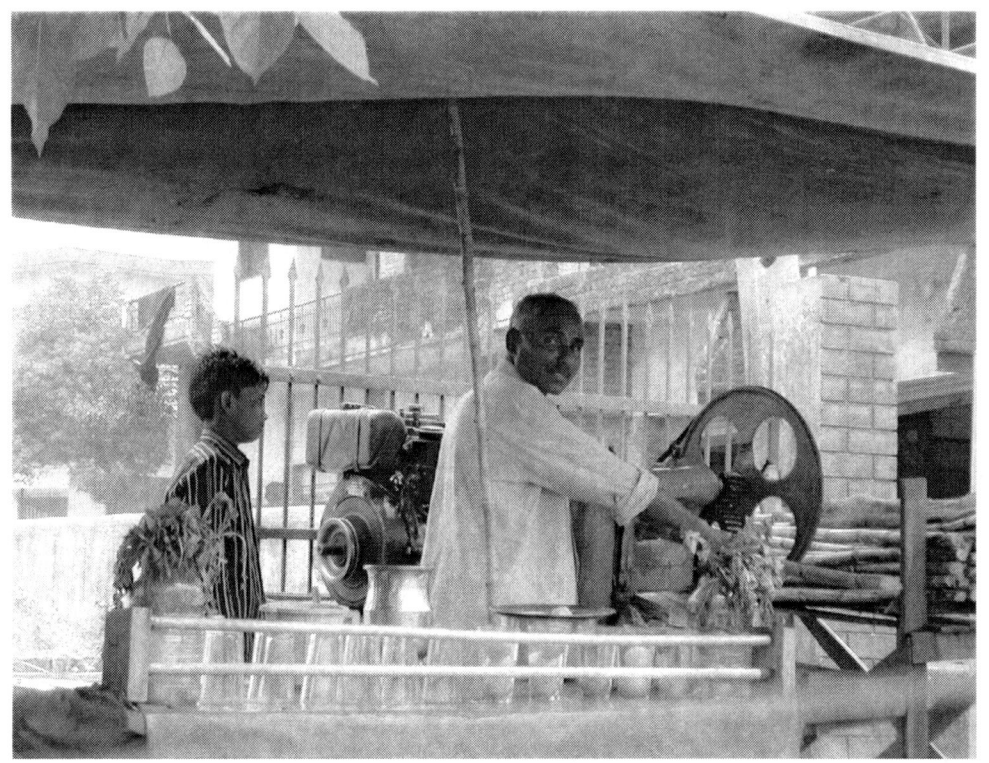

Sugarcane juice vendor

All bottled juices are vata promoting and if taken regularly over a long period of time, they vitiate vata. This is the reason that in India, the bottled drinks are not much popular, and freshly pressed juices are sold almost everywhere.

Beverages

Fresh juices are specially recommended for sick and convalescent persons. Carrot juice is particularly recommended for those who have problems with their vision. Pomegranate juice is rejuvenating and brings balance of the three energies in the body. Juice from sweet apples does the same thing. Sugarcane juice purifies the urinary system. It is often made with a bit of lemon, ginger and peppermint to balance its sweet rasa (see the picture above). Sour juices should be avoided.

SHARVATS AND OTHER DRINKS

Spicy Lemon Drink

This is not a traditional recipe; I have made it specially to help against dry throat in hot weather and to re-establish an equilibrium after the loss of vitality due to sweating. This syrup is equally good when mixed with hot water and used as a hot drink for winter evenings. It is thirst quencher, promotes appetite and helps digestion. It cures loss of appetite and imbalance of vata. Its hot drink helps cure bad throat.

Ingredients for about two bottles of syrup:

Sugar	1 ½ kg (4 pounds)
Lemon juice	200 ml (1 cup)
Fennel seeds	2 tablespoons
Long pepper	5*
Black pepper	1 teaspoon
Dried ginger (powdered)	1 tablespoon
Ajwain	1 tablespoon
Liquorice (powdered)	2 teaspoons
Cloves	1 teaspoon
Cardamom powder	1 tablespoon

Powder all the spices together except cardamom. Powder the cardamom and keep it separately. Add the spice mixture in about 800 ml (4 cups) of water and cook covered for about 10 minutes on low heat. Add sugar into it and stir. When all the sugar is dissolved, let the whole thing cook uncovered on low heat for about half an hour. Keep stirring from time to time until it becomes thick syrup. Add powdered cardamom and cook for another five minutes. Let it cool down and then add lemon juice. Mix juice and syrup well. Filter the syrup through a strainer. Put it in clean and dry glass bottles with tightly closed lids. The syrup can be stored without a refrigerator for several months.

---

* Take half a teaspoon of pepper more if you do not find Long pepper.

To make a drink, add the syrup in hot or cold water according to your need. In 200 ml (one cup) of water, generally 1½ to 2 tablespoons of syrup are required. You can add the quantity of syrup according to your taste.

Almond Sharvat

This syrup is used to make a cold drink or it is added in cold milk to make almond milk. In addition to almonds, the syrup has poppy seed extract, which is cold in its Ayurvedic nature, small cardamom, and some pepper.

Ingredients for about two bottles of syrup:

Sugar	1 ½ Kg (4 pounds)
Almonds	100 gm (½ cup)
Poppy seeds (white)	50 gm (1/4 cup)
Cardamom seeds	10 gm (2 teaspoons)
Pepper	5 gm (1 teaspoon)

Put about 800 ml (4 cups) of water in a pot and add sugar. Cook on medium heat while stirring. When all the sugar is dissolved, continue to cook for half an hour on low heat and keep stirring from time to time. When the syrup is cooled down, filter it through a strainer.

Separately, soak the almonds over night and peel them. Put in wet grinder and make a purée. Keep it separately. Similarly, make purée from the poppy seeds by adding a little water into them in a wet grinder. Filter through a muslin cloth and take out the extract. If the purée is too thick, add a little more water.

Take cardamoms out of their pods and grind them very fine along with the pepper. You can use the electric grinder for it. Add into the syrup the cardamom and pepper powder, the purée of almonds and the extract of poppy seeds. Stir everything together and heat the pot again. Keep stirring and put the heat low so that the syrup does not boil over. Cook for about five more minutes. Let it cool down and store in clean and dry bottles which can be closed tightly. If it is too hot and humid, the sharvat should be stored in the refrigerator. Before mixing it with milk or water, always shake the bottle to make the contents homogeneous. Normally, 1 to 1½ tablespoon of syrup may be added to 200 ml (1 cup) of water or milk but adjust the quantity according to your taste.

Saffron Milk

Saffron milk can be made both hot and cold. In winter, hot milk is recommended whereas in summer cold milk is to be preferred.

Ingredients:

For two drinks, you require:

Milk	½ litre (2 ½ cup)
Candy sugar	2 teaspoons or according to taste
Saffron	250 mg (a pinch)
Finely chopped almonds	2 tablespoon

For hot milk, heat up the milk and add all the other ingredients. Stir with a spoon until the saffron is dissolved. Pure saffron dissolves slowly and does not colour the milk immediately as does the synthetic saffron which is sold very often for genuine saffron.

For cold milk, take a few spoons of milk and heat it. Dissolve in it the ingredients as above. Let it cool. Add this to the cold milk and stir well. You can also add ice cubes in it, but that changes the consistency of the milk.

Almond Milk

Almond milk is made the same way as saffron milk. Replace saffron with 3-4 crushed cardamoms and double the quantity of almonds from the above recipe.

Similarly, you can make **Almond-pistachio milk** with half the quantity of almonds and half the pistachio nuts. Add cardamom and sugar. Both milk drinks can be served cold or hot.

Rose Milk or Kewara Milk

Rose and Kewara are the flowers from which an extract is made through distillation. Extracts are available in Ayurvedic medicines and food shops. The reason they are important is that they are good for balancing the three energies of the body. They can be used in desserts which are consumed cold. Similarly, they can be taken with cold milk.

There are many kinds of roses but the one used to make the extract is *Rosa centifolia*. The Kewara tree is called Screw pine in English and *Pandanus odoratissimus* in Latin.

The milk is sweetened, cooled and then one of the two extracts is added into it. About a teaspoon of extract is added in about a litre (5 cups) of milk.

Lassi

Lassi is a general name for drinks made by whipping milk or yoghurt and then adding water to it.

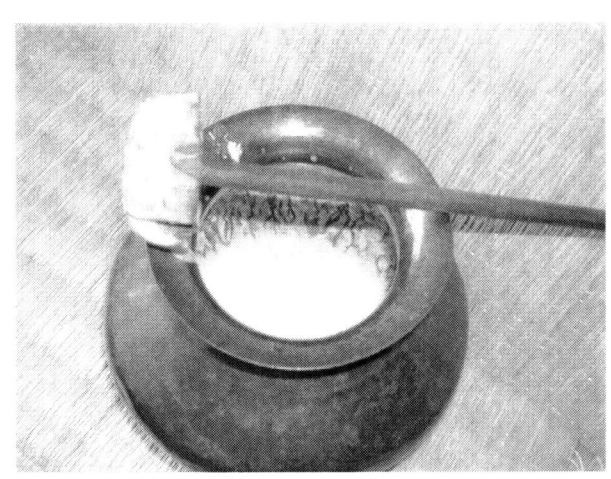

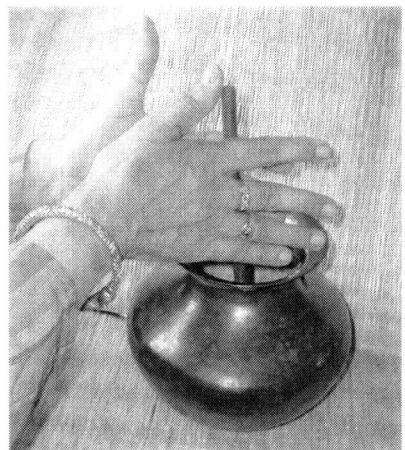

Sweet lassi

Ingredients:

For 3 portions, you require:

Yoghurt	200 gm (1 cup)
Sugar	3 tablespoons or according to taste
Water	400 ml (2 cups)
Rose water	1 teaspoon

Whip the yoghurt with the sugar and then add water. Use a hand mixer or a blender. Add water and whip again. In the end, add rose water and serve.

Beverages

Salty lassi

Ingredients:

For 3 portions, you require:

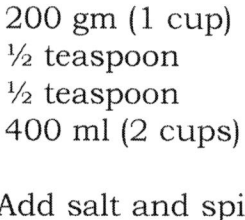

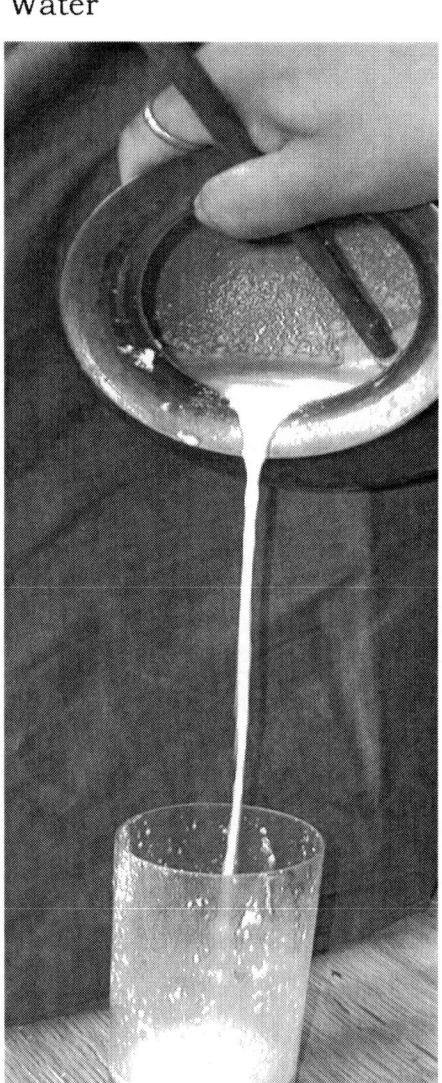

Yoghurt	200 gm (1 cup)
Salt	½ teaspoon
Mixture H	½ teaspoon
Water	400 ml (2 cups)

Add salt and spice mixture into yoghurt and whip. Add water and whip again.

It is traditional to pour lassi into a glass from a distance to serve it foamy. The cream of the yoghurt appears on the top.

I have described above the traditional way of making lassi. You may make the lassi faster with modern equipment by using a hand mixer. You may also make **fruit lassi** by adding bananas, homemade sweet fruit jams or other crushed fruits like papaya or mango.

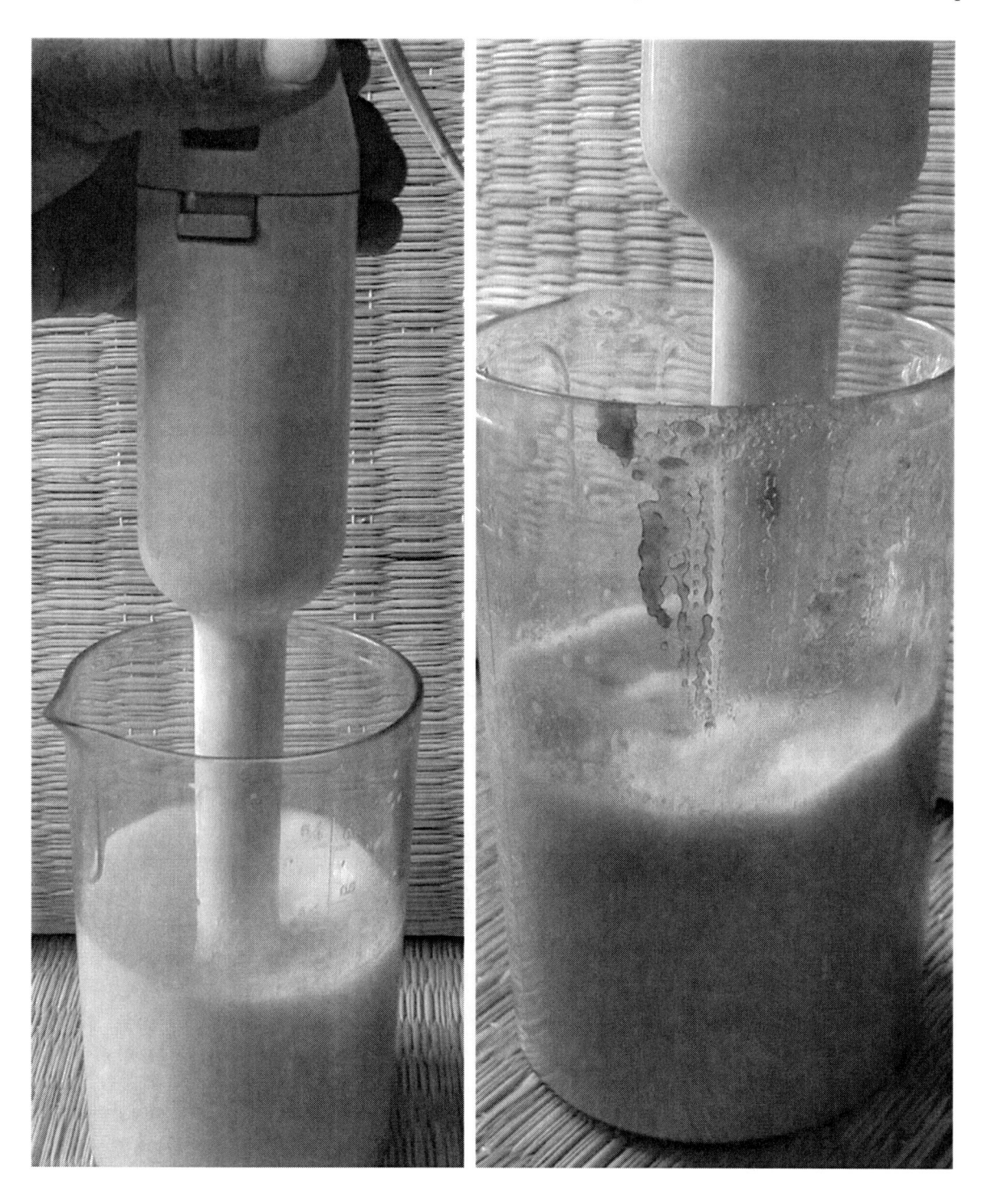

Ayurvedic Food Culture and Recipes

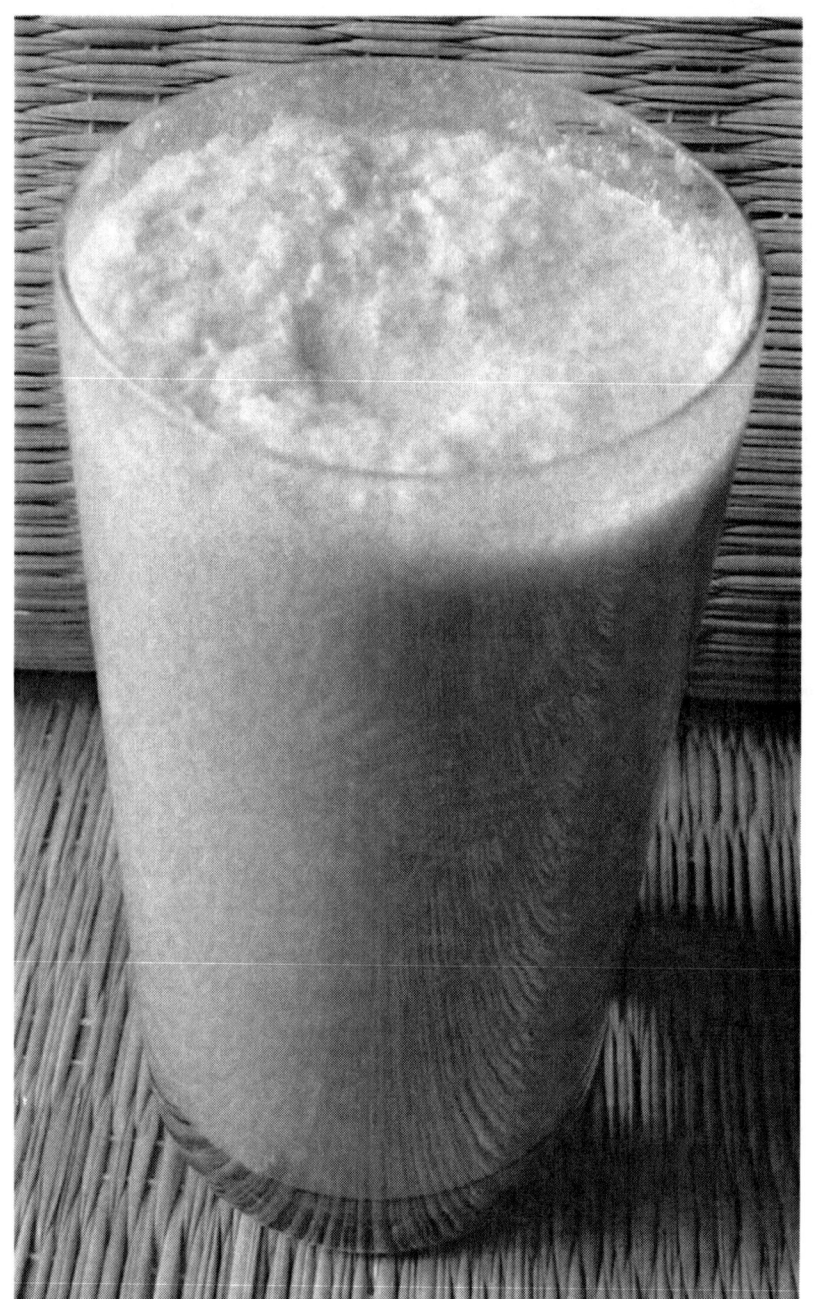

To make a rich preparation of lassi for breakfast, you may add almond or cashew powder into it.

Saffron Lassi

This preparation is made by adding saffron into the sweet lassi. However, the saffron does not dissolve into a cold preparation. You should dissolve it in a little hot water or hot milk and cook for about two minutes. Let it cool and then add to the lassi.

Traditional Ayurvedic Sweet Lassi without water

This recipe has been described by Charaka and is still available in some shops in Varanasi. Freshly made curd is whipped for a very long time with a wooden instrument for whipping as shown in previous pictures. Whipping makes the curd or yoghurt liquid. Sugar, rose water or kewara are added to it and whipped once again. No water is added into this preparation. For serving, it is poured into to a glass or an earthenware from a height as shown in picture on page 108.

BREAKFAST RECIPES

In the tradition of Ayurveda, breakfast was limited to drinking something and then there was an early lunch and an early dinner. As stated earlier, upon getting up in the morning, it is advised to drink hot water. During the night, energy channels of the body (*srotas*) are closed. Upon getting up in the morning, they open gradually and one should act according to the natural body rhythm. Thus, according to the Ayurvedic food culture, it is not recommended to eat breakfast immediately after getting up like many westerners do. Besides that, dried cereals with cold milk or 'muesli' may vitiate vata and eating cold grains in the morning is hard on the body when the body channels are gradually waking up.

After drinking hot water, it is recommended to go for a walk or do yoga and so on. After evacuation, bath and other daily rituals, people drank something like milk or yoghurt drinks in the North or coconut water in the South. There used to be an early lunch. In our modern life-style, our system of working does not allow us to do that. A light breakfast is essential for those who go out of the house to work somewhere else and have to spend a substantial amount of time commuting. However, your breakfast should be according to the type of work you do. Those of you whose work involves physical labour will need breakfast with grains like the recipes of porridge and semolina given below. Others who have mainly sitting jobs and have less physical exercise should take light breakfast like yoghurt or simply fruits. Those who tend to put on weight or are over-weight should also limit themselves to fruits for breakfast. Persons who are thin and feel weak need carrots or porridge breakfast with nuts and raisins. Persons who are normally healthy and neither too fat nor too thin, may make alternatively different breakfast recipes given on the following pages. It is also recommended to alternate the breakfast according to your state of health and weather etc. For example, if you have symptoms of vata vitiation, eat warm breakfast. If kapha is vitiated, the recipe with chickpea flour is recommended. For pitta vitiation, cold milk and sweet fruits like papaya and banana should be eaten. Carrot breakfast is always good to have equilibrium. Those suffering from constipation and headaches related to digestion should eat germinated chickpea breakfast.

WHEAT PORRIDGE OR *DALIA*

This porridge is made out of crushed and roasted wheat. From an Ayurvedic point of view, the best would be to soak the wheat 24 hours in water and when it is about to germinate, put it in a strainer and dry it. When it is completely dry, you can crush it in a coffee grinder. It should be carefully crushed so that it is granular and not powdered. This can be stored. In the Indian grocery stores abroad, *dalia* can be bought ready made. In Turkish grocery stores, a similar product can be bought by the name of *Bulgar*.

Ingredients:

For one person, you require:

Wheat porridge	3 tablespoons
Ghee	1 teaspoon
Cardamom	2-3
Water	300-400 ml (1 ½ to 2 cups)
Milk	200 ml (1 cup)
Sugar	according to taste
Chopped dried fruits like almonds, raisins, cashew nuts, pistachio etc.	1-2 tablespoons (optional)

Heat the ghee a little and add *dalia* into it. Roast it while stirring on the medium fire. When it is slightly brown, add water and crushed cardamoms after removing the pods. Bring it to boil and let it cook on low fire until the wheat softens. It may take about 10 minutes. The crushed wheat or *dalia* will absorb all the water. Add milk, sugar and nuts and cook for a minute or two. You may increase or decrease the quantity of milk and water according to the consistency you wish to have. It is nicer to keep the *dalia* a little liquid.

Dalia is a rich breakfast. It is very sustaining and energy giving. It is specially recommended to those who have rather late or uncertain lunch timings. If you wish a light breakfast, you may eat a small portion of it.

Suggestions: You may leave out ghee, nuts and milk in case you are trying to lose weight. *Dalia* can be cooked in water.

SEMOLINA PORRIDGE

Ingredients:

For one person, you require:

Semolina	2 tablespoons
Ghee	1 teaspoon
Sugar	1 tablespoon or according to taste
Cardamom	2
Water	200-300 ml (1- 1½ cup)
Almonds	5 to 10*
Raisins	one teaspoon*

*These two ingredients are optional.

Put the pot on fire and add ghee into it. When the ghee melts, add semolina and peeled off and crushed cardamoms. Fry on low fire for about a minute while stirring constantly. Add sugar, stir briefly and add 250-300 ml (one cup) of water. Add also the fruits and keep stirring and cook for a minute after it comes to a boil.

This preparation is lighter than *dalia*. If you wish even more light breakfast, take it without almonds and raisins.

Suggestions: You may use other dry fruits like cashew nuts, walnuts, coconut, pine nuts and dates. You may add milk instead of water. It will be a good breakfast for children and for those who are doing physical work.

BESAN (CHICKPEA FLOUR) HALVA

Halva means a sort of purée. It is a general word to signify the preparations which are made in the form of purée. A halva can be made from potatoes or carrots or semolina or from many other things. Some dictionaries do not indicate the meaning of this word correctly.

This is a rich breakfast and is specially recommended for children for two reasons. Firstly because it is rich in protein which growing children need. Secondly, because childhood is kapha dominating and besan is very good to cure any disorders due to kapha. Besan is strength promoting.

Ingredients:

For one person, you require:

Besan	2 tablespoons
Ghee	1 tablespoon
Sugar	1 tablespoon (or according to taste)
Water	200 ml (1 cup)
Cardamom	2-3
Dried fruits finally chopped	1 tablespoon (optional)

Breakfast Recipes

Put the ghee in the heated pan and add besan and pealed and crushed cardamoms into it. Fry the besan, while stirring constantly. Keep the fire low. When it is slightly roasted, add sugar and continue stirring for half a minute. Now add water and keep stirring very carefully so that the preparation does not get knots. Add the dried fruits, stir a little more and it is ready.

POTATO HALVA

This halva is also recommended for children as potatoes are hot and a copious food. Besides that, children like potato preparations.

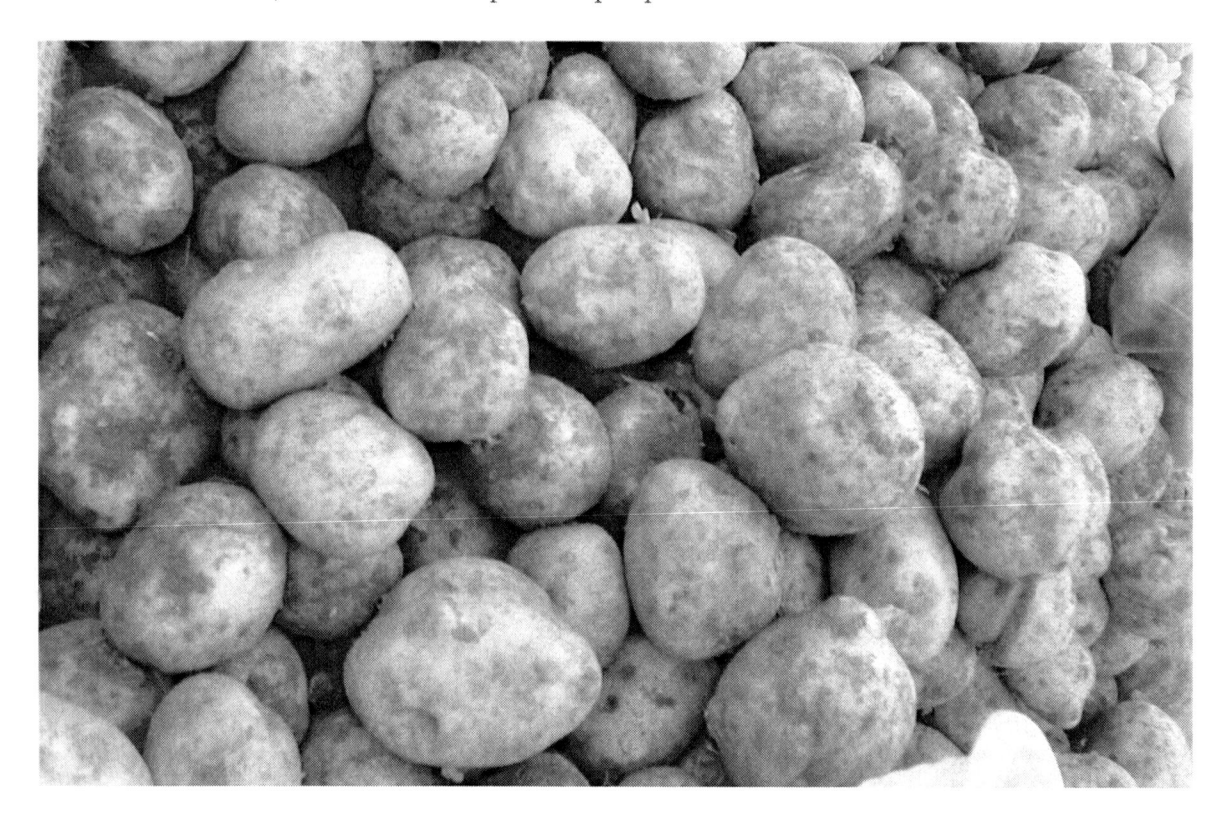

Ingredients:

For 1-2 persons, you require:

Potatoes	3 medium sized
Ghee	1 tablespoon
Sugar	1 tablespoon or according to taste
Cardamom	2

In this preparation, you need boiled potatoes. The potatoes should be always boiled with their skin. Boiled potatoes may be kept in the refrigerator for 2-3 days. Peel the potatoes and mash them properly. You may do that with a hand mixer. Heat ghee in a pan and fry mashed potatoes in it while stirring constantly. Keep the fire low so that the potatoes do not stick to the surface of the pan. When the potatoes are light brown, add sugar and cardamom (taken out from pods and crushed) and keep frying for another 2 minutes. Potato halva is ready.

CRUSHED GERMINATED WHEAT PORRIDGE AND WHEAT-MILK PORRIDGE

In Section I, it has been explained about the germination. The best germination according to Ayurveda is just the beginning of the germination. You require soaking wheat in water for about 24 hours to begin the process of germination (see Chapter 3 of Section I for details). Crush the germinated wheat in the wet grinder. Do not crush fine for the first recipe. For the wheat-milk porridge, you need to crush the wheat very fine and then extract the wheat starch from it through a strainer. That means you are not using the husk of the wheat. This recipe is specially recommended for weak and convalescent persons.

For crushed germinated wheat porridge, use the same recipe as for the wheat porridge described earlier.

For wheat-milk porridge, use the recipe given below.

Ingredients:

For one person, you require:

Germinated wheat	4-5 tablespoons
Ghee	1 teaspoon (optional)
Sugar	1 tablespoon or according to taste
Cardamom	2-3
Almonds (peeled off and chopped)	5-7

Crush the germinated wheat into a very fine paste in the wet grinder. You may have to add a little water in it so that it becomes like a purée. Take it out from the grinder and add some water so that it becomes semi-liquid. Filter it through a strainer to extract the starch out. This starch is called wheat-milk.

Normally this is cooked for about five minutes with cardamom and ghee and in the end sugar and almonds are added. Cook another 2-3 minutes after adding sugar and cardamom.

CARROT-MILK PREPARATION

Ingredients:

For one person, you require:

Carrots	2 medium sized
Ghee	1 teaspoon
Milk	about 200 ml (1 cup)
Cardamom	2-3
Sugar	1 to 2 teaspoons (according to taste)
Almonds, raisins or other dried fruits	optional

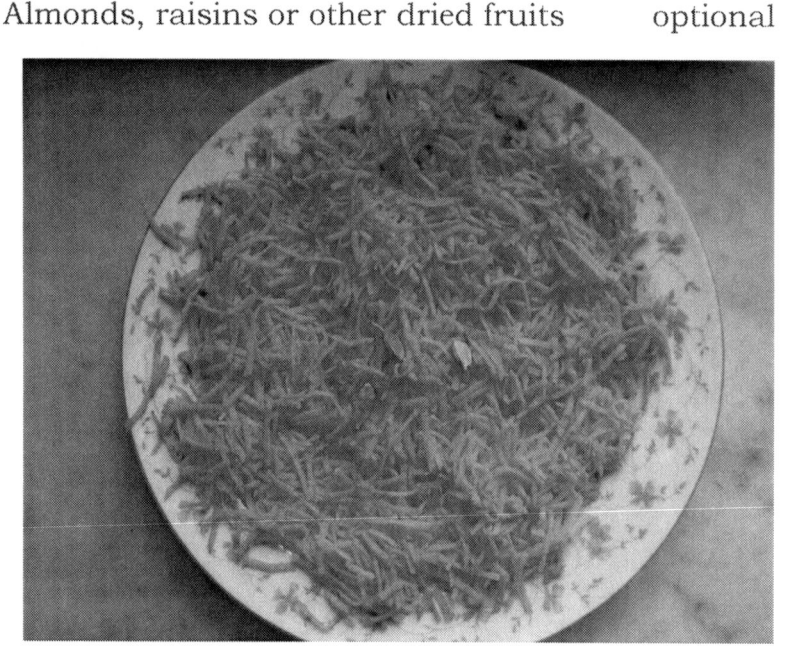

Grate the carrots and put them into the pot with pre-heated ghee. Stir a little and cook on low heat with the lid on the pot. Let them cook for about 10 minutes or until the carrots are soft. Keep stirring and if you feel that they are sticking on the bottom, you may add a spoon or two of water. Add sugar and cardamom and stir well for about a minute. Now add milk and let everything cook together. You may add some dried fruit as mentioned above.

Suggestions: You may make this preparation without milk. That means, you may not add any milk but do add chopped almonds and raisins.

This is a very healthy breakfast. It is good for your complexion and vision.

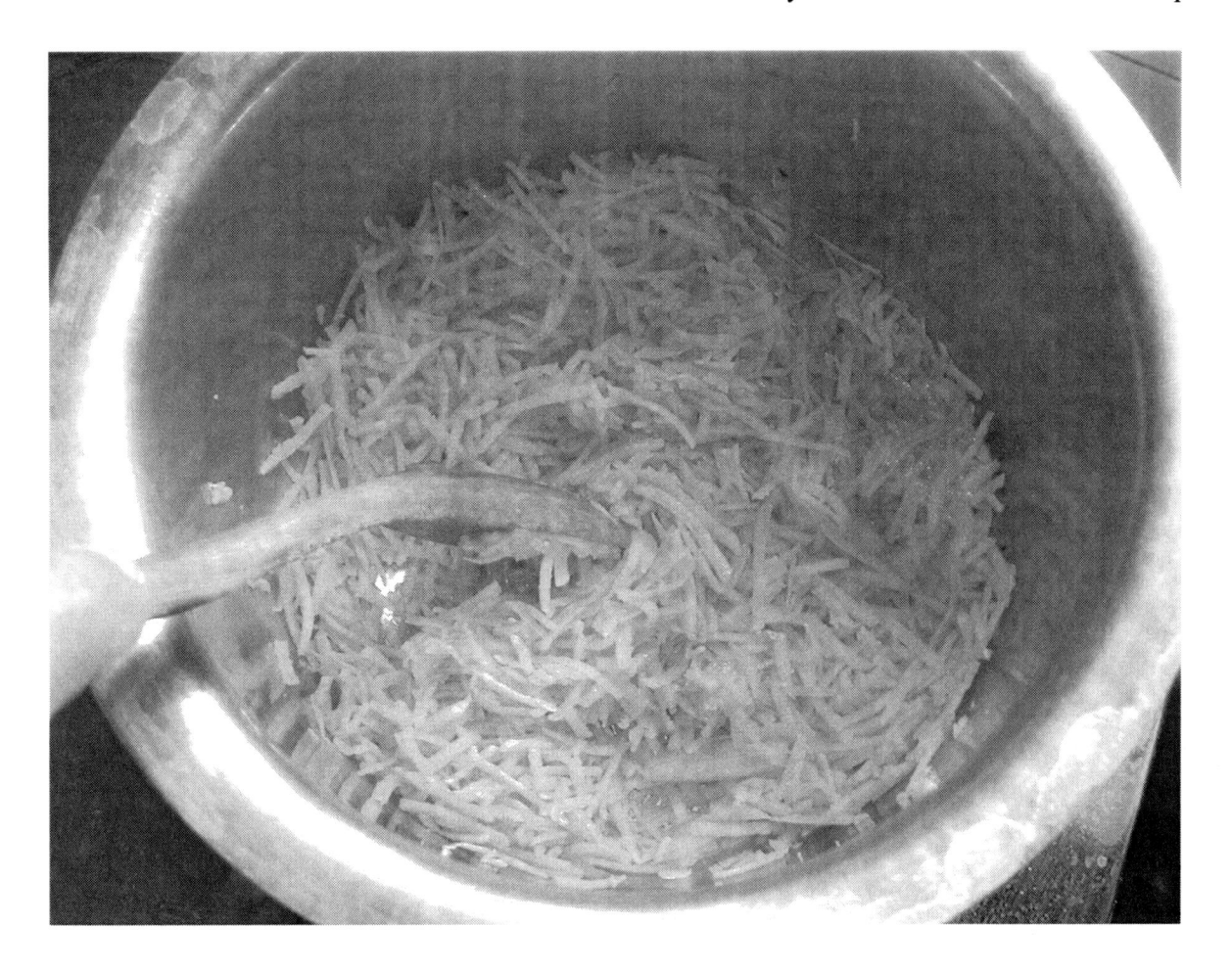

FRESH YOGHURT AND FRUIT BREAKFAST

This breakfast is suitable for pitta persons. If you are vata and tend to yawn during the day, take a warm breakfast. For a kapha person, too much yoghurt is not recommended.

You are not supposed to have tea or coffee with this breakfast. Take your tea or coffee or other hot drink at least half an hour before the yoghurt and fruit breakfast.
Fresh homemade yoghurt is recommended. You may add sweet fruits like Banana, sweet apple, sweet grapes etc. into your yoghurt. Melons should be avoided with yoghurt. Papaya can be eaten separately as its taste does not match with the taste of yoghurt.

Caution: People with joint pains and any other inflammation in the body should not take yoghurt.

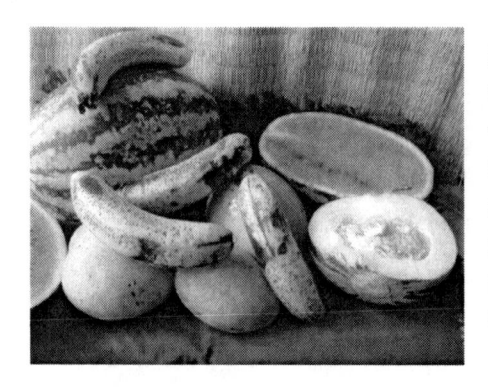

Breakfast with only fruits is especially good for those who want a light breakfast and want to lose weight. Papaya is a highly recommended fruit for this purpose. You may mix different fruits but avoid eating sour fruits in the morning. Sour fruits of citrus variety or other sour tasting fruits are better after meals rather than empty stomach early morning.

GERMINATED DARK CHICKPEA BREAKFAST

This breakfast is specially recommended to those who suffer from constipation and headaches generally related to digestion. In Ayurvedic tradition, they say that this breakfast makes one strong like a horse. In fact, dark chickpeas, which are slightly smaller in size than the normal chickpeas but similar in shape and are brown in colour, seem to be the favourite diet of horses. In France and perhaps also in other European countries, they can be bought at horse shops.

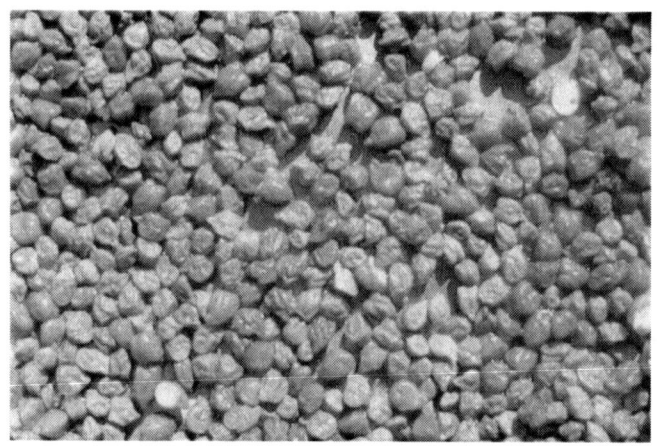

Ingredients:

For one person you require:

Black gram or dark chickpeas   3 to 5 tablespoons

Soak the chickpeas in water for 24 hours. They begin to germinate and become soft and edible. Wash them with water and eat them. Chew them properly In case you find it very hard to eat the raw chickpeas, you may divert slightly from the Ayurvedic tradition and fry them with little ghee, salt and cumin seeds. They are delicious.

FRUIT PRESERVATION RECIPES

Ayurveda has a tradition of preserving fruits in sugar syrup. There are medicinal as well as other fruits and even some vegetables like carrots that are preserved in sugar syrup.

Carrots and apples in syrup

Ingredients:

Carrots or apples	500 gm (one pound)
Sugar	300 gm (1 ½ cup)
Water	100 ml (½ cup)
Cardamom (pealed and powdered)	10
Powdered ginger	1 teaspoon
Powdered black pepper	¼ teaspoon

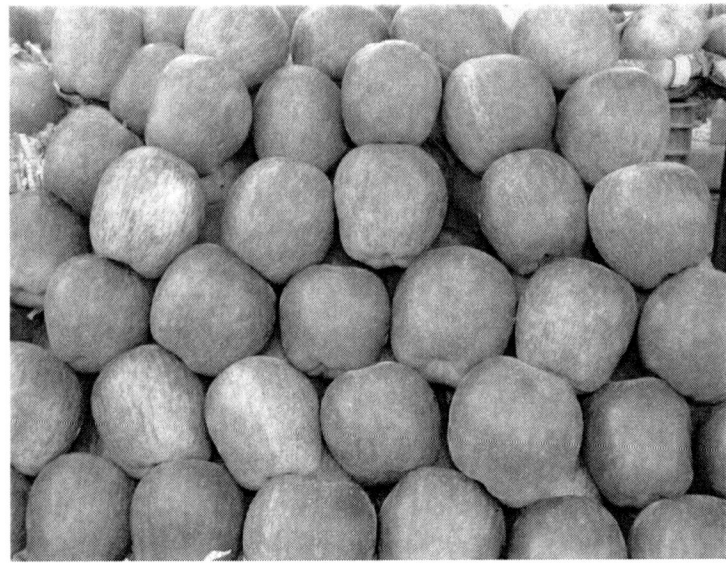

Peel and chop the fruits. Carrots may be cut finger shaped and apples can be cut in roundels. Put a few spoons of water in a pot and add the fruits. Add carrots or apples and cook on a low fire with the lid on. Carrots will take generally 10 minutes to cook whereas for apples, five minutes are enough. The fruits should not be too soft. In other words, they should be slightly steamed. Separately, prepare the sugar syrup by cooking the sugar with 100 ml (½ cup) of water and add also the spices in it. Cook all this on a slow fire and keep stirring from time to time. Cook until it makes a thread. Filter this syrup with a thin muslin cloth. Heat up once more the filtered syrup and add to the steaming carrots or apples. Cook them together another two minutes. Store it in a dried jar and it can be preserved for several weeks in the refrigerator.

Suggestions: These fruits can be also served for dessert with little fresh cream and some nuts on the top.

FRUIT JAMS, JELLIES AND MARMALADE

Jams, jellies and marmalades are a good way to preserve fruits and can be used for breakfast not only with bread but also to sweeten the yoghurt. These preparations can also be used for desserts along with other things like fresh cream and almonds. However, excess of pure sugar is not recommended and it should be balanced from an Ayurvedic point of view. Too much of sour in some fruits will also give rise to an imbalance from an Ayurvedic point of view. The recipe varies according to the nature of the fruit. Fruits like berries or grapes with seed or guavas, it is better to cook them with a little water and take out their pulp through a strainer. For the other fruits, prepare the pulp, and use the following recipe for preparing a jam or a jelly.

Fruit pulp	500 gm (2 ½ cup)
Sugar	300 gm (1 ½ cup)
Fresh ginger, grated	2 tablespoons
Or ginger powder	1 tablespoon
Pepper	½ teaspoon

Cook the fruit pulp with sugar. Keep stirring in between and cook on a slow fire. Add ginger and pepper after about 15 minutes. The total cooking time should be about an hour. But cook always on a very low heat. It is important to cook this for a long time. If you cook for a shorter time, the preparation is vulnerable to get fungus.

Marmalade: For the preparation of marmalade from citrus peels, buy organically grown fruit and always remember that the more sour the fruit, the less bitter the peels. Nevertheless, the peels should be boiled and first water should be thrown out. Then cook them until they are soft. Crush them properly. You may use the wet grinder for this purpose. But do not make a purée out of it. Just run the grinder briefly. Cook the pulp with sugar. Do not add ginger and pepper in this recipe. Add instead five tablespoons of lemon juice. Cook on low heat and with the lid on. Stir from time to time. Store the preparation in tightly closed dry jars and keep them in the refrigerator.

MAIN MEALS

SOUPS

The beginning of the meal should be slow and with a light dish. Soups are highly recommended as they bring fluid to the body. Salads are usually not recommended to begin the meal accept when it is extremely hot and dry climate. Raw vegetables, especially leafy, uncooked vegetables are hard to digest and it is suggested that we activate the stomach functions gradually with something warm, fluid and light to digest. In windy weather, which is vata, soups are highly recommended. For those who are of vata constitution, have any kind of malaise due to vata vitiation, suffer from sleep disturbances or have constipation, soup is highly recommended for dinner. You will see that in Ayurvedic cooking, besides soups, there are also other dishes which are prepared in liquid form. Dals, beans, green peas and several other vegetables are prepared with plenty of fluid sauce. Remember, in Ayurveda it is recommended to drink one hour after the food. In fact, when the meal is fluid, one does not feel the need to drink during the meal any way.

DAL-PALAK SOUP (SPINACH-MUNG DAL SOUP)

Spinach is astringent and gives rise to distension. That is why spinach recipes are prepared with some specific ingredients which create an equilibrium of this rasa.

Ingredients:

For 2 to 3 portions you require:

Fresh spinach	200 gm (½ lb.)
Carrot	2 medium sized
Mung dal*	100 gm (½ cup)
Water	500 ml (2 ½ cup)
Fresh lemon juice	1 tablespoon
Salt	¼ teaspoon or to taste

---

* Mung dal is mung beans split, and without husk. It is available in the shops as mung dal. It has yellow colour.

Main Meals

Pepper	a pinch
Mixture B	1 teaspoon
Turmeric	1 teaspoon
Ghee	1 tablespoon
Chopped basil	1 tablespoon

Add in pot chopped spinach and carrots, cleaned and washed mung dal, mixture B and about 300 ml (1½ cup) water. Cook for about 20 minutes to half an hour, on slow fire, half covered and stir from time to time. Make sure that the dal is very well cooked as the time of cooking may vary according to the quality of the water. In the end, add some more water to make it fluid and bring it to boil. The quantity of the water you add depends upon the consistency of the soup you will like to have. After having cooked, add salt, pepper and lemon juice. You may decide to blend it with a hand blender or serve it as such. Add ghee before serving. The quantity of ghee may be increased according to your dietary need and according to the other items of your menu. Add chopped basil on the top before serving.

Suggestions: Those of you who do not like sour may leave out lemon juice. In a preparation without lemon juice, the ghee can be replaced with little fresh cream. But make sure that one of them should be there as spinach is astringent in nature and ghee, cream or milk helps to balance it. That is the reason for adding carrots in the recipe. Pure spinach may give distension, bloating and stomach-ache.

CARROT SOUP

Ingredients:

For 2 or 3 portions you require:

Carrots	½ Kg (1 lb.)
Potato	1 medium sized
Water	400 ml (2 cups)
Chopped green herbs	4 tablespoons
Mixture A	¾ teaspoon
Salt	¼ teaspoon
Turmeric	½ teaspoon
Ghee or butter	1 tablespoon
Fresh cream (optional)	1 tablespoon
Mixture G	1 teaspoon

Wash, peel and chop the carrots and the potato. Put them in a pot along with water. Bring them to boil and add spices and salt. Cook them covered on a low heat until the vegetables are soft. Blend the cooked contents with the hand mixer and add green herbs. Cook for a minute again. Add ghee or butter before serving. You may enrich this soup by adding cream. Alternatively, you may leave out ghee or butter and add only cream. Add mixer G on the top before serving.

Suggestions: This soup is easy to digest and helps establish equilibrium in the body. It may be given to sick and weak persons but in that case, reduce the quantity of mixture A to ¼ of a teaspoon. Those with weak digestion should not use mixture A. Instead, they should use ½ teaspoon each of cumin and ajwain.

MIXED VEGETABLE SOUP

Mixed vegetable soup may be prepared with different vegetables of your choice like green peas, carrots, broccoli, spinach, tomatoes, cabbage and so on. You may add little of each vegetable.

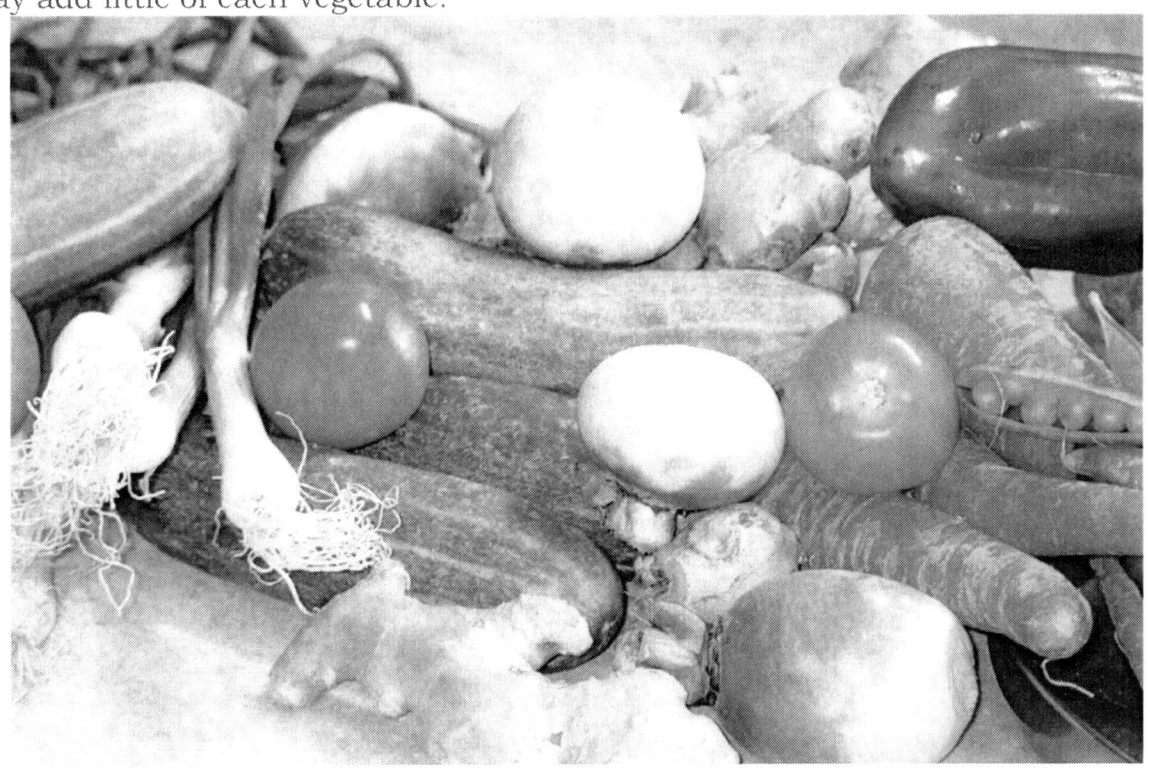

This soup can be prepared in two forms, either mixed with a blender or keeping the pieces of the vegetables. In the second case, you will have to work hard on cutting the vegetables into tiny pieces so that the soup has a good appearance.

Ingredients

For 2 to 3 portions, you require:

Carrot   1 medium sized

Main Meals

Broccoli	100 gm (¼ lb.)
Potato	1 medium sized
Green peas	3 tablespoons
Tomatoes	2 medium sized
Water	300 ml (1 ½ cup)
Salt	¼ teaspoon
Pepper	a pinch
Nutmeg	¼ of a nut (freshly grated)
Mixture C	½ teaspoon
Cumin	½ teaspoon
Mixture G or	½ teaspoon
Fresh herbs chopped	1 tablespoon
Ghee or butter	1 tablespoon

Cut all the vegetable into fine pieces and put them all except tomatoes in a pot and cook them for about 15 minutes on low heat after it comes to boil. Keep the pot covered. Add tomatoes, salt and the spices except nutmeg and cook for another 10-15 minutes on reduced heat and with the lid on. Add the nutmeg in the end. Add ghee or butter before serving and decorate it with either fresh herbs or with mixture G.

Comments: Mixed vegetable soup can be made with different kinds of vegetables of your choice. Some varieties of beans need slightly longer time to cook. Vegetables like aubergine are not suitable for making soup. In case you use zucchini, it is better to blend the soup with the hand mixer. When you plan to blend the mixed vegetable soup, you need not cut the vegetable into very fine pieces as is said in this recipe. Nevertheless, the vegetables should be always cut into small pieces to reduce the cooking time and the cooking should be done on low heat.

RED LENTIL (MASOOR DAL) SOUP

Ingredients:

For 3 to 4 portions you require:

Red lentils	150 gm (¾ cup)
Carrots	4 medium sized
Tomatoes	5 medium sized
Onions	2 medium sized
Garlic	4 to 6 cloves
Water	1 Litre (5 cups)
Mixture A	1 teaspoon
Salt	1/3 to ½ teaspoon

Mixture B	½ teaspoon
Mixture C	½ teaspoon
Turmeric	1 teaspoon
Butter or ghee	2 tablespoon

Wash and soak the lentils for about 10 minutes in water. Take a big pot of two litres so that it is half full when you add water. Bring the water to boil and add lentils after draining out the water in which they were soaking. Add turmeric and bring it to boil. Go on adding carrots cut into small pieces and when everything is boiling, reduce the heat and let it cook slowly for 15 minutes. Then add to it tomatoes cut into small pieces and onions in lamellae. Add also the rest of the spices and salt except garlic. Let everything cook for another 15 minutes on low heat after it comes to boil. Depending on the quality of water, you may have to cook a little longer or add a little more water. Add garlic when the soup is ready and turn off the fire. Add butter or ghee in the end before serving.

Comments: This soup is rejuvenating and rich in different rasas. It is a meal by itself. It makes a good meal with hot flat bread (in India, Tandoori roti or nan) with a little butter on it.

PANEER SOUP

Ingredients:

For 4 portions you require:

Freshly made paneer from milk	1 Litre (5 cups)
Lemon juice	2-3 tablespoon
Finely chopped onions	3 medium sized
Fresh finely cut ginger	2 tablespoons
Tomatoes	5-6 medium sized
Salt	½ teaspoon
Mixture A	1 teaspoon
Ajwain	1 teaspoon
Cumin	1 teaspoon
Kalonji	½ teaspoon
Ghee	2 tablespoons
Jaggery or crystal candy	1 teaspoon
Garlic	4 cloves (optional)
Chopped Coriander or Persil leaves	3 tablespoons

Pour all the milk in a big pot, boil and add lemon juice to make Paneer as has been explained previously. Leave this pot as such. Separately, put the ghee in another pot and heat it on medium fire. Put finely cut onions and ginger into it and fry while stirring. When they are sauté, add all the spices and stir together

Main Meals

for about a minute. Add tomatoes cut into small pieces and stir everything together. Put the lid on, reduce the heat and let tomatoes cook gradually. It will take about 10 minutes until they are completely cooked. Keep stirring in between so that they do not stick to the bottom of the pot. When your sauce is ready, pour the entire contents into the Paneer pot, stir everything together and cook for about 10 minutes on a low heat. Add also jaggery or crystal candy at this time. Put off the fire and add chopped garlic and herbs into it. If you have something else on the menu with garlic, you may leave out garlic in this recipe.

Comments: This is another rich soup, which is an entire meal by itself. Cumin and Ajwain is added in this recipe because some people may have problem digesting due to the sour medium of the soup. Remember there was the lemon juice and then many tomatoes were added. That is the reason to add sugar.

PUMPKIN SOUP

This is very simple soup to make. The choice of pumpkin is important, as according to Ayurveda, young pumpkins are cold whereas overripe are hot in their Ayurvedic nature. Try to choose a ripe pumpkin.

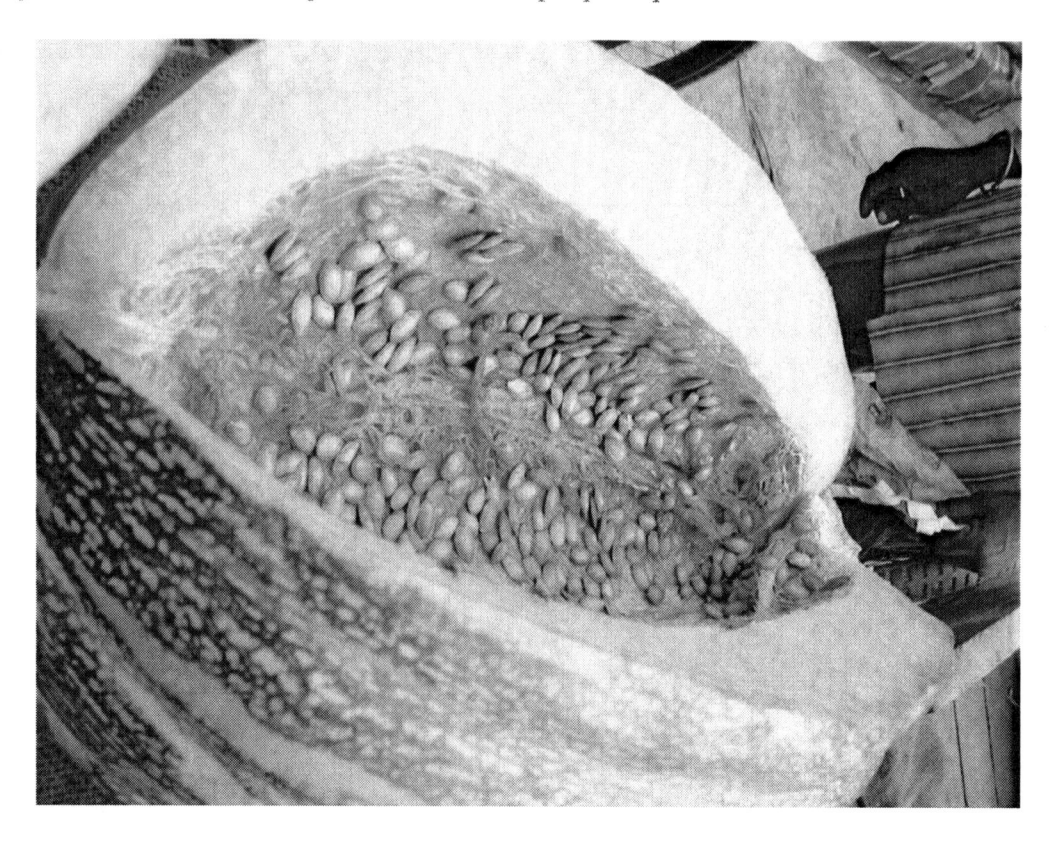

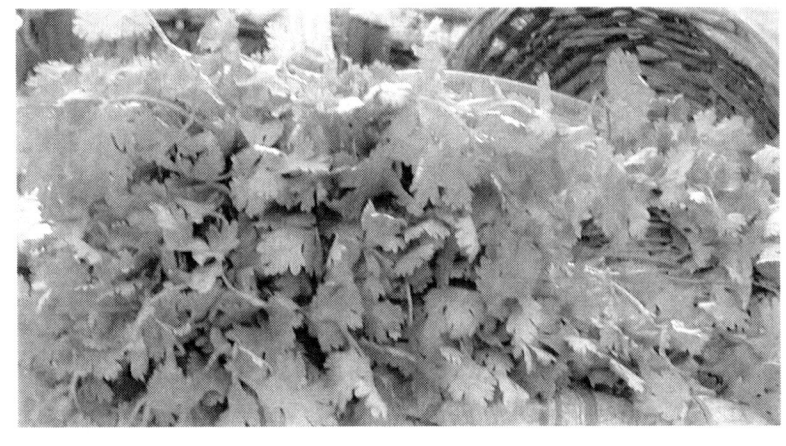

Ingredients:

For 2 to 3 portions you require:

Pumpkin	400 gm (1lb.)
Water	200 ml (1cup)
Salt	¼ teaspoon
Cumin	½ teaspoon
Small cardamom	4
Pepper	6-7 seeds
Dill seeds	¼ teaspoon
Milk	100 ml (½ cup)
Butter (optional)	1 to 2 teaspoons

Peel and cut the pumpkin into small pieces and cook it in water with the lid on and on low heat until it is completely soft. Remove the pods of the cardamom and powder all the four spices in a mortar. Add the spices and the salt into the pot and cook for another 2 minutes. Add milk, stir everything together and bring it to boil. Let it cool a little and mix it with a hand mixer. Add a little butter in each portion before serving.

GREEN VEGETABLE SOUP

There are different kinds of green leafy vegetables available in every country. One can mix different green vegetables and make soup. There are certain leaves like from radish, beetroot and turnip, which are generally thrown away can be used for making soup. The best is to mix various kinds of edible green for this purpose. There is a vegetable called *Bathua* in Hindi (called Lamb's quarters in English and *Chenopodium album* in Latin), which is a healthy vegetable from an Ayurvedic point of view as it brings equilibrium of the three energies of the body. If you can find it and grow it in your region, it is good for making soup as well as green vegetable with mixture B (see the recipe for cabbage with mixture B later in the book).

Main Meals

Ingredients:

For 2 to 3 portions you require:

Mixed green vegetables	200 gm (½ lb.)
Water	300 ml (1 ½ cup)
Potato	2 medium sized
Mixture C	1 teaspoon
Cumin (powdered)	½ teaspoon
Black Pepper	a pinch
Mace (powdered)	a pinch
Salt	¼ teaspoon
Butter or ghee	1 tablespoon

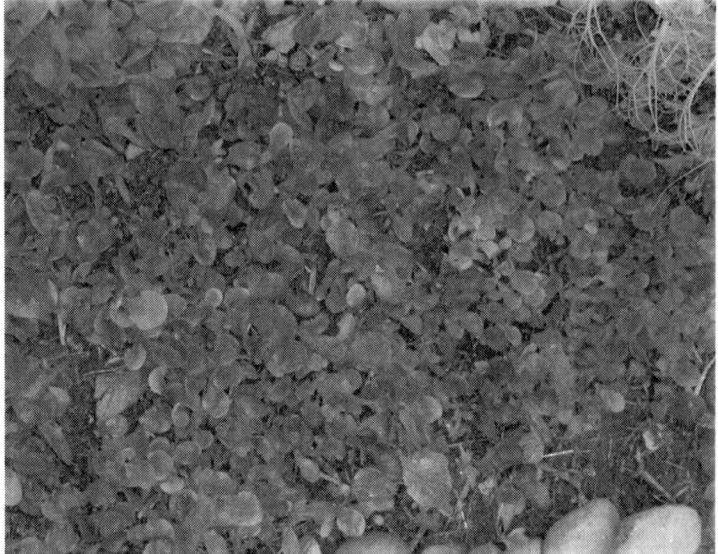

Wash and cut the mixed green vegetables. Peel the potatoes and cut them into small pieces. Cook everything in water on a low heat and with the lid on. Depending upon the quality of the vegetables and season, it may take up to 20 minutes until they are cooked properly. Add all the spices and cook for another 5 minutes. Blend everything well with the hand mixer and serve it after adding butter or ghee.

Comments: Instead of potatoes, you may add 1 to 2 tablespoons of maize flour or semolina and cook it along with the green vegetables.

SPINACH SOUP

You may use the same recipe for spinach soup but take special care to add potatoes and in the end some milk or cream. This is because spinach is astringent and if proper care is not taken, it will cause distension. Another alternative is to add a tablespoon of Soya bean flour.

Ingredients:

For 2-3 portions you require:

Spinach	200gm (½ lb.)
Water	300 ml (1 ½ cup)
Mixture C	1 teaspoon
Cumin (powdered)	½ teaspoon
Ajwain (powdered)	½ teaspoon
Salt	¼ teaspoon
Pepper	a pinch
Ghee or butter	1 tablespoon
Soya bean flour	1½ tablespoon

Wash the spinach and cook it in 200 ml (1 cup) of water for about 15 minutes. Cook it covered and on low heat. Add the spices and the salt and cook another 5 minutes with the lid on. Separately, heat ghee or butter in a wok or in a pan and add Soya bean flour into it. Stir and fry the flour for about a minute on low fire. Go on adding water into it and stirring. Add about 100 ml (½ cup) of water and stir well so that it is homogenous. Add this into the cooked vegetables, stir and mix everything together. Use the hand blender to mix everything together. You may add some water and cook a little after mixing up if the soup is thick in consistency.

LEEK SOUP

Leek is a very tasty vegetable to make soup. It is not as strong as onions although it is from the same variety of vegetables. Leek is cold in its Ayurvedic nature and thus makes a very good combination with potatoes and is prepared like this in many countries in Europe.

Ingredients:

For 2 to 3 portions, you require:

Leeks	2
Potatoes	2 medium sized
Water	½ Litre (2 ½ cups)
Salt	¼ teaspoon
Pepper	a pinch
Nutmeg (grated)	¼ of a nut
Mice (powdered)	a pinch
Mixture C	½ teaspoon

Main Meals

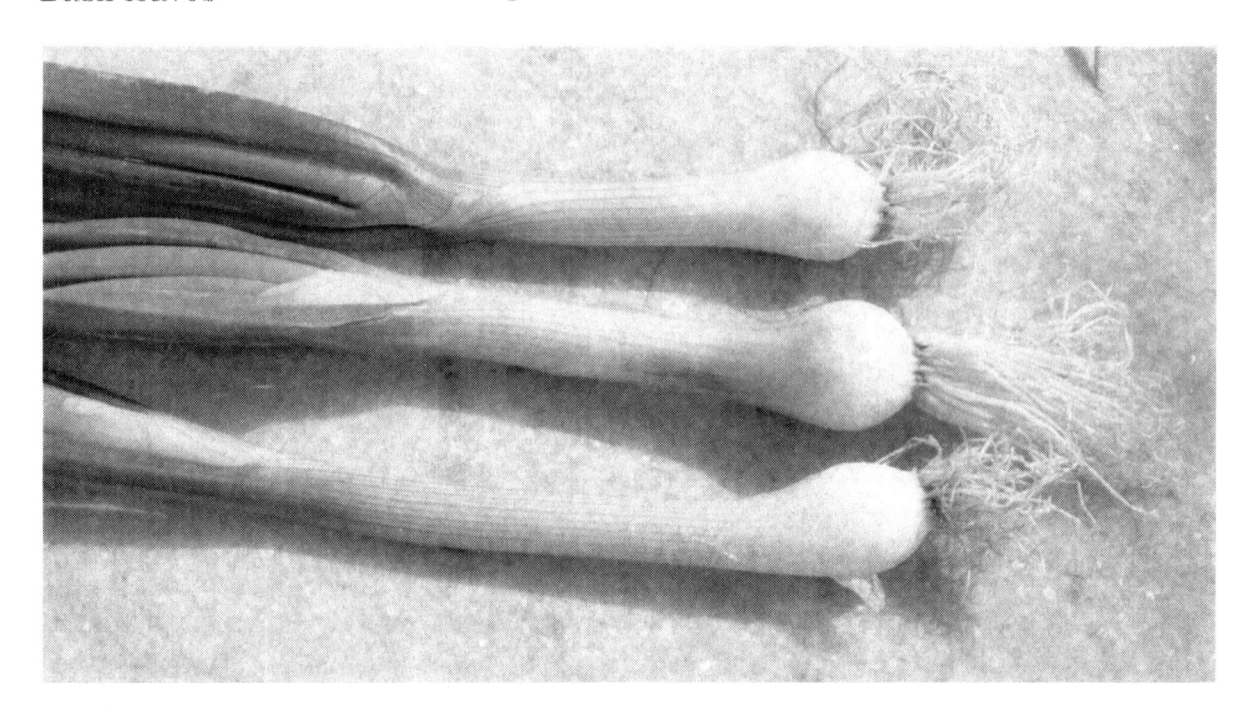

Fresh Cream	2 tablespoons
Mixture G	½ tablespoon
Basil leaves	6

Wash and cut the leeks into small pieces. Peel the potatoes, wash and cut them also into small pieces. Bring the water to boil and put all the vegetables in it. Reduce the heat and let the vegetables cook slowly for about 20 minutes or until they are completely soft. Wait until they are little cooler and blend them with the hand mixer properly. Now, add all the spices except mixture G and basil leaves, mix everything well and cook for another 5 minutes. Add the cream just before serving. Decorate the soup with mixture G and finely chopped fresh basil leaves.

Suggestions: In case you do not have cream, cook the vegetables with half the quantity of water and replace the other half with fresh milk. But add the milk later after blending. Cream may be also replaced with butter but the soup does not taste as nice as with the cream.

WARM STARTERS

As I have already stated above for the soups, in Ayurveda, it is generally recommended to begin the meal with something warm and easy to digest. Cold starter like salads, especially leafy salads are not recommended. Keeping in mind the Western tradition of starters other than soups, I am giving below some recipes.

ROASTED PANEER

Ingredients:

For about 4 persons, you need:

Milk	1 litre (5 cups)
Lemon juice	1 tablespoon
Cumin	½ teaspoon
Ajwain	½ teaspoon
Pepper	a pinch
Salt	a pinch
Ghee or butter	a teaspoon

Make paneer from a litre (5 cups) of milk for about 4 persons. Hang the paneer until most water is drained. Roast cumin on a hot frying pan. It takes about 30 seconds on a real hot pan. Mix the roasted cumin, other spices and salt with the paneer. Put the contents back in the cloth and flatten it by putting some weight on it as has been explained previously. After a little while, remove the weight and cut the flattened paneer into pieces. Take a non-stick pan and smear it with some ghee. Roast the pieces of paneer on it. When one side is light brown, turn around and roast the other side.

Suggestion: You may serve the roasted paneer with roundels of tomatoes and cucumber around it.

Main Meals

FLAT BREAD WITH ALMONDS AND RAISINS

Ingredients:

For 2-3 persons, you require:

Flat breads	2
Butter or ghee	1 teaspoon
Mixture G	½ teaspoon
Ajwain	a pinch
Salt (if the bread is unsalted)	a pinch
Peeled almonds	15
Raisins	1 tablespoon

Crush almonds and raisins together in a mortar or in a wet grinder but do not make a fine paste. Almonds should be left in small pieces. Heat the ghee or butter a little and put mixture G and ajwain in it. Add also salt if your bread is unsalted. Mix them all together. Heat the bread on a pan and smear on it the herbal butter or ghee you have prepared. Then put thin layer of the paste of almonds and raisin.

APPETISING CAULIFLOWER DISH

Ingredients:

For 2 to 3 portions, you require:

Cauliflower	1 medium-sized
Paprika	1
Cucumber	1
Beetroot	1
Grated ginger	1 tablespoon
Fresh lemon juice	1 tablespoons
Dill seeds	½ teaspoon
Mixture C	1 teaspoon
Salt	1/3 teaspoon
Pepper	½ teaspoon
Raw sugar	½ teaspoon
Ghee or cooking oil	1 tablespoon

Wash and cut the cauliflower into small pieces (about an inch, 2-3 cm). Take a pot that can be covered properly. Add one tablespoons of water in the pot. Put it on low heat, add the cauliflower into it and put the lid on. Stir it after about two minutes. The cooking time is dependent upon the quality of your vegetable, season etc. You have to cook just enough to bring the vegetable in a half-cooked state. If there is too much water, remove the lid and stir so that the water evaporates. Add salt, pepper and sugar in the lemon juice and mix well all the ingredients.

Cut paprika, cucumber and boiled beetroot in small pieces. Add half of the above-prepared lemon juice with spices to these chopped vegetables. Heat ghee or oil in a pan and put ginger into it. Add to it the steamed cauliflower and stir. Add dill seeds and Mixture C and cook all this for three minutes while stirring. Add the rest of the spiced lemon juice and stir again. For serving, decorate the colourful raw vegetables in a circle in the plate and spread nicely the cauliflower preparation in the middle.

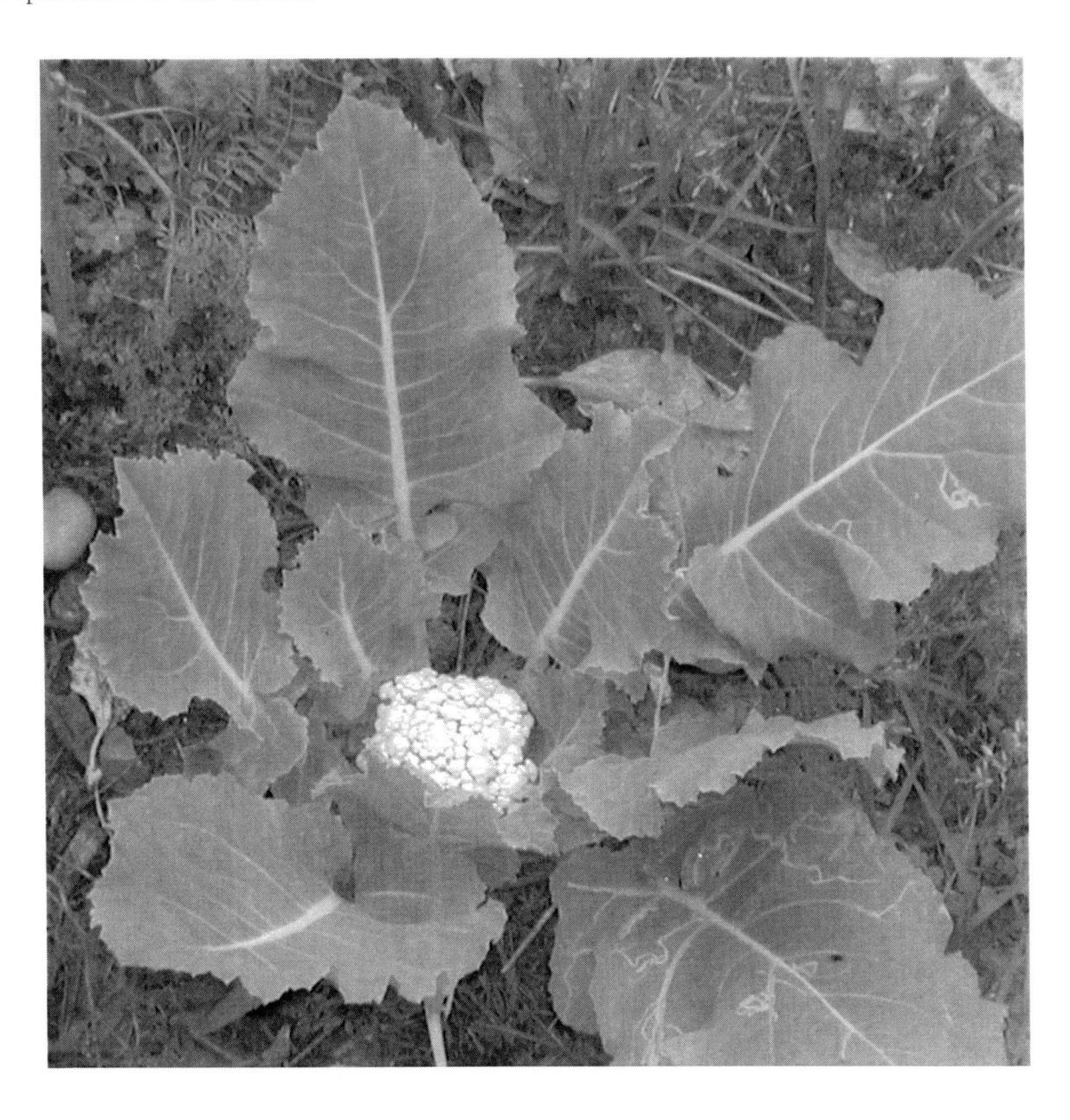

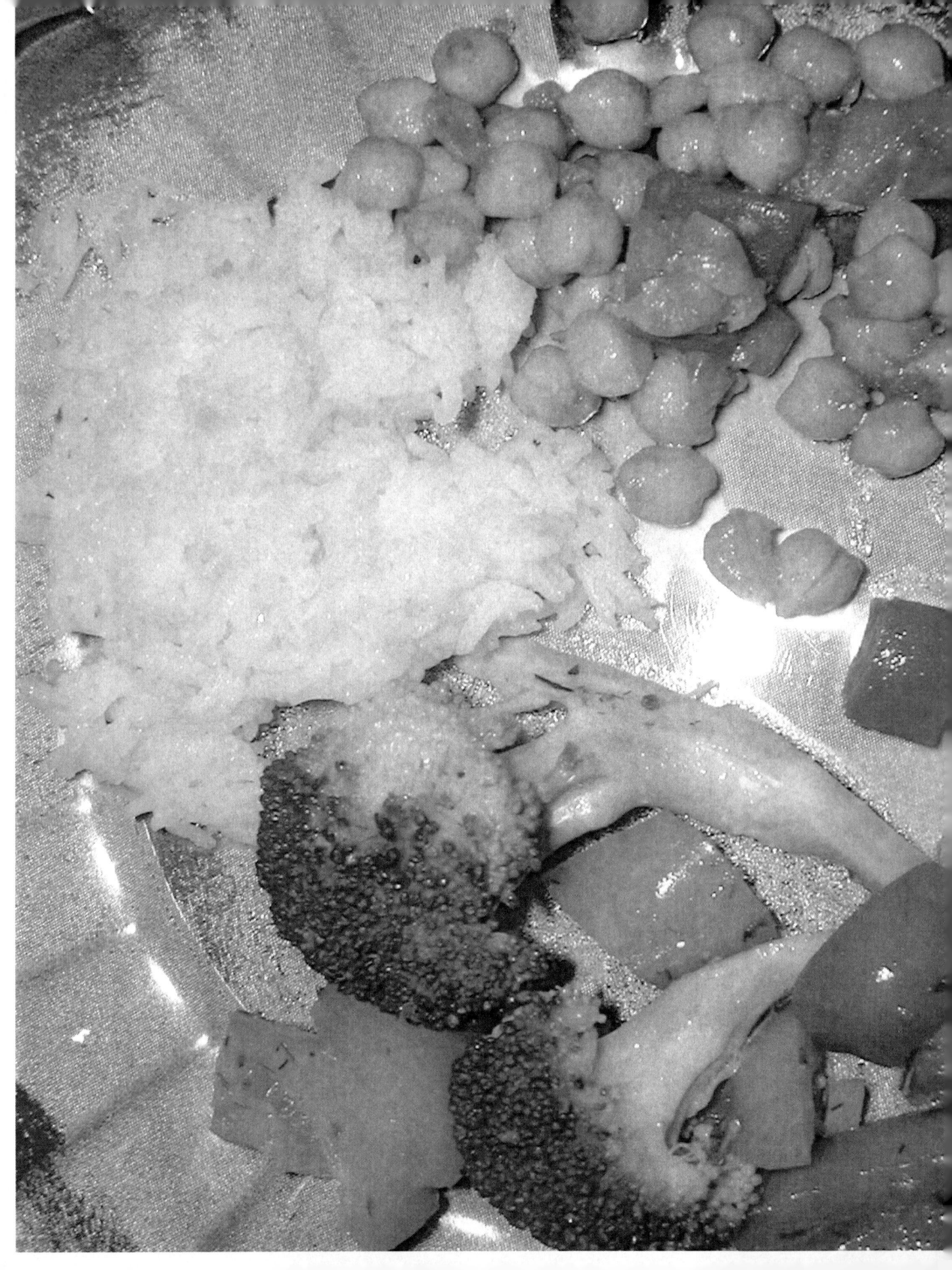

MAIN COURSE

PASTA

Pasta of different shapes and forms and from different kinds of grains is made all over the world. Italian pasta is especially good as it is mostly made fresh. Pasta is generally made from wheat flour but in Asia, there is also rice pasta. Pasta made with different vegetables and herbs makes a delicious food. Besides, pasta can be prepared quickly and it can replace bread, which is a *basa* food from Ayurvedic point of view.

It is better to use whole grain pasta. Do not get fooled by words like 'brown flour pasta'. Generally the colours are added in the white flour in such products. Read always the contents carefully before making a choice of pasta.

What recipe you make from pasta depends upon your menu. If you have vegetable soup and a salad and are looking for something more filling, then you make the following simple recipes. Later, I have given some complicated recipes with cheese, paneer etc., which are more copious and make an entire meal.

CUMIN PASTA

Ingredients

For 2-3 portions you require:

Pasta	200 gm (½ pound)
Salt	¼ teaspoon
Cumin	1 teaspoon
Fennel	¼ teaspoon
Chive (finely chopped)	1 tablespoon
Butter or ghee	1 tablespoon
Salt	¼ teaspoon

Cook the pasta with the salt and drain out the water. Melt butter or ghee in a pan and add spices and herbs into it. Stir for about two minutes on very low heat and add the cooked pasta. Mix everything together.

Main Meals

PASTA WITH ONIONS AND GARLIC

To have a little variation from the above recipe, you may fry an onion cut into small pieces. Leave out the chive in this case. Use the same spices as above. Add 3 to 4 cloves of garlic towards the end.

PASTA WITH ARUGULA (Rocket Salad)

Arugula or Rucola is a very good green vegetable. It provides us the bitter rasa, which is usually missing in modern cooking. Due to dominant bitter rasa, it is a cold vegetable from an Ayurvedic point of view. Since pasta is also cold in its Ayurvedic properties, we will add some hot spices to create the balance.

Ingredients:

For 2-3 persons, you require:

Pasta	200 gm (½ pound)
Salt	¼ teaspoon
Arugula	100 gm (¼ pound)
Dill seeds	¼ teaspoon
Spice mixture F	½ teaspoon
Cardamom	4
Butter or ghee	1 tablespoon

Cook pasta with a pinch of salt and drain out the water.

Wash and chop arugula leaves and fry them in ghee along with salt and spices. Do not add cardamom at this stage. Arugula cooks quite fast and normally the tender leaves are cooked in about 5 minutes. However, if the leaves are slightly over-ripped, the cooking time may be a little longer. Powder the cardamom seed and add in the vegetable along with the pasta. Stir everything together for about a minute.

PASTA WITH SPINACH

I will give below different recipe ideas for making pasta with spinach.

A. Use the above recipe by replacing arugula with spinach and add also ¼ teaspoon of Mixture C in addition. In the end, add a tablespoon of fresh cream. Remember spinach is astringent and to create a balance, the cream is added. In case you do not want cream, add some paneer or mozzarella.

B. Fry an onion in ghee, add two tomatoes, salt and Mixture A. Cook well until the sauce is ready. Add cooked and puréed spinach. Cook all the vegetables together for about 5 minutes and add the sauce on the pre-cooked pasta. Separately, put a spoon of cumin seeds on a hot pan and heat for about ½ a minute while stirring. Powder this cumin and add on the top of the preparation for a distinct flavour.

C. You may add paneer in preparation B. Make the paneer in small cubes as has been told earlier. Roast it slightly on a non-stick pan smeared with little ghee. Then add these pieces to the above preparation at the last minute.

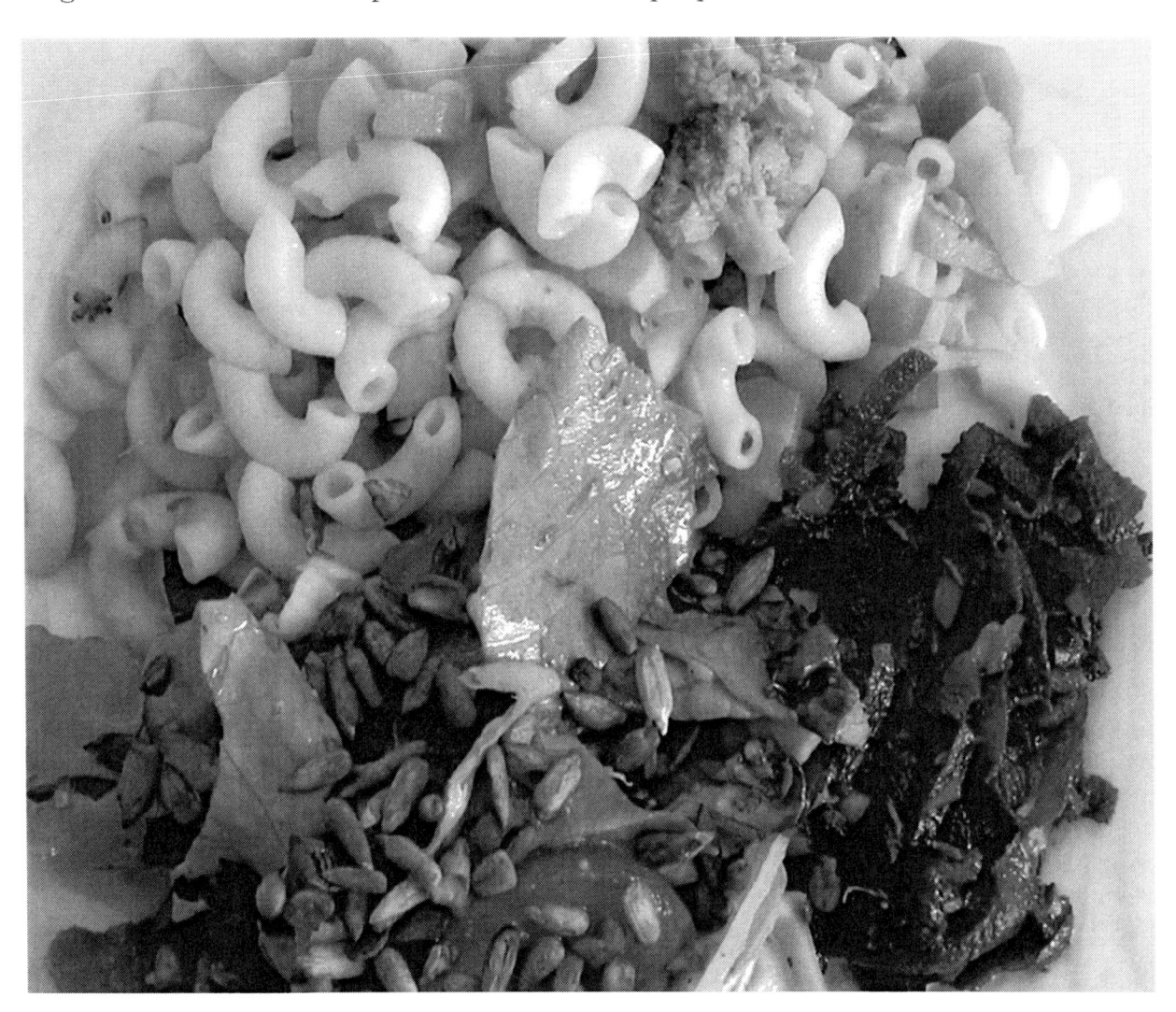

Main Meals

BASIL PASTA

Ingredients:

For 2-3 portions, you require:

Pasta	200 gm (½ pound)
Tomatoes	4 medium-sized
Onions	2 medium-sized
Parmesan	100 gm (¼ pound)
Paprika	1
Mixture C	1 teaspoon
Ajwain or thyme	1 teaspoon
Pepper	1 fourth teaspoon
Ghee or butter	2 tablespoons
Fresh basil leaves	about 20
Sesames seeds	one teaspoon
Chilli (optional)	half green chilli
Salt	half teaspoon or according to taste

Cook the pasta with a pinch of salt and drain out the water.
Chop onions in lamellae and fry them in 1 tablespoon of butter or ghee until they are golden brown. Add tomatoes and paprika, which should be cut in small cubes. Stir and let them cook on a low fire for about seven minutes while stirring them from time to time. Add Mixture C, salt, ajwain, pepper and chilli. Continue cooking for another ten minutes. Add garlic in the end and remove the pot from the hotplate. After adding garlic, the vegetables should not be cooked.

Heat half a tablespoon of ghee in a pan and add pasta to it. Stir constantly until the pasta is hot. Serve the hot pasta in plates in a circle, put the vegetable preparation in the middle and then grated Parmesan on the top. Very finely chopped basil leaves should be put on the central heap of the plate.

VEGETABLE AND MINT PASTA

Ingredients:

For two persons, you need:

Pasta	200 gm (½ pound)
Onions	2 medium-sized
Courgette (Zucchini)	1, cut into small pieces
Tomatoes	4 medium-sized, cut into small cubes
Fresh ginger	finely chopped, 1 tablespoon full

Garlic	2 cloves, finely chopped
Ajwain, dill seeds, cumin	½ teaspoon of each
Pepper	a pinch
Salt	½ teaspoon
Olive or sesames oil	2 tablespoons
Fresh mint leaves	10-15

A special spice mixture with following ingredients:

Cardamoms	4
Cloves	3
Mace	a pinch
Dried basil	½ teaspoon

Grind all the four ingredients together after taking out the seeds of the cardamoms out of their pods. Cook the pasta with a pinch of salt and drain out the water.

Put oil in a pan and add onions cut into lamellae and ginger. Fry them until they are slightly golden. Then add on to it the courgette. Fry for 4-5 minutes while stirring and then add salt, pepper, ajwain, dill seeds and cumin. Stir everything together and fry for another minute. Now add tomatoes and stir them well into the rest. Cover the vegetables and let them cook on slow fire until the tomatoes are completely cooked. Keep stirring from time to time. In the end, add the special spice mixture and garlic and turn off the heat.

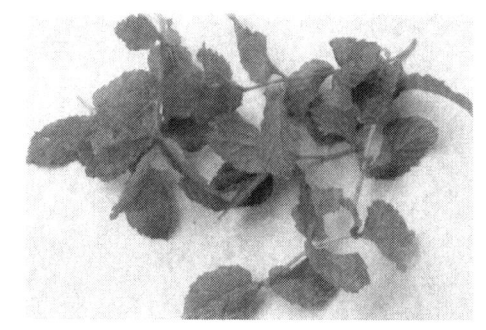

Add 1 tablespoon of oil in the pan and when it is hot, add the pasta into it. Stir gently and heat the pasta. Serve the pasta in plates in the middle and the vegetable preparation around it. Decorate the plate with finely chopped mint leaves and put four entire mint leaves on four sides.

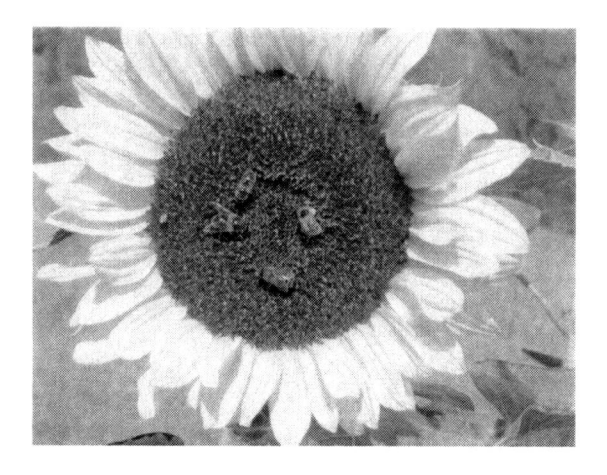

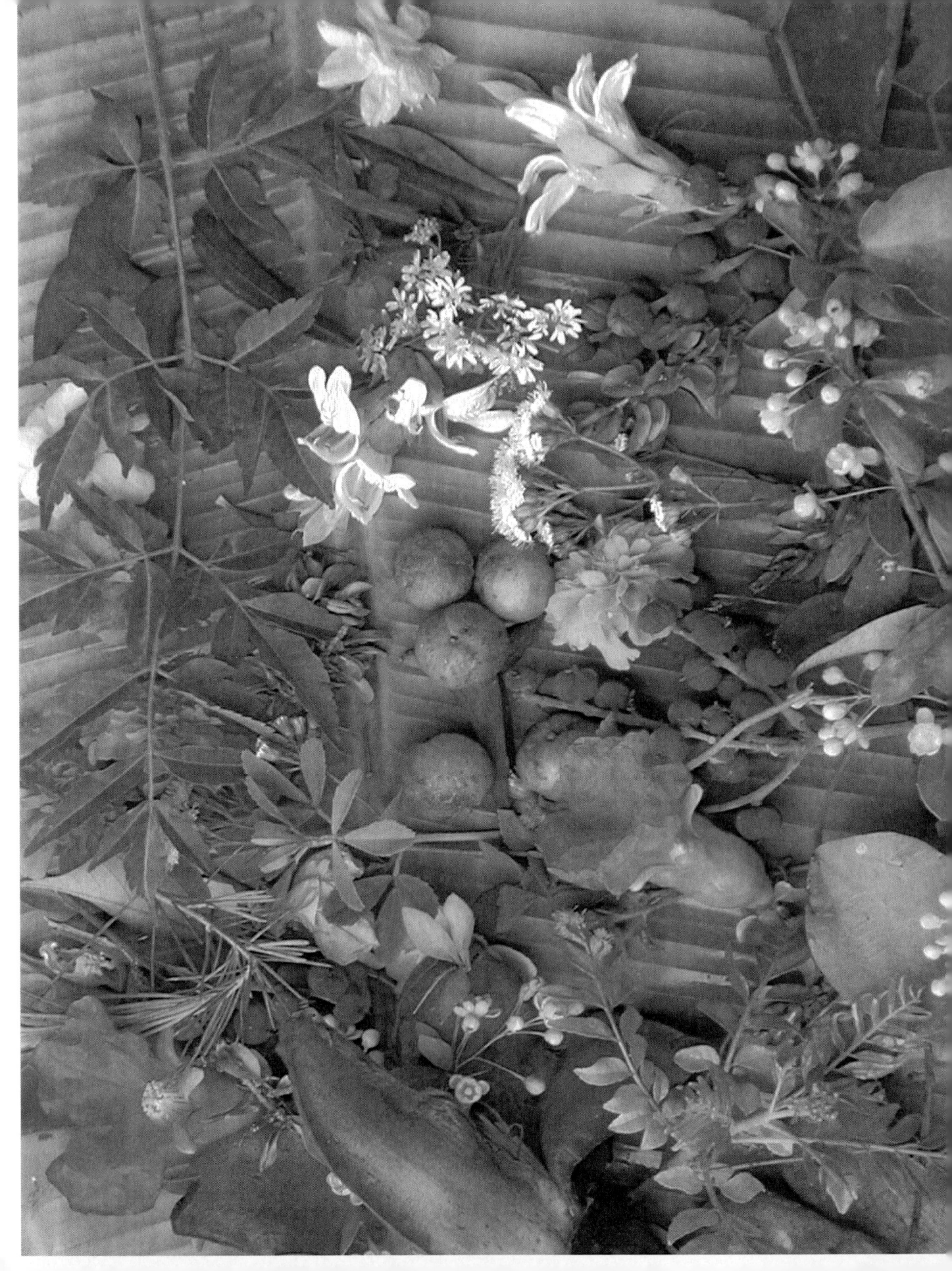

RICE

There are numerous varieties of rice in this world, and rice is a staple food for the majority of the world population. In the West, it is not eaten so frequently but many people are taking to vegetarian diets now and are eating rice. You can make a variety of dishes from it. My recipes below are for Basmati rice. *Shali* rice, which is highly recommended in Ayurveda, is grown only in some parts of the Himalayan Mountains and its production is depleting due to the popularity of the Basmati rice. Since it is so rare, I am not giving the specific recipes for it. Normally shali rice needs 2 ½ times the quantity of water in proportion to the rice whereas the Basmati rice needs twice the volume of water than the volume of rice.

PLAIN RICE

Ingredients:

Basmati rice	1 cup or whatever measure you use (about 200 gm)*
Water	2 cups (or twice the quantity of the rice with the measure you have used)
Cardamom	3
Clove	5

You always need double the amount of water to cook rice. You may measure your rice with any glass or cup and simply take double the quantity of water. Wash the rice properly and then soak it in water from 10 to 15 minutes. For plain rice preparation, put the water in a pot with a thick bottom. Add cardamom after removing the pods and cloves. Cover the water, bring it to boil and then add the soaked rice in it after draining out completely the water they were soaked in. Do that with a strainer. When all the rice is in boiling water, reduce to very low heat and put the lid on. Let the rice cook very slowly. After about 8 minutes (or a little more, depending upon the quality and age of rice and quality of water), you will smell the fine perfume of Basmati. Put off the heat and let the pot remain as such. Put a little weight or a napkin to cover the lid so that the vapours do not escape. Let it lie for about five minutes like this before serving. Rice should always be cooked a little before they are served.

---

* Rice is not taken by weight but by measure (volume). If you wish to cook 200 gm of rice (half pound), which is generally enough for three persons, measure it with a glass or any other container and measure the quantity of the water with the same container. You always require twice the volume of water to cook rice.

Main Meals

Suggestions: This preparation does not have any salt. You can taste the pure flavour and taste without salt. Normally, this rice is eaten with other vegetable preparations. Rice leftover can be cooked with milk and made into a dessert (see recipe in the dessert section).

Quantity of rice: Depending upon the other courses in the meal and appetite of persons, an average quantity of rice falls between 50 to 75 gm (¼ to 3/8 of a cup) per person. However, persons involved in physical labour and those who eat it as staple food, normally consume large quantities of rice.

SAFFRON RICE

To make saffron rice, in the above preparation, replace all the spices with 250 mg (¼ of a gram or a pinch) of saffron. The rice gets a very delicate taste of the saffron and is coloured lively yellow.

SALTY RICE WITH ONIONS

Ingredients:

Basmati rice (about 200 gm)	1 cup or any other similar measure of your liking
Water	2 cups or twice the quantity of the rice
Onions	2 medium sized
Cardamom	3 pods
Clove	5
Laurel leaves or Cinnamon leaves	2-3
Cumin	1½ teaspoon
Cooking oil or ghee	1 tablespoon
Salt	1/3 teaspoon or according to taste

Wash the rice three to four times and soak it in water for 10 to 15 minutes before preparation. Cut the onions into lamellae. Heat the oil in a pot and add spices after having taken out the cardamom from their pods. Add immediately the onion and stir-fry until the onions are slightly brown (sauté). Add salt and mix it well with onions and then add rice after draining out the water in which it is soaked. Stir the rice gently with the rest and keep the heat low. Prior to that, boil the measured quantity of water and add it to the pot after having stirred the rice very gently for about a minute with onions and spices. Keep the heat very low. After having added water, cover the rice with a lid without any holes in it. Cooking time is about 8-9 minutes but it varies with the quality of rice, type of water and intensity of heat. Therefore, try to put off the heat as soon as you have a nice perfume of Basmati. Keep the rice covered for 5 minutes after removing from the stove. Put a napkin on the lid of the pot so that it retains its heat for this time.

Suggestions: Slightly over-cooked rice is ruined as it becomes sticky and loses its shape and form. Under-cooked rice vitiates vata. Therefore, the rice should be cooked very carefully. After a little practice, you will learn to adjust the cooking time in your particular situation. Adding boiling water instead of cold is a trick, which is very helpful for cooking good rice.

This kind of rice makes a complete meal when served with a mixed salad. It is usual to serve different kind of rice preparation with yoghurt sauce called *rayata* during lunchtime. However, at night yoghurt has ill effects and it is not recommended. Recipes for different kinds of rayatas are given later in this section.

MIXED VEGETABLE RICE

Ingredients:

Basmati rice	½ cup (100 gm)
Water	1 cup (200 ml)
Paprika	1 big or two small
Green peas	6 tablespoons
Onions	1 medium-sized (in lamellae)
Carrots	2 medium-sized (grated)
Cumin	1 teaspoon
Cardamom	3
Clove	5
Pepper	¼ teaspoon
Salt	¼ teaspoon or to taste
Cooking oil or ghee	1 tablespoon
Raisins	1 tablespoon
Coriander leaves or Celery leaves (chopped)	1 tablespoon

Heat the cooking oil or ghee in a pot and add spices and salt in it. Add the onions immediately and fry them for a minute on medium fire. Add young and tender green peas and cook another 2 minutes while stirring from time to time. Add paprika and grated carrots. Mix everything by stirring and cook all these vegetables with the lid on for another 2 minutes. Add the washed and soaked rice in this preparation after draining out the water. Stir the rice gently with vegetable preparation for about a minute. Reduce the heat. Separately, boil the water and add into this preparation. Put the lid on and cook it on gentle fire. As said above, cooking time is around 8-9 minutes; judge it by the perfume of the

Main Meals

Basmati rice. Continue to keep the lid on for another 5 minutes and cover the pot with a napkin during this time.

Serve this preparation with chopped herbs on the top.

MUSHROOM AND TOMATO RICE

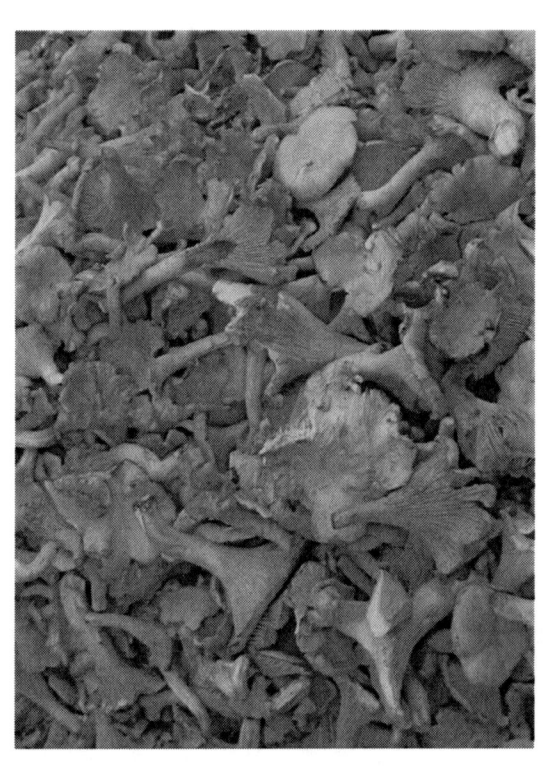

Ingredients:

Basmati rice	½ cup (about 100 gm)
Water	1 cup or 200 ml
Mushrooms	½ cup or 50 gm of chopped mushrooms
Tomato	2 medium sized cut into small pieces
Garlic	3 cloves
Salt	1/3 teaspoon or to **taste**
Cooking oil	1 tablespoon

Special freshly ground spice mixture:

Coriander	½ teaspoon
Cumin	½ teaspoon
Clove	5
Pepper	10 seeds
Nutmeg	¼ of a nut

Grind all these spices together a little before use.
Fry mushrooms in oil for about 5 minutes on a medium heat and keep stirring. Add spice mixture and salt and stir well. Add finely chopped tomatoes and stir them with the rest. Cook for about 3-4 minutes and stir from time to time. Now add washed and soaked rice into the pot after draining out the water it was soaked in. Mix the rice gently with the ingredients in the pot and cook for a minute while stirring. Put the fire low and add boiling water. Stir everything together and then put the lid on the pot. Let it cook on gentle fire. As indicated previously, the cooking time for the rice is 8-9 minutes and switch off the fire when you smell the nice perfume of Basmati. Quickly uncover the lid and sprinkle finely chopped garlic on the rice. Replace the lid and put a napkin on the pot after putting off the fire and wait until 10 more minutes before serving.

Suggestions: It is recommended to serve this dish for lunch with cucumber *rayata* for which the recipe is given later in this Section.

SOUR, SWEET AND SPICY RICE

Ingredients:

Basmati rice	½ cup (about 100 gm)
Water	1 cup or 200 ml
Ginger (finely chopped)	2 tablespoons
Green chilli	1 finely sliced
Carrots	2 medium sized, grated
Spinach	Few leaves, finely chopped
Ghee	1 tablespoon
Mixture C	1 teaspoon
Salt	1/3 teaspoon
Raisins	2 tablespoons
Garlic	3 cloves finely chopped
Lemon juice	1 tablespoon

Heat the ghee and add ginger, paprika, carrot and spinach. Stir-fry all these vegetables and if they stick on the bottom, reduce the heat and place the lid on the pot. If needed, add a tablespoon of water but not more than that. Cook for about 5 to 7 minutes. After the vegetables are sauté, add salt and spices and stir. Now add the washed and soaked rice after draining out their water. Stir the rice and the vegetables gently and add boiling water after a minute. Reduce the heat and place the lid on the pot. Let the whole preparation cook gently. After about 7 minutes, add raisins and garlic and stir gently only from the top layer of rice and replace the lid immediately. Put off the heat after 2 minutes and keep the preparation covered as such for another 5 minutes. Put a napkin on the pot as has been described above. Add lemon juice before serving.

Suggestions: You may serve this rice with banana *rayata* (the recipe is described later in this section) during lunchtime. If you wish to serve this rice for dinner, you may serve it with sweet and sour chutney or with a little fruit marmalade. It may be also served with the slices of fresh, sweet and juicy fruits like mango, apple, peaches, pineapple etc.

GREEN RICE

Ingredients:

Basmati rice	½ cup (about 100 gm)
Water	1 cup (200 ml)
Different green, leafy vegetables	200 gm (½ pound)
Onion	1 medium sized
Cumin	1 teaspoon

Main Meals

Mixture C	1 teaspoon
Salt	¼ teaspoon or to taste.
Ghee	1 tablespoon

Wash and soak the rice for at least 10 minutes as in all the rice recipes described above. Fry the onions in ghee briefly and then add the cumin, mixture C and salt. Stir everything together and go on adding green vegetables while stirring. Cook the vegetables on low fire with the lid on the pot for about five minutes. Uncover and stir again in order to get rid of excessive water if any. Add washed and soaked rice into the vegetables after draining out the water. Stir gently and add boiling water. Put the lid on and cook on a low heat. After about 8 or 9 minutes, when you have the perfume of the basmati rice, turn off the heat and leave the preparation as such for another 5 minutes. Put a napkin on the pot so that it maintains its heat. This preparation looks green due to the predominant colour of the green vegetables.

FRIED RICE PREPARATIONS

Let this name not remind you of the rice in some oriental restaurants, soaked with fat and flooded with spices. In Ayurvedic cooking, we use rather small amount of fat and the quantity of the spices is always moderate. Unlike the previous recipes with rice and vegetables, the following recipes are prepared with pre-cooked rice, which I have described above as plain rice. Plain rice can be kept in the refrigerator for up to two days. Therefore, you can try different recipes with it. These preparations of rice taste different than when rice is cooked along with the vegetables like in the recipes given above.

PAPRIKA, BROCCOLI AND GINGER RICE

This recipe is very quickly done if you have already the pre-cooked rice.

Ingredients:

For two portions, you require:

Cooked plain rice	2-3 small bowls (something like a soup bowl)
Broccoli	100 gm (¼ lb.)
Paprika	2 medium-sized
Fresh ginger, chopped	1 tablespoon
Cumin	½ teaspoon
Mixture A	½ teaspoon
Ghee or cooking oil	2 tablespoons
Salt	¼ teaspoon

Cut broccoli into very tiny pieces, almost like chopped herbs. Put ghee or cooking oil in a pan or a wok and add broccoli into it. Stir-fry for a few minutes and then add ginger and the spices. Stir for a minute and add paprika chopped into thin and long pieces. Cook everything together for few minutes while stirring. Now add rice into the pan little by little while stirring gently. Reduce the heat, as the rice will tend to stick to the bottom. When all the rice is added and the contents of the pan are well mixed, cover the preparation and let the rice heat with the vapour from the vegetables on a very low heat for a minute.

GREEN PEAS RICE

Ingredients:

For two to three portions you require:

Cooked plain rice	2-3 small bowls
Green peas	1 bowl
Onion	1 medium-sized
Salt	¼ teaspoon
Cumin	1 teaspoon
Mixture H	½ teaspoon
Ghee or cooking oil	2 tablespoon

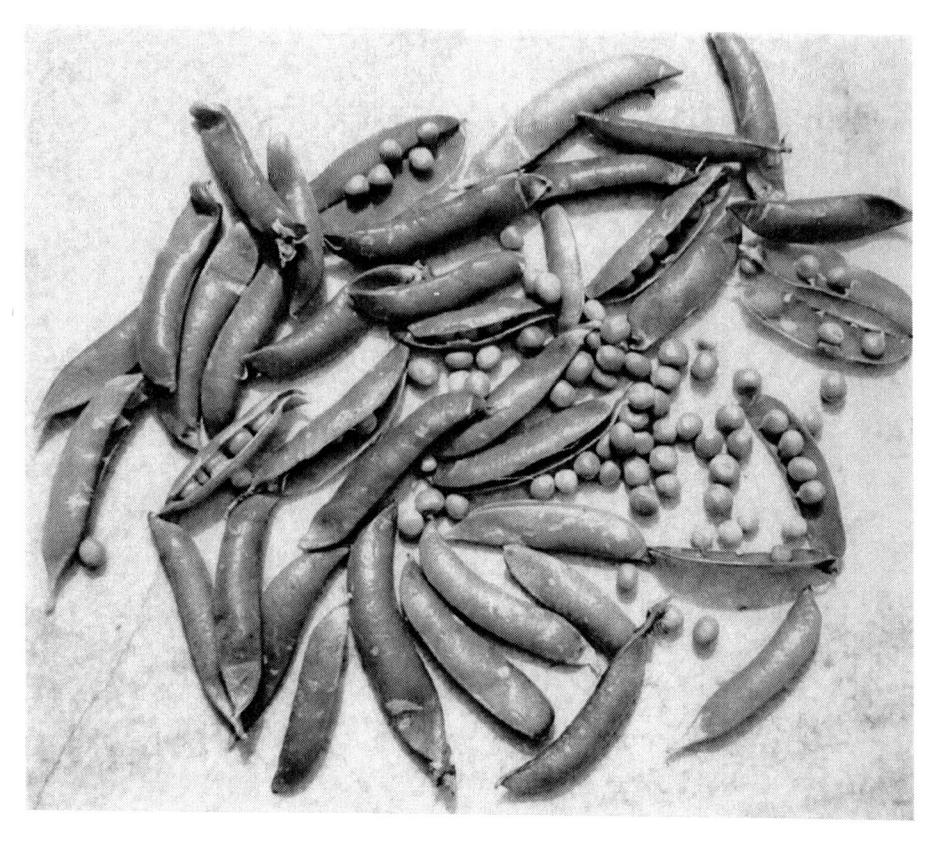

Main Meals

Add ghee or oil in a wok or pan and heat it. Add cumin and salt into the hot oil and then onions cut in lamellae. When onions are fried a little, add tender peas. Stir everything together and cook with the lid on. The tender variety of peas (young peas) will take about 3 minutes to cook whereas the bigger and ripe peas require longer or sometimes pre-cooking is required. Then go on adding rice slowly while stirring gently. Reduce the heat and put the lid on for just a minute like in the previous recipe.

Comments: The quality of the green peas is important. If the peas are over-ripped, they are highly vata. In case you do not have young peas and you wish to make your preparation with ripe or over-ripped peas, then pre-cook them with half a teaspoon of ajwain until they are soft. You may also use a little garlic in a salad with this meal to avoid the vata effect of these peas. In any case, the recipe tastes better with young peas.

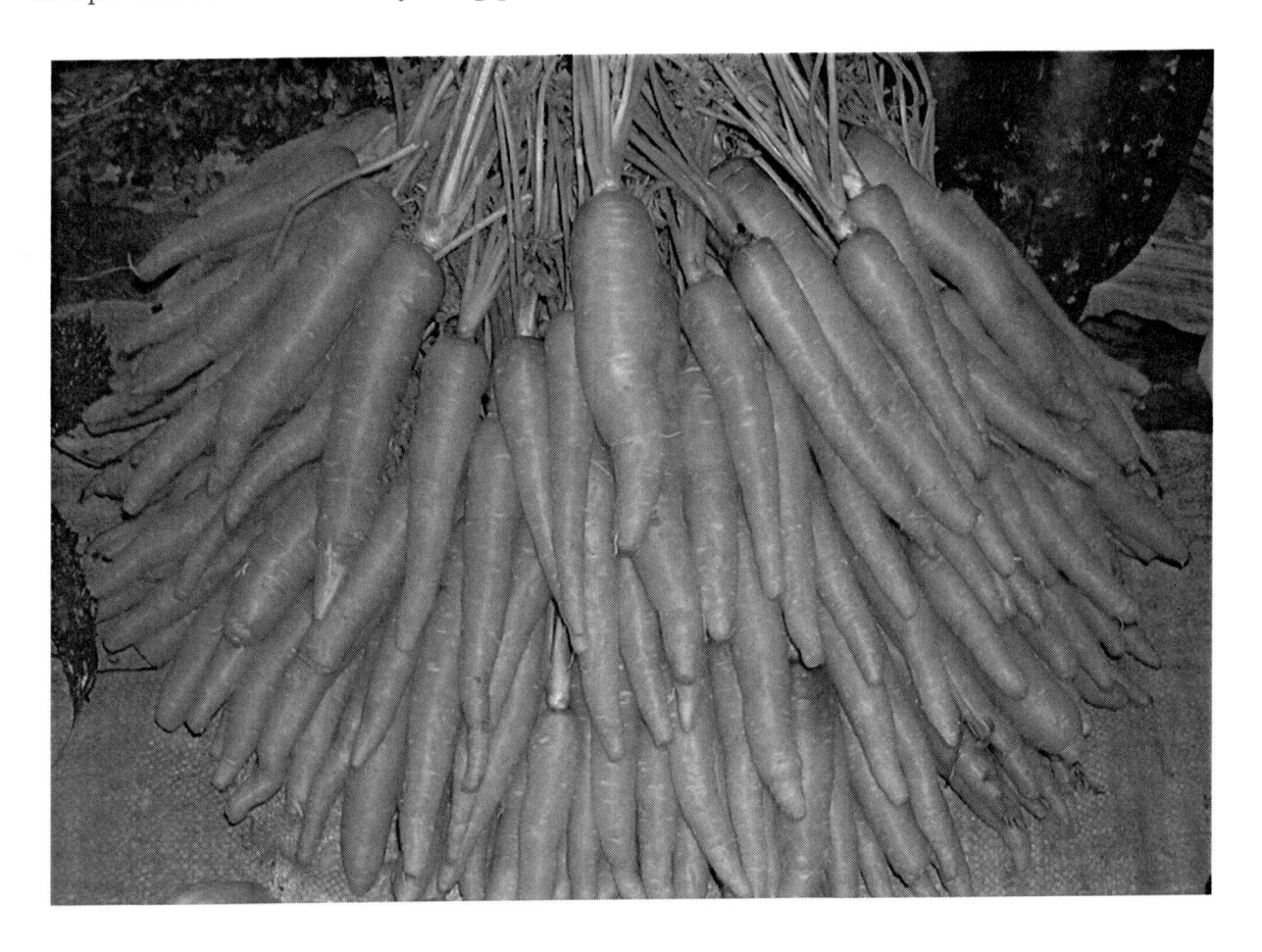

SOME OTHER GRAINS

I have described many different preparations with rice and various vegetables together. There are also other grains one can prepare in a similar manner. Many of you who use this book may not be rice eaters. As in Ayurvedic food culture the use of pre-prepared bread should be kept to a minimum (specially the bread with yeast), it is important to learn those preparations where we can use the wheat grains or other grains like millet and eat them fresh and warm. Later in this Section, I have given many recipes for breads for the same purpose. But grains and vegetable preparation together is quick to make and therefore depending upon the time schedule, one has the freedom to organise oneself.

I have mentioned dalia in the breakfast recipes. Dalia can also be prepared with different vegetables or without vegetables with different spices and grains to replace bread. The essential preparation method for dalia dishes is the same as for the rice, but dalia dishes are not so delicate in terms of precision in cooking time as the Basmati rice preparations. One has to only take care that there is enough water and the grains are well cooked.

DALIA WITH SESAME SEEDS

Ingredients

For two portions you require:

Dalia	100 gm (½ cup)
Water	300 ml (1 ½ cup)
Salt	a pinch
Cumin	½ teaspoon
Ghee	1 teaspoon
Sesames seeds	1 teaspoon

Heat the oil in a pot and add cumin seeds first and then few seconds later add dalia. Roast dalia by stirring it for a minute or two on medium heat. Add water and salt and reduce the fire. Let the preparation cook for about 10 minutes on low fire. Add sesame seeds, stir a little and cover the preparation again. Cook until the grains are soft. Like rice, consider measuring dalia rather than weighing it and take three times the water with the same measure. It may be possible that the dalia or the bulgar you have has bigger grains or is of another variety. Keep in mind that the grain should be soft. Uncooked grain vitiates vata.

Main Meals

Suggestions: You may try the other recipes given for rice to make dalia preparations. Only take care that each time your grain is soft. You can taste at the end of the preparation and add a little more water if needed.

Germinated wheat grains can also be cooked like this. It is a very healthy food and that is why I have given many recipes from it. Whole grains cooked like this are harder to digest as compared to the flat bread recipe from the crushed germinated wheat, which is given later in the book. Add always some ajwain in it. Those of you with weak digestion or suffering from digestive disorders may not eat the wheat cooked like this.

Finger millet or some other grains may be prepared in a similar manner. Take care to find out the Ayurvedic nature of the grain you are using. Make the choice of your spices accordingly. Also observe the reaction of a particular grain on you. Avoid eating it if it gives you a heavy feeling. Alternatively, try adding some rock salt, ajwain, ginger and lemon juice in the preparation.

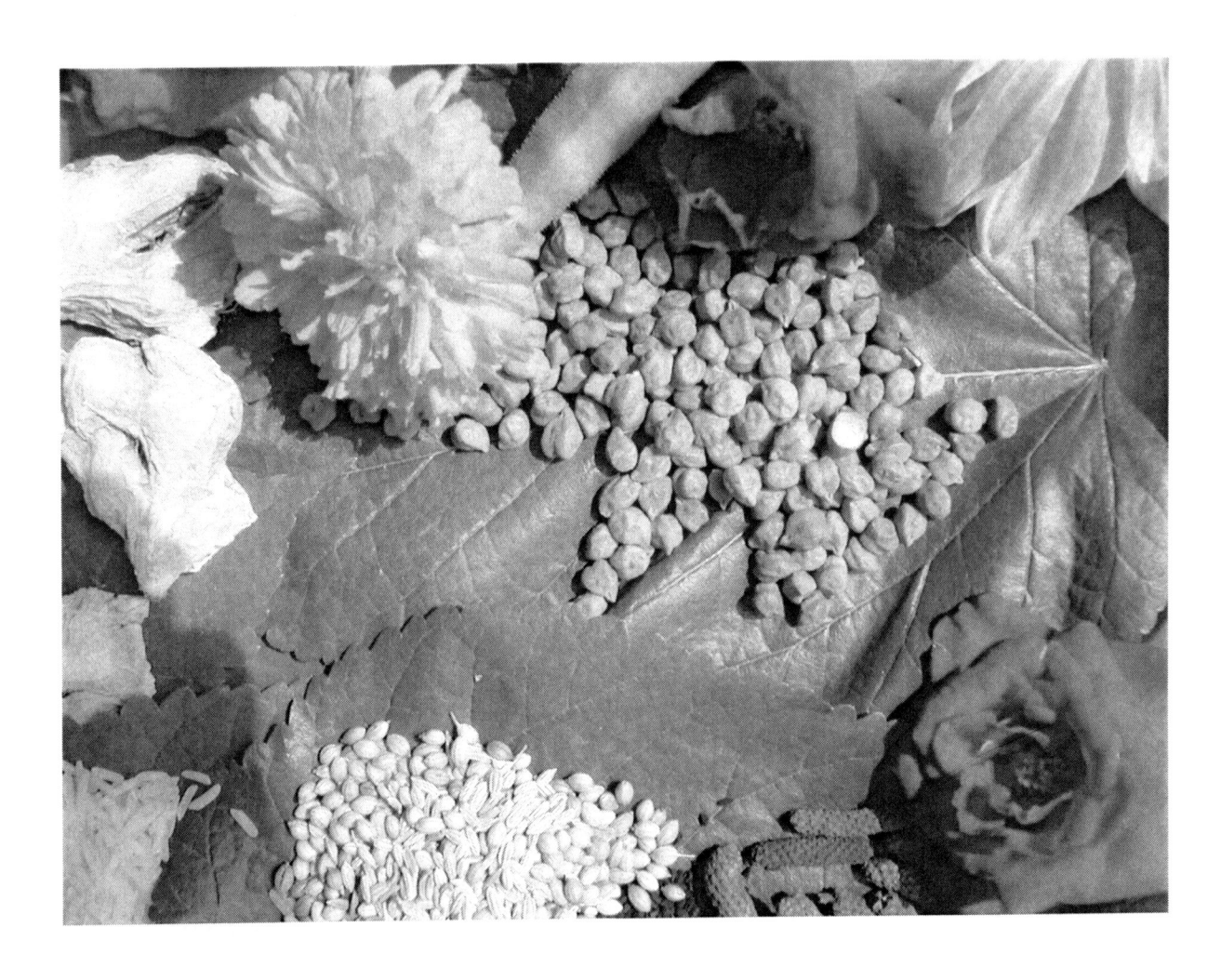

VEGETABLE PREPARATIONS

Different vegetables can be prepared on the stove in a wok or in a pot with the lid on or are baked in the oven. Vegetable prepared on the stove may be eaten with some kind of flat bread or plain rice whereas the baked vegetable may be served as a second course to soup or a starter. From an Ayurvedic point of view, different vegetables should be mixed together to obtain all the different rasas. In case you are eating a single vegetable preparation like the baked potatoes, think of making a mixed vegetable salad or any other preparation where several different vegetables are used.

MIXED VEGETABLES WITH GINGER

This is a mixed vegetable recipe that is without salt. Generally people are extremely sorry when they are supposed to eat food without salt due to an ailment or regiment. Try this recipe and you will realise that sometimes vegetables without salt can taste better than with salt.

Ingredients:

For two to three persons, you require:

Carrots	3 medium-sized
Green peas	4 tablespoons
Beans	100 gm (¼ lb.)
Cauliflower	100 gm (¼ lb.)
Paprika	1 medium-sized
Ginger (chopped)	3 tablespoons
Cumin	½ teaspoon
Fennel	½ teaspoon
Cardamom	4
Clove	4
Ghee or cooking oil	2 teaspoons
Raisins	1 tablespoon

Cut the vegetables into small pieces but keep them separately. Paprika should be cut into long pieces. Grind all the four spices together and remove the cardamom pods before that. Heat the oil in a pot and add beans into it. Stir a little and then put the lid on and reduce the heat. Beans take longer to cook than the rest of the vegetables and that is why they need prior cooking. After about 10 minutes, add carrots, peas, cauliflower and ginger into it. Stir everything together and cook for another 10 minutes with the lid on. Keep stirring from time to time. The vegetables cook with their own vapours when cooked with the lid on and on low heat. Add the powdered spices and raisins and stir everything together. Cook for another two minutes and it is ready.

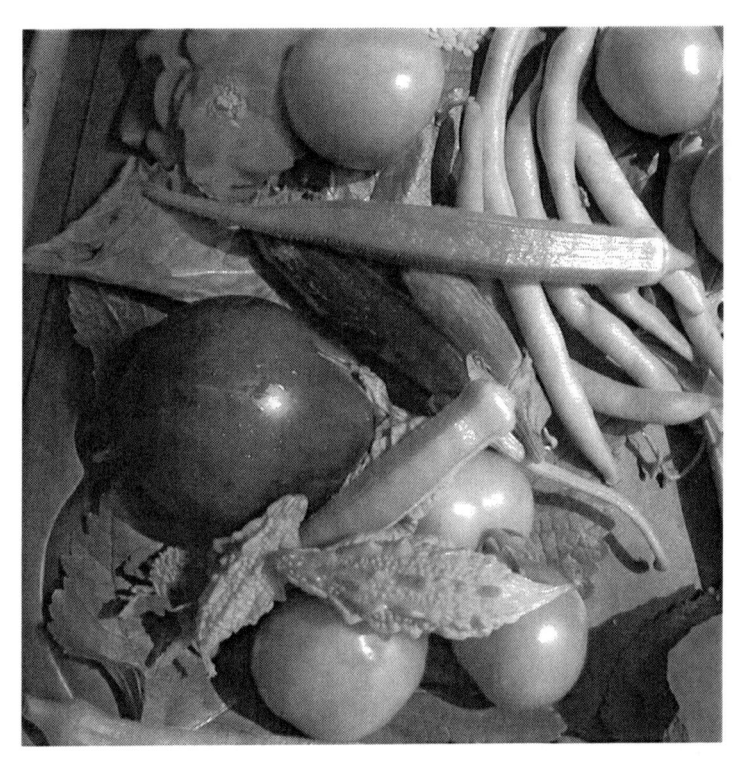

STRING BEANS WITH GINGER

This is a simple recipe meant specially for those who have to watch their weight because there is no fat at all in this preparation. However, it is suggested that you eat these with something that has a little fat. It is not advisable to have the entire meal without fat. For example, potatoes fried on a non-stick pan with only half a teaspoon of oil will make a nice combination with this preparation.

Ingredients:

For 2 to 3 portions:

String beans	200gm (½ lb.)
Water	100 ml (½ cup)
Tomatoes	2 medium-sized
Salt	¼ teaspoon
Ginger (small pieces)	1 tablespoon
Cumin	½ teaspoon
Cardamom	4

Put the water into a pot and bring it to boil. Cut the beans into small pieces and put them in boiling water. Cook for 15-20 minutes on low heat with the lid on. Stir from time to time and add a little more water if needed. Add tomatoes, ginger and spices and cook for another 10 minutes. Carda-moms should be added after taking them out from the pods and crushing a little.

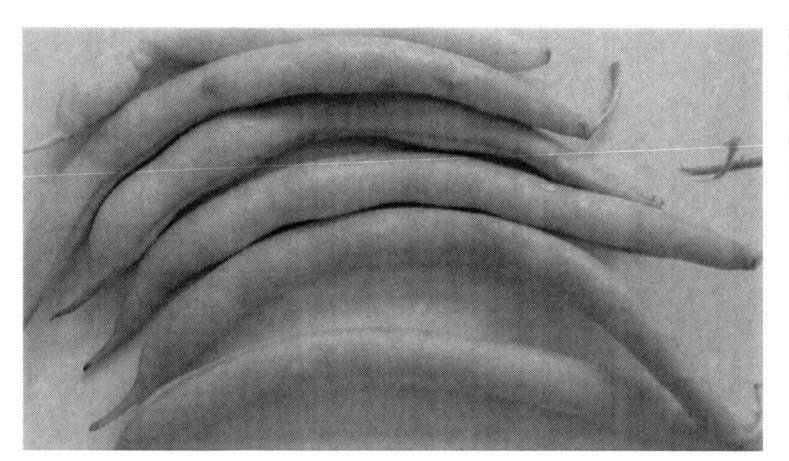

CABBAGE WITH MIXTURE B

There are many vegetables, which can be cooked quite simply and quickly by using mixture B.

For two to three persons, you require:

Green cabbage	about 600 gm (1 ½ lb.)
Cooking oil	2 tablespoons
Salt	1/3 teaspoon or to taste
Mixture B	1 tablespoon
Green chilli	½ to 1 (optional)
Fresh lemon juice	1 teaspoon (optional)

Heat the oil in a pan or a wok on medium fire. When it is hot enough, add mixture B. After few seconds, add salt and chilli and then immediately after the finely chopped cabbage. Go on adding cabbage and stirring so that the spices can mix well with the vegetables. Cook uncovered for first five minutes while stirring from time to time. Depending upon the season and the quality of the cabbage, you may put the lid on. Fresh cabbage has lot of water and you need not cover. If the cabbage is hard, you will require cooking it on low heat with the lid on. In the end, when the cabbage is soft, remove the lid and stir to make the vegetable crisp. You may add lemon juice in the end and stir. However, the addition of lemon juice is optional. Some of you may not like it sour and may leave out the lemon juice. For those who have a little problem in digesting cabbage should add lemon juice.

Main Meals

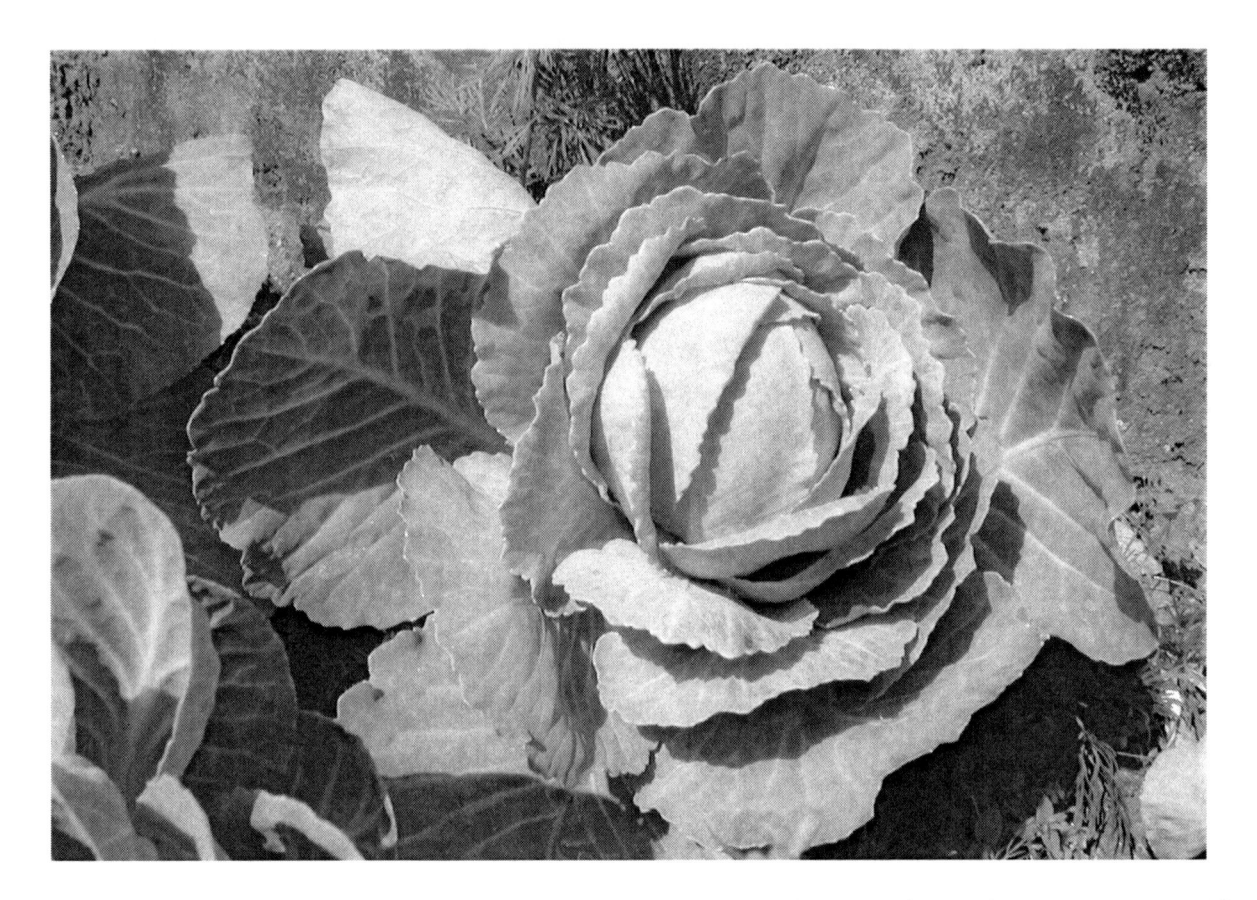

Suggestions: This recipe can be used to cook other leafy and green vegetables. Cauliflower or broccoli also makes delicious preparations with this method. Potatoes can be cooked like this but they should be first boiled with their skin. The skin should be removed after boiling and then they should be cut into small pieces. The above recipe is applied to potatoes but the cooking time is reduced in this case. Mixed vegetable is another very good preparation with this method. You may add carrots, paprika, green peas, potatoes and cauliflower in your mixed vegetable preparation.

AUBERGINE PURÉE (BHARTHA IN HINDI)

In many countries in the world, the purée of aubergine with onions, tomatoes or garlic etc. is prepared in different forms. In North India, it is a classical dish but with time people have adopted different modes of preparations diverting from Ayurvedic principles. The essential in aubergine preparation is that when the whole vegetable is baked, it makes a balanced preparation.

The big and round variety of aubergine is used for this purpose. The entire aubergine is either baked on the fire directly or is baked in the oven. After baking, it is turned into a purée. You may take off the peels if your vegetable is not organically grown. It is easy to make the purée with the hand blender. Once you have the purée, make the basic sauce with onions and tomatoes and mix everything together.

Ingredients:

For 3 to 4 portions, you require:

Aubergine	2 medium-sized
Onions	3 medium-sized
Garlic	6 cloves
Ginger	3 tablespoons finely chopped
Green chilli	1 (optional)
Fresh coriander leaves	a bunch
Tomatoes	5 medium sized
Mixture A	1 teaspoon
Cumin	1 teaspoon
Fennel	½ teaspoon
Mixture C	1 teaspoon
Turmeric	1 teaspoon
Ghee or cooking oil	2 tablespoons
Salt	½ teaspoon
Raw sugar or jaggery	1 teaspoon

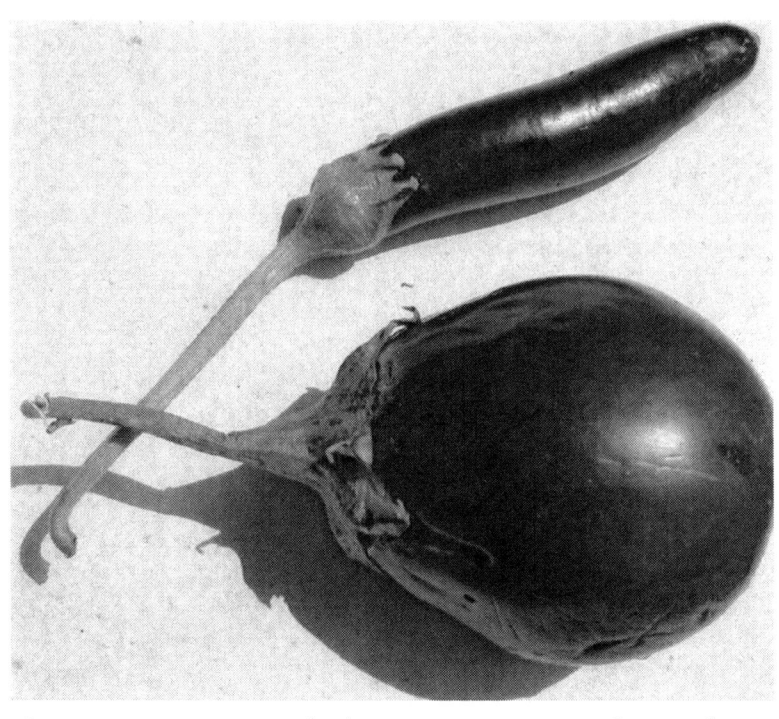

This recipe has two parts. The first part is to make purée from aubergine after roasting and the second part is to make the **basic sauce** with which the purée is combined later. You can make many diverse preparations with the basic sauce you will learn to make here.

Purée from aubergines: Bake the aubergines directly on gas or in the oven. You need a high temperature in the oven and let the aubergine bake until they are completely soft. Take them out, remove their upper stem and cut them into small pieces. Make purée from them with hand mixer. Leave them on one side.

Main Meals

Basic Sauce

Add ghee in a wok or a pot and when hot, put finely chopped onions into it. Fry the onions while stirring. When the onions are sauté, add turmeric and stir for about a minute. Add the other spices and salt. Stir everything together and cook for about another minute. Now add tomatoes, which should be cut into small pieces beforehand. Stir the tomatoes with the rest and let them cook for a while until they turn completely soft and the whole preparation looks like a sauce. Add a spoon of raw sugar and stir. It is better to cook the tomatoes with a lid on and stir from time to time. Keep the heat low. When the tomatoes are completely mashed, your sauce is ready.

Bhartha preparation: Add the aubergine purée into the sauce, stir well and cook for about 15 minutes while stirring from time to time. Peel garlic, take out the coriander leaves and crush all these along with ginger and chilli in a stone mortar or an electric wet grinder. Add this paste into your preparation just 1 to 2 minutes before finishing the cooking. Stir everything well and your Bhartha is ready.

Suggestion: Bhartha is best served with flat bread and rayata dish (see later in this Section for these recipes). If it is for dinner, serve with a mixed salad instead of rayata.

PREPARING OTHER DISHES WITH THE BASIC SAUCE

The basic sauce you have learnt to make above can be used for making many different vegetable, egg and meat dishes. I will give you some ideas in this direction. One fundamental factor to remember is that the proportion of the sauce and the ingredients you put in it should be about one to two. For the quantity of the sauce we have prepared above for the purée of two aubergines, I will give you the quantities of other ingredients you can prepare in that sauce.

Potatoes: Take 5 medium-sized potatoes and boil them with the skin. Peel off the skin and cut them into small cubes. Add the cut potatoes in the basic sauce. Cook for about 5 minutes while stirring from time to time. Then add about 300 ml (1½ cup water), stir to mix and bring it to boil. Let the whole thing cook for 15 minutes on slow fire. Put the lid on and stir occasionally. The potatoes should be extremely well cooked in this preparation. They should become almost like a part of sauce but yet not like a purée. Mash them with the help of a wooden spoon.

Potatoes and green peas: In this recipe, potatoes are not dissolved like in the above. You require two potatoes and 100gm (¼ lb.) of young and tender green peas. Peel and cut potatoes into very small pieces. Fry them in a non-stick pan with a very little fat on the surface of the pan until they are light brown. Add potatoes and green peas in the basic sauce. Stir to mix and cook for five minutes while stirring from time to time. Add 300 ml (1½ cup) water, stir and let it cook for 15 minutes on slow fire with the lid on. Stir from time to time to make sure the vegetables do not stick to the bottom.

If your peas are not tender, you need to cook them in water before hand. In the sour medium of the basic sauce, it is not possible to cook the hard and over-ripped peas.

Remember always, in all these recipes to add the mixture of garlic, ginger and herbs at the last minute.

Paneer and green peas or paneer alone: Make paneer from half a litre of milk and press to make pieces. Smear ghee on a pan and roast the pieces a little. Add 100 gm (¼ lb.) green peas to the basic sauce and cook for few minutes. Add 300 ml (2 ½ cup) water and let the preparation cook for 15 minutes. Add paneer pieces in the end and cook only for a minute or two after adding them. Remember to add your mixture of garlic, ginger and herbs in the end.

Eggs: With basic sauce, you can prepare delicious scrambled eggs. The amount of sauce prepared above is good for 5-6 eggs. When the sauce is ready, break eggs into it and go on stirring fast. You require cooking for about two minutes after the addition of eggs.

Eggs are hot in their Ayurvedic nature and therefore garlic should be left out. However add finely cut ginger pieces in the sauce before putting the eggs inside and decorate the preparation with chopped green herbs.

Chicken: Take 5 to 6 pieces of chicken drumsticks and fry them in a pan with a little butter or ghee. Make them slightly brown. Turn them around a few times so that all sides are well cooked. Add these to the basic sauce, stir and cook them with the lid on for about 5 minutes on low heat. Add 100 ml (½ cup) water in it to keep the sauce fluid and cook for another 20 minutes with the lid on while stirring the preparation from time to time.

Main Meals

FRIED AUBERGINE WITH OTHER VEGETABLES

This is a quicker recipe for aubergine than the bhartha. I am giving five different versions of this preparation with slight variations.

Version A

Ingredients:

For two portions, you require:

Aubergine	1 medium-sized
Paprika	2 medium-sized
Ginger, long cut pieces	2 tablespoons
Tomatoes	2 medium-sized
Salt	¼ teaspoon
Mixture A	½ teaspoon
Cumin	¼ teaspoon
Fennel	¼ teaspoon
Dill seeds	¼ teaspoon
Mace (powdered)	1 pinch
Fresh herbs (chopped)	1 tablespoon
Ghee or cooking oil	1 to 2 tablespoons

Cut the aubergine, paprika and tomatoes into roundels but keep them separately. Heat a non-stick pan with a little ghee or oil on it. When hot, put in one layer of aubergine pieces. Keep the heat medium. When the pieces are brown on one side, turn them around. Smear a little more fat on the bottom of the pan if required.

Now fry the next series of aubergine pieces taking care that you use minimum fat. This is the reason for using a non-stick pan. Like this, fry all the aubergine pieces and keep them on a plate. Add a little more ghee or oil in the pan and fry the paprika and the ginger for about three minutes stirring gently. Add all the spices and the salt and stir and cook for another two minutes. Take this preparation also out from the pan. Reduce the heat to very low and spread a layer of fried aubergine pieces in it. On the top of it, put a layer of spicy paprika and ginger you have just prepared and then put a layer of the roundels of tomatoes, which are still uncooked. Now add another layer of paprika and then another layer of tomatoes. The top layer should be of aubergine.

After you have laid out all the layers, put the lid on and let everything cook at a very low fire for about five minutes. This last part is better done on an electric stove than on gas. If you are using gas, put the pan off the fire in between and put it on again after a while. The last part can be done also in an oven on medium heat; your dish should then be covered with aluminium foil or a lid. Before serving, stir gently and mix all the vegetables so that you see all the colours on the top. Decorate them with the chopped herbs.

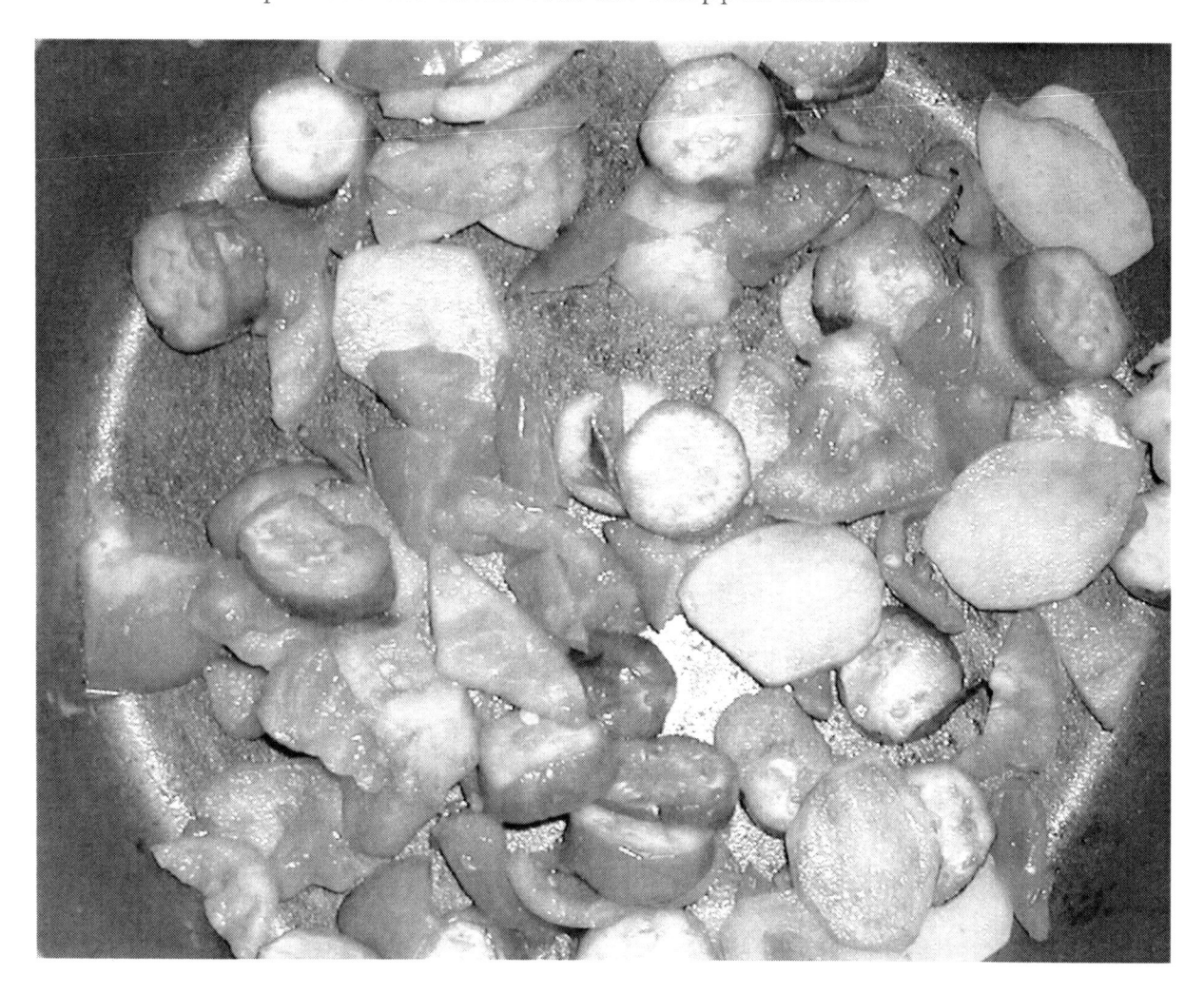

In this recipe, the advantage is that you use the minimum of fat. Most of the time, when aubergine is cooked, it is full of fat. This is because aubergines soak up fat. With the slow cooking process and on the non-stick pan, we try to limit the use of fat to the minimum. The second advantage of this recipe is that it has the freshness of half-cooked tomatoes.

Version B

In this version of the recipe, we add onions and garlic. Fry the roundels of the onions along with the paprika. The tiny pieces of garlic or crushed garlic should be added in the end when you are mixing all the vegetables together. You may use 2 medium sized onions and about 4 cloves of garlic.

Main Meals

Version C

For this recipe, add two medium-sized carrots to Version B. Cut the carrots into pieces of about finger long but flat surfaced. Fry the carrots for about five minutes and then add onions, ginger and paprika. Then proceed with the recipe as you have done in version A.

Version D

The above three recipes are meant to be served with rice, bread (or meat for those who eat it) or with some other kind of staple food. But in this version of the aubergine recipe, we will add potatoes making it a meal by itself. Since potatoes are used, we will have to increase the number of spices, and therefore I am rewriting the ingredients of this recipe. I am writing the addition of potatoes to Version A, but you may also prepare Versions B and C with potatoes.

Ingredients:

For two portions, you require:

Aubergine	1 medium-sized
Potatoes	3 medium-sized
Paprika	2 medium-sized
Ginger, long cut pieces	2 tablespoons
Tomatoes	3 medium sized
Salt	½ teaspoon
Mixture A	1 teaspoon
Mixture C	½ teaspoon
Cumin	½ teaspoon
Fennel	½ teaspoon
Dill seeds	¼ teaspoon
Mace (powdered)	1 pinch
Fresh herbs (chopped)	2 tablespoon
Ghee or cooking oil	2 tablespoons

For making this version with potatoes, fry the roundels of the potatoes in a similar manner as you have done with the aubergine. Cut them thin so that they do not take too long to cook. Turn them when one side is brown. When all of them are fried, put half the amount of salt on them in such a manner that all the pieces get equally salted. Do the rest in the similar manner as described for Version A. At the end, put a layer of potatoes between the layers of paprika and tomatoes.

Paprika

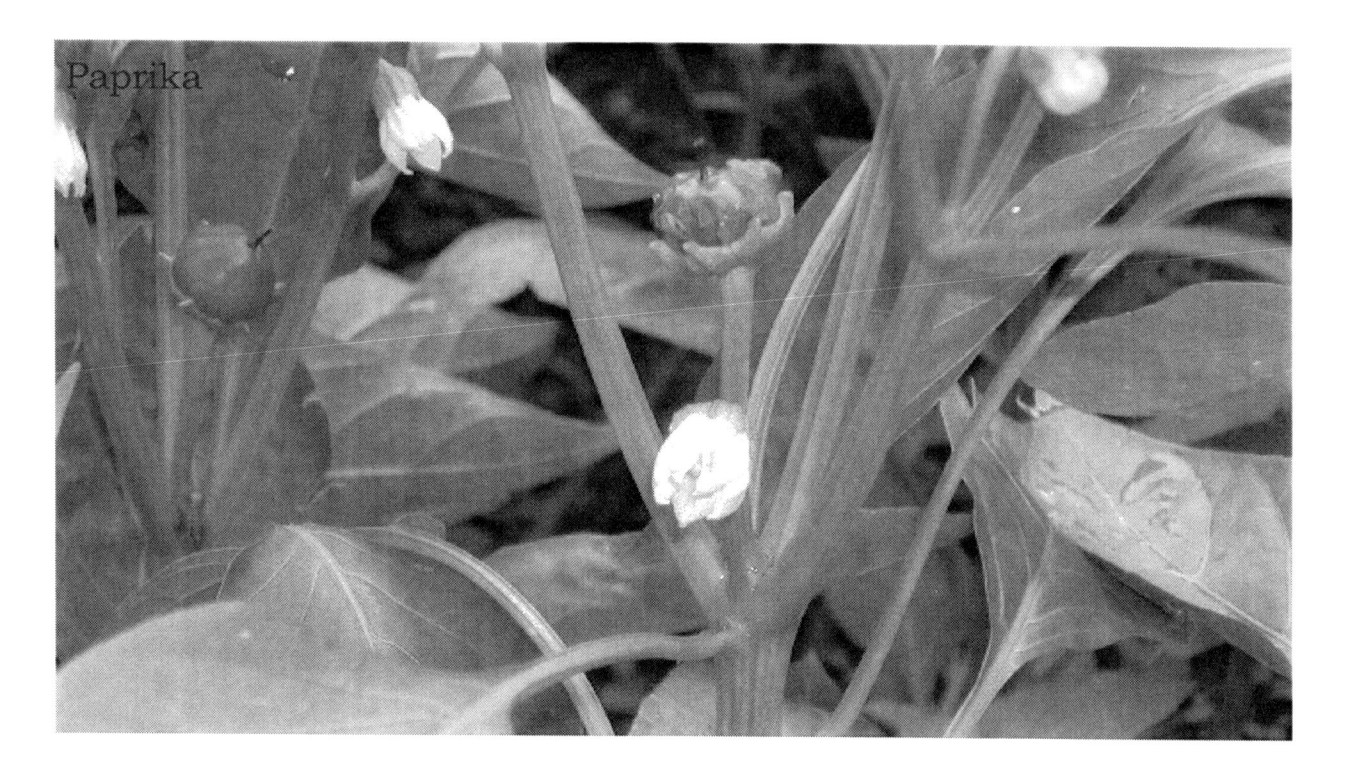

Version E

In this recipe, the potatoes of Version D are replaced by slices of paneer. Unlike potatoes, you do not need to fry paneer. When you are frying paprika and ginger, put the paneer pieces in them towards the end. This way, the paneer will be heated and when you are making layers of paprika and aubergine, the paneer pieces will be evenly distributed in the dish. Like the preparation of Version D, this preparation also makes an entire meal.

Comments: Please note that with the addition of the potatoes, I have increased the amount of spices but not the amount of dill seeds. Potatoes are hot and dill seeds are very hot. I have added the cooling mixture C into this preparation to create a balance.

Suggestions: All the above dishes may be served with little pieces of sweet and juicy fruits on the side of the plate. The fruits suggested are mango, pineapple, nectarine, apple and so on.

Main Meals

CARROTS AND GREEN PEAS

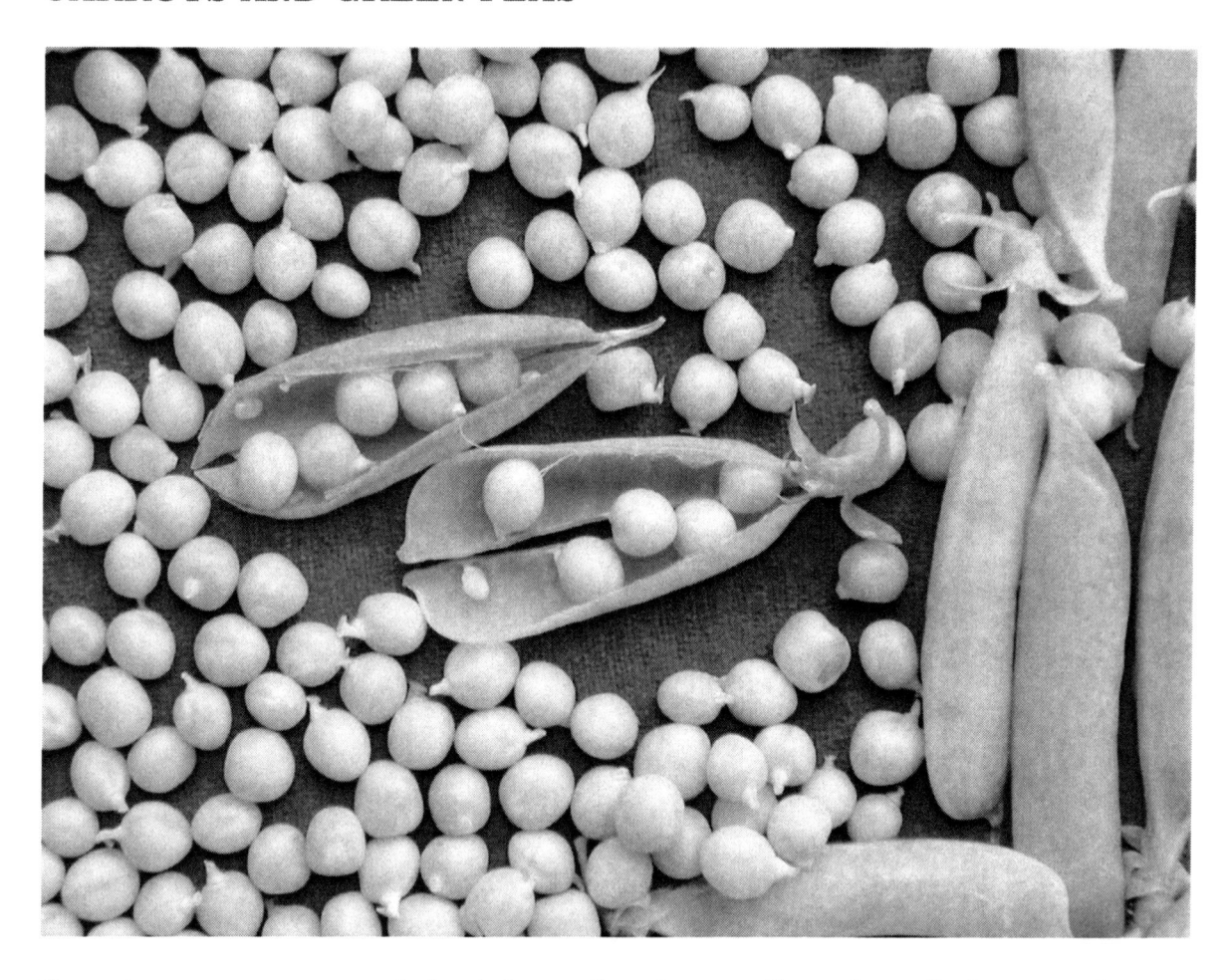

Carrots are a very good food from the Ayurvedic point of view as they create equilibrium of the three energies of the body. Besides, carrots are always available in abundance. I highly recommend eating carrots in diverse forms. This recipe tastes good and looks beautiful.

Ingredients:

For two portions, you require:

Carrots	4 medium-sized
Young green peas	100 to 150 gm (½ to ¾ Cup)
Onion	1 medium-sized
Ginger	1 tablespoon
Turmeric	¼ teaspoon
Salt	a pinch
Cumin	½ teaspoon
Mixture A	½ teaspoon
Ghee or cooking oil	1 tablespoon

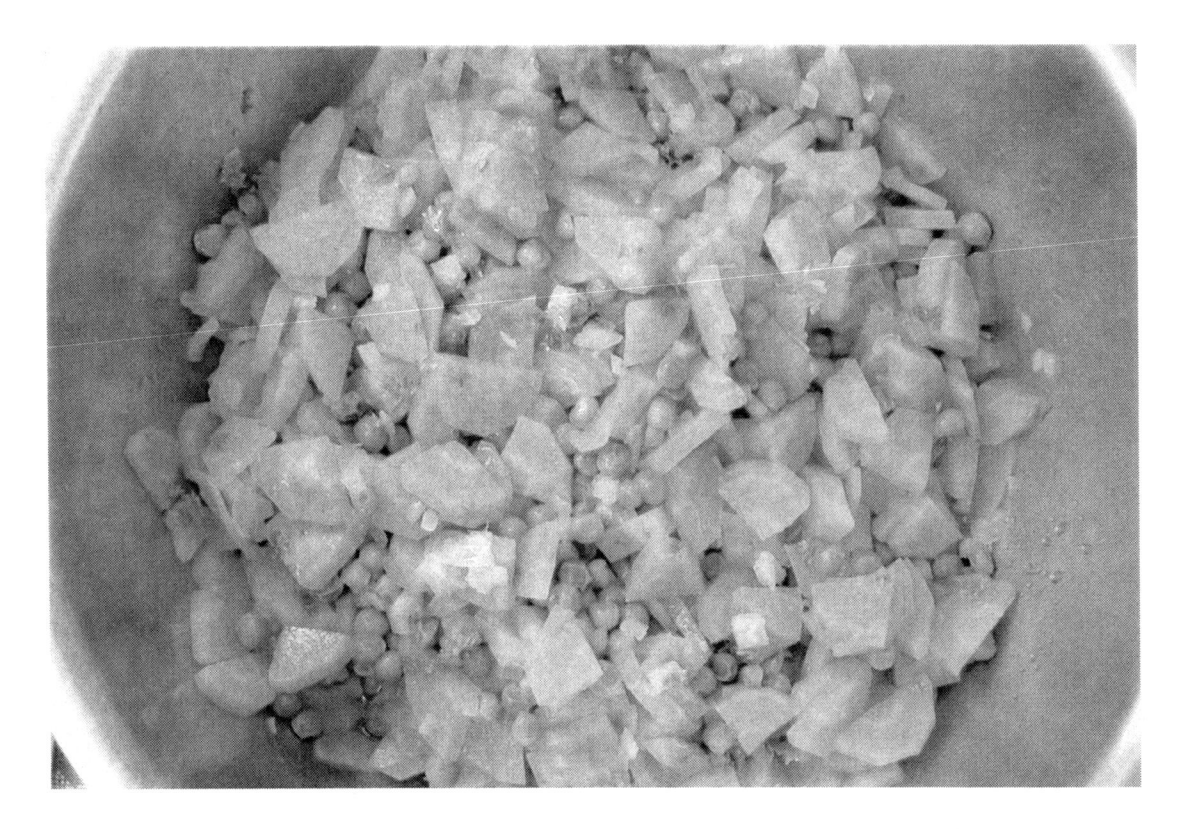

Cut the ginger and the onions into small pieces and fry them in ghee or oil. When the onions are sauté, add all the spices and the salt and stir everything together. Add carrots cut into small pieces and young green peas. Stir to mix everything together. Reduce the heat and cook the vegetables with a lid on the pot. The cooking time is about 15 minutes. Keep stirring from time to time.

CARROTS AND FENUGREEK LEAVES

Fenugreek leaves (methi) is a winter vegetable in India. In the West, dried leaves are available in Indian grocery stores. You can easily grow fenugreek seeds yourself to obtain the tender leaves. They can be even grown in pots. The leaves are blood purifier and strength promoting. Thus, along with carrots, it is a healthy combination.

Use the same recipe as above. Green peas are replaced with a handful of fenugreek leaves. If fresh, fenugreek leaves have to be plucked from stems and chopped finely.

Main Meals

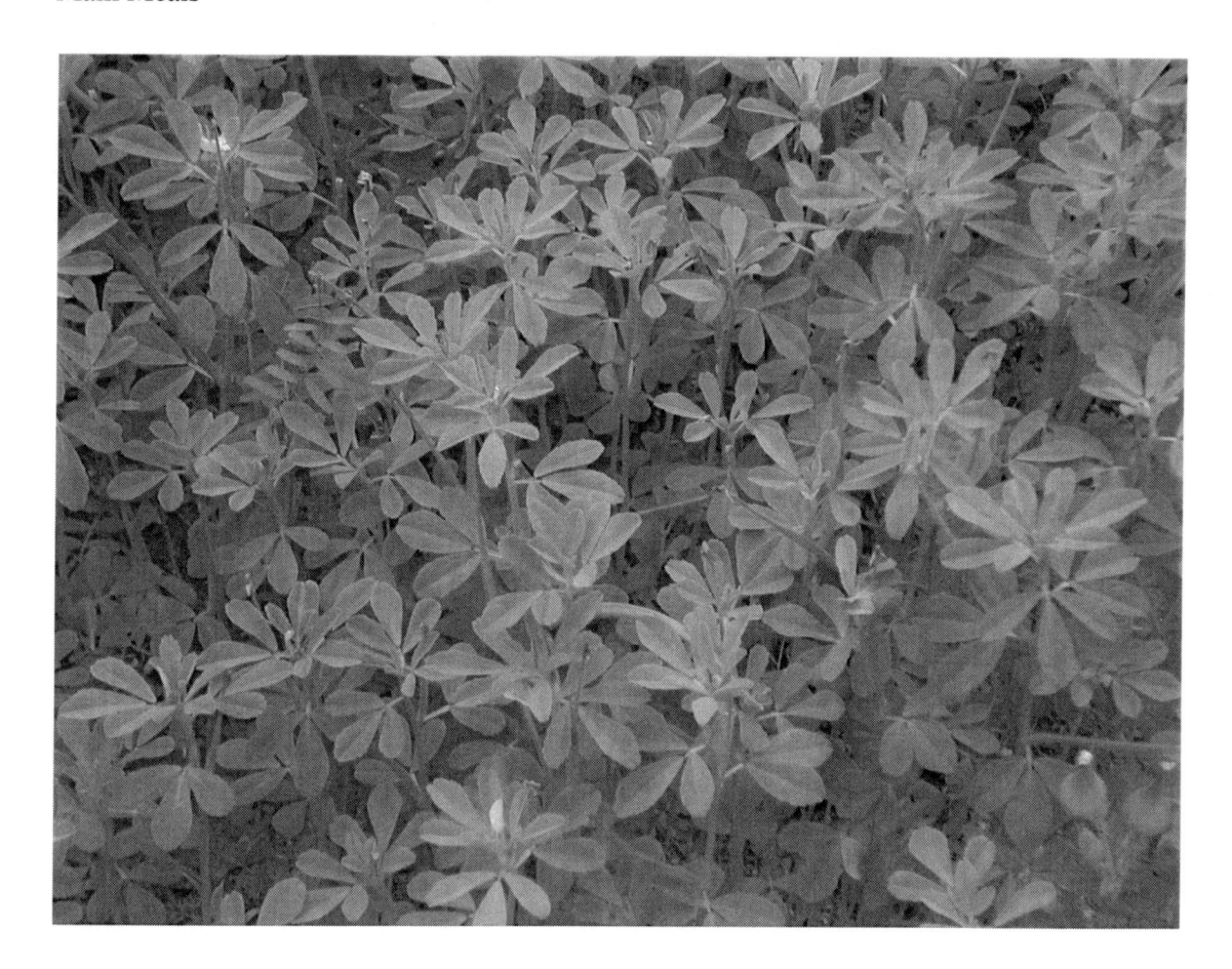

PUMPKIN

Here is one very simple recipe for pumpkin. Since pumpkins are easy to grow in varied climatic conditions and the crop is always in abundance, one can make a variety of preparations from them. Unlike the pumpkin soup recipe given earlier, the following recipe is sour and with spices.

Ingredients:

For 2 to 3 portions, you require:

Pumpkin	about 1kg (2 lb.)
Cooking oil	1 tablespoon
Mixture B	1 teaspoon
Salt	¼ teaspoon or according to taste
Turmeric	1 teaspoon
Mango powder or	1 teaspoon
lemon juice	1 tablespoon
Green chilli (optional)	½ to 1

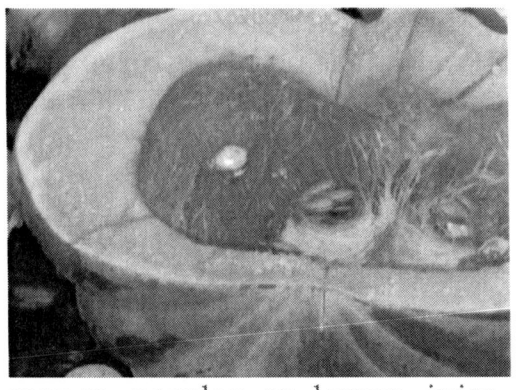

Peel, clean (get rid of the seeds etc.) and cut the pumpkin into small pieces. Heat oil in a wok or a pot and add the spices and the salt (except mango powder or lemon juice). Add the pumpkin pieces and mix everything together. Put the lid on and reduce the heat. Cook for about 15 minutes. Stir once or twice in between. Normally pumpkin has plenty of water. Cook until the pumpkin pieces are completely soft. Remove the lid and add mango powder or lemon juice. Stir and cook for another 5 minutes. This preparation should not be very watery. Depending upon the quality of pumpkin, there is sometimes lot of water and one has to cook a little longer in the end while stirring so that the water evaporates.

The taste of the pumpkin depends upon how ripe the vegetable is and how long it has been kept after plucking. If it is over-ripped or has been kept longer after plucking it is sweeter than pumpkins normally are. This recipe is sweet and sour tasting. In case your pumpkin is raw and it does not taste sweet, you may add a little raw sugar into it.

TURNIP

Turnip, like carrot, is another vegetable that brings equilibrium in the body. You may prepare it in the following three manners.

Version A
Peel and cut the turnips into small pieces and prepare it with Mixture B in the same manner as has been described earlier for cabbage.

Version B
The second method to prepare turnips is as follows:

Ingredients:

For 2 portions, you require:

Turnips	4-5
Onion	1 medium-sized
Ghee	1 tablespoon
Salt	¼ teaspoon or to taste
Mixture A	1 teaspoon
Turmeric	½ teaspoon
Cumin	½ teaspoon

Main Meals

Cut the onion into small pieces. Peel and cut the turnips also into small pieces. Heat the ghee and add onions into it. When onions are sauté, add the spices and salt and stir. Add turnips now and mix everything well. Reduce the heat, put the lid on and let them cook for about 10 minutes. Stir from time to time to make sure that the preparation does not stick to the bottom.

Version C

The third recipe to prepare turnips is in basic sauce with tomatoes, onions, garlic etc. I have already given the recipe for making the basic sauce (see page 150). Take one medium-sized turnip per serving. Peel them and cut them into cubes of 2-3 cm (1 inch). Put a little ghee in a non-stick pan and fry them until they are brown. Make sure that the turnip cubes are well roasted from all the sides.

Prepare the basic sauce now as has been explained earlier in the Aubergine recipe. When the sauce is ready, add 200 ml (1 cup) water into the sauce, stir and bring it to boil. Then add the roasted turnip cubes into the sauce and cook everything together on a low heat for about 15 minutes. Stir from time to time and in the end add the paste of ginger, garlic and herbs as described earlier in the recipe of the basic sauce.

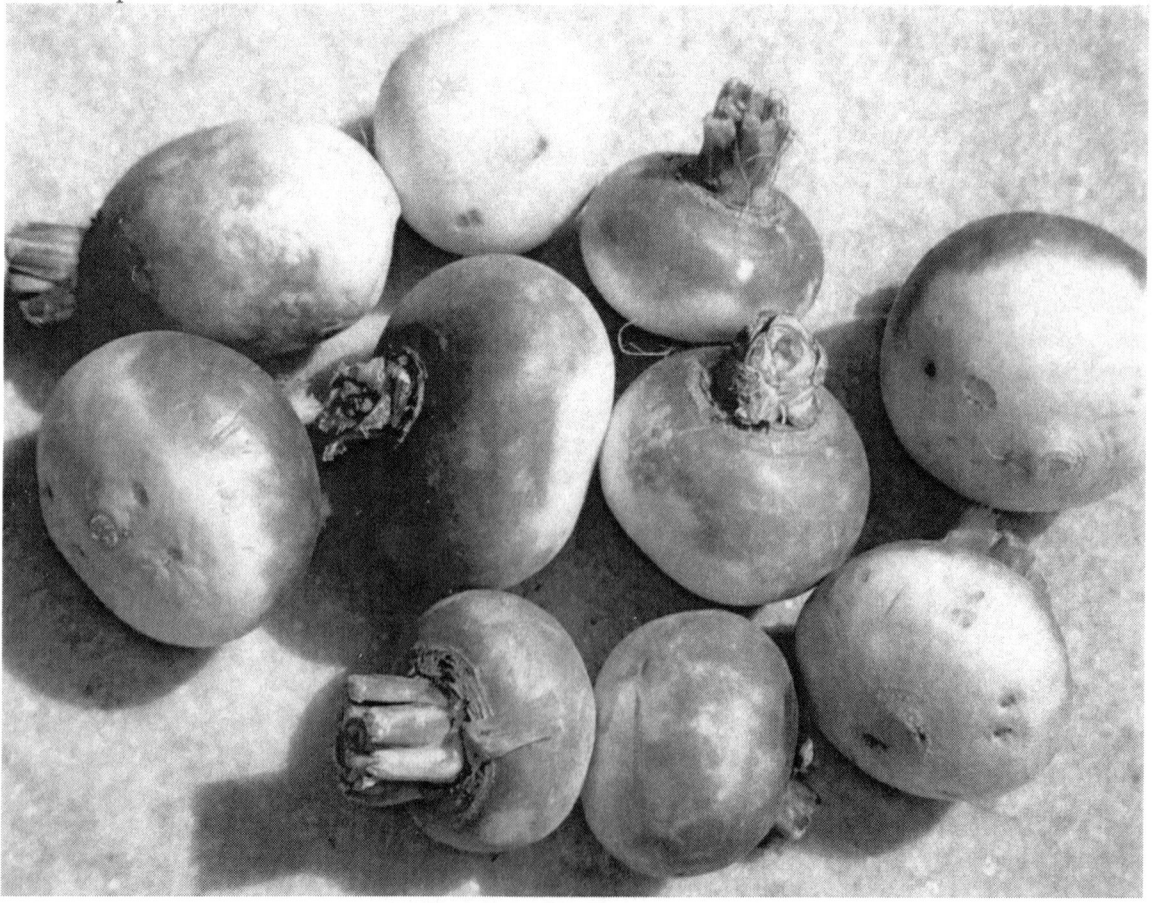

Suggestions: You may add 100 gm (½ cup) green peas into this recipe. Add them at the same time when you add the turnip pieces. If your peas are not young and tender, you have to pre-cook them in a little water.

GINGER-PANEER

This is a rich dish as there is a large amount of paneer in it. But it is not difficult to digest as we have plenty of ginger in it.

Ingredients:

For 3-4 portions, you require:

Paneer	200 gm (½ lb.), that is the amount from 1 litre (5 cups) of milk
Ginger (thin and long pieces)	2 tablespoons
Tomatoes	7-8 medium sized
Ghee or butter	1 tablespoon
Mixture A	1½ tablespoon
Small cardamom	5 crushed after removing the pods
Salt	1/3 teaspoon
Raw sugar or jaggery	1 teaspoon
Chopped coriander leaves	1 tablespoon

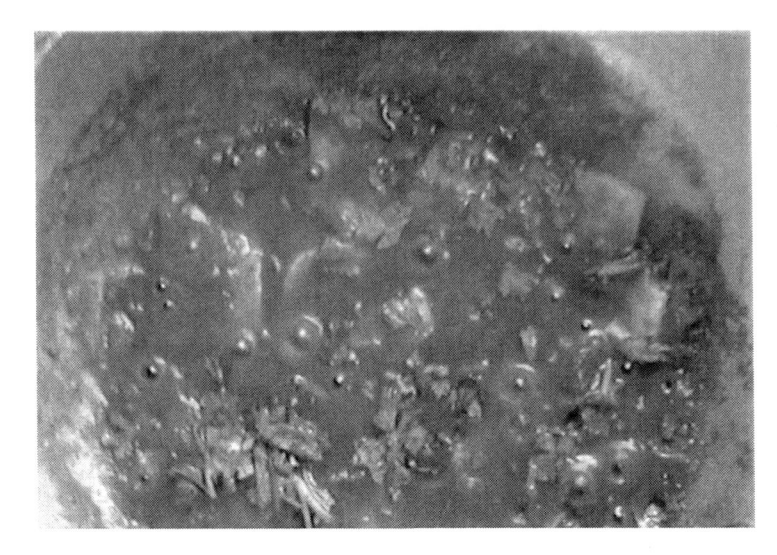

Make the paneer and press it so that you obtain a solid piece. Cut this piece into pieces.

Peel off the skin of the tomatoes by putting them briefly in very hot or boiling water. Cut them into small pieces. Heat the ghee or butter in a pan or wok, add ginger pieces and fry for about a minute. Add the spices and salt and cook for another 30 seconds while stirring. Take care that the cardamoms are not crushed too fine. Add the tomato pieces, stir and let everything cook on a low heat until the tomatoes turn into a purée. Add raw sugar. The amount of sugar depends upon the acidity of the tomatoes. If the tomatoes are very sour, you can add a little more sugar. In the end, add the pieces of paneer and stir them very delicately with the sauce. Cook for a minute after adding the pieces. Decorate the preparation with coriander or other chopped green herbs.

Main Meals

SPINACH

For cooking spinach, one has to take special care, as it is astringent. If you do not do something to create the equilibrium, you will get a bloating feeling in the stomach and distension as I have already pointed out in the recipes of spinach soups. People may not realise the logic of it, but in most spinach recipes around the world, milk, cream or tomatoes are added.

Spinach is two kinds: one has triangular and smaller leaves and the other has rounded, bigger, thicker and shiny leaves. In my opinion, the one with smaller leaves tastes finer. In any case, spinach is a delicate and fine vegetable and one can make many delicious dishes out of it.

Version A: Spinach with potatoes

Ingredients:

For 3 portions, you require:

Spinach	200gm (½ lb.)
Onion	1 medium-sized
Ghee	1½ tablespoon
Potatoes	2 medium-sized
Mixture A	1 teaspoon
Fennel	½ teaspoon
Turmeric	½ teaspoon
Green chilli	½ (optional)
Salt	a pinch
Fresh cream	1 tablespoon
Raw sugar	½ teaspoon

Peel and cut the potatoes into small cubes and fry them in a pan by adding ½ tablespoon of ghee. Stir them from time to time and cook until they are well-roasted and light brown. Wash and cut the spinach into small pieces. Fry finely cut onions in a tablespoon of ghee and when sauté, add turmeric, salt and other spices. Add also green chilli cut into small pieces. Fry everything together for about two minutes and add spinach. Stir well, and when the vegetable is mixed with the spices, put the lid on, reduce the fire and let it cook for about 10 minutes. Stir from time to time to make sure it does not stick to the surface. When the spinach is well cooked, take away the lid and stir for a while. It should not be watery and if there is any water, cook on a medium fire while stirring. Add the roasted potatoes into this preparation and stir together for about two minutes. Mix sugar with cream and add to this preparation before serving.

Version B: Spinach with paneer

This recipe is prepared nearly in the same manner as above except that the potatoes are replaced with paneer pieces. Do not fry the paneer. Add the paneer pieces towards the end and stir gently to mix them with spinach. After adding the paneer pieces, cook for about 2 minutes. You should not add cream in this recipe. It will taste good with cream but it will be too rich.

Alternatively, one could prepare this dish in a purée of spinach with paneer pieces in it. For that, cook the spinach first in water and make a purée. Then fry onions, add spices and cook together with the spinach purée. After cooking for some time, add the paneer pieces in the end like stated above.

Version C: Spinach with tomatoes

Either make spinach purée after cooking spinach in water for about 15 minutes and mixing it with hand mixer or cook the chopped spinach as such. Make the basic sauce (see page 150) with onions, tomatoes etc. and add the cooked spinach into it. Cook spinach with the sauce for about 10 minutes. Add crushed ginger, garlic and herbs in the end.

COURGETTE OR ZUCCHINI

Courgette or zucchini is found almost everywhere in the world. In India, we have also some other vegetable which is quite similar to courgette or zucchini and is called *Lauki* in Hindi. *Lauki* can be round or elongated, broader at one end. This latter variety is sometimes big and can weigh several kilograms. It is also sold at Indian grocer's abroad. The courgette variety of vegetables brings balance of the three energies in the body and is highly recommended. You can always add them in mixed vegetable preparations or mixed vegetable soups. However, they are usually not put in mixed vegetable rice because they become too soft too quickly and do not look appealing in such preparations. In any case, there are several different preparations, which can be made from this variety of vegetables.

Version A

This is a simple preparation of this vegetable with tomatoes.

Ingredients:

For 3 portions you require:

Main Meals

Courgette	4
Ginger (small pieces)	1 tablespoon
Tomatoes	4 medium-sized
Water	200 ml (1 cup)
Salt	¼ teaspoon
Mixture B	½ teaspoon
Mixture F	½ teaspoon
Mixture G	½ teaspoon
Ghee or butter	1 tablespoon (optional)

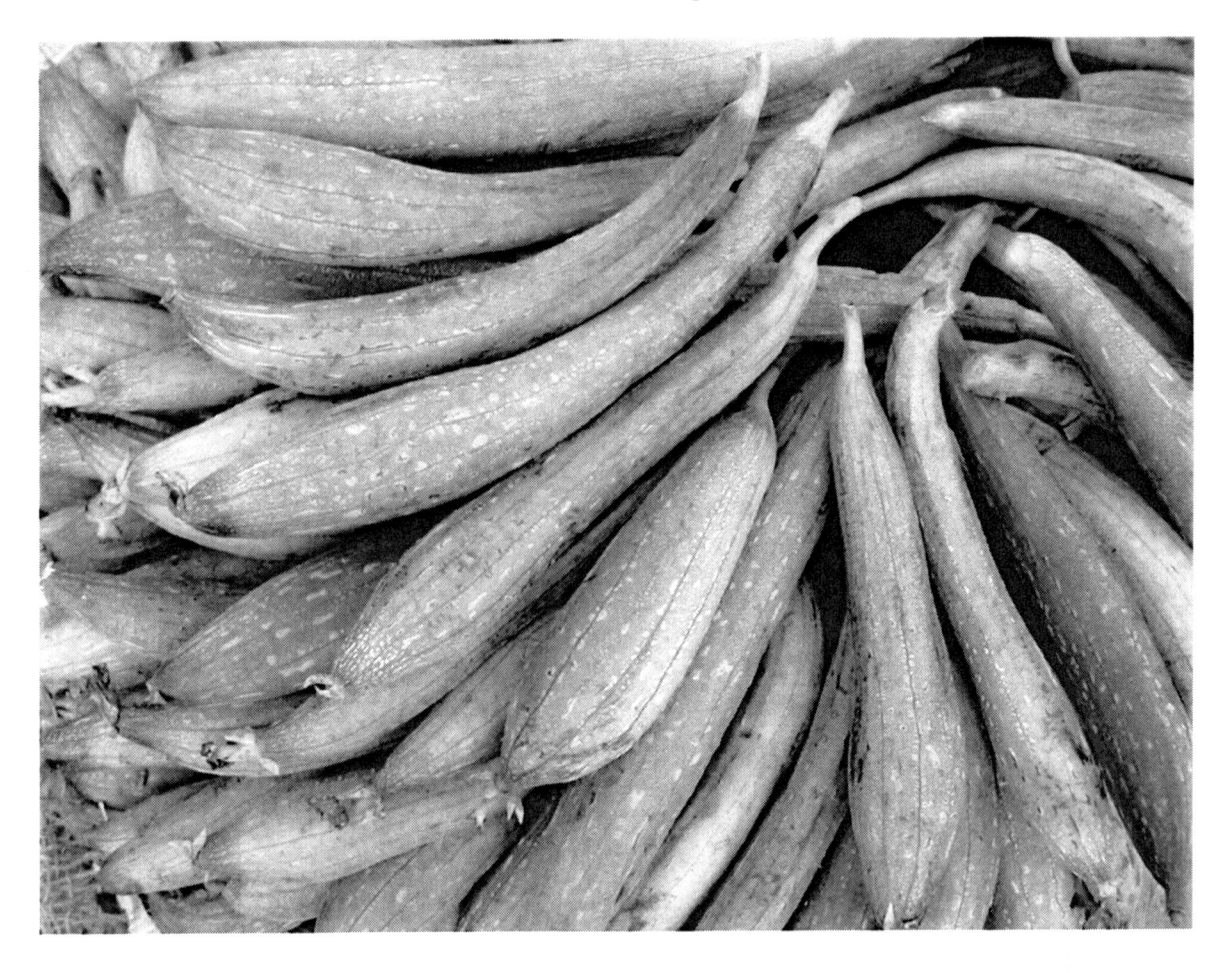

This is a kind of recipe you can make when you are short of time and are unable to pay full attention at each step of the preparation. Cut all the vegetables into small pieces and put everything in a pot excluding ghee. Put water in the pot first, then courgette. Sprinkle the pieces of ginger on the top of courgette, then all the spices including salt. Cover the spices with the pieces of tomatoes and put the lid on. Let everything cook on a low heat for about 20 minutes. Stir once after about 15 minutes. The cooking time I have given is after the vegetable is boiling. Thus, in the beginning, you can use a high flame or more heat and once it is near boiling, reduce the heat and let it cook alone for about 20 minutes.

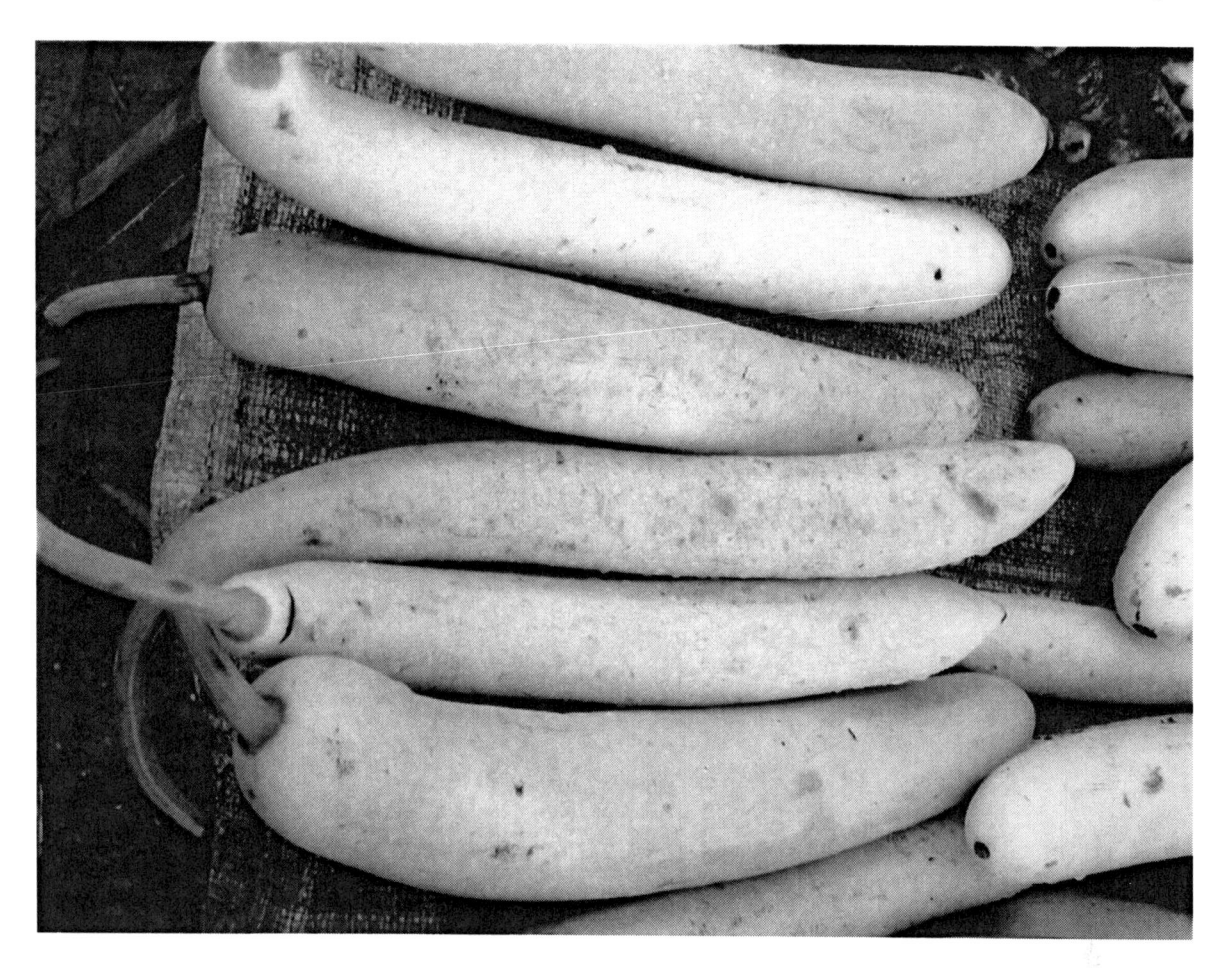

Add ghee or butter in the end if you wish. The preparation tastes also good without any fat. The advantage of this preparation in the family is that one can add ghee for those who want or who need. Adults with less physical work need only a little fat whereas growing children need some more.

Suggestions: You can also make this preparation of courgette mixed with other vegetables like aubergine, onions, carrots etc. Easy recipe like this is sometimes handy when you have leftovers of various vegetables.

Version B

This recipe is done with the described on page 150. Roast the courgette pieces in a non-stick pan by adding a little ghee or cooking oil and add these to the Basic sauce. After putting the pieces into the sauce, cook them for 10 to 15 minutes with the sauce so that the vegetable pieces are well soaked in the sauce. The reason it is essential to pre-cook the vegetable before adding it to the sauce is that the vegetables do not cook well in a sour medium.

Main Meals

Version C

Ingredients:

For 3 portions, you require:

Courgette (grated)	3
Onion (finely chopped)	1 medium-sized
Ginger (finely chopped)	1 tablespoon
Mixture B	½ teaspoon
Mixture E	1 teaspoon
Ajwain	1 teaspoon
Salt	1/3 teaspoon
Besan	about 150 gm (¾ cup)

Mix all the ingredients well. The quantity of besan can be increased or decreased in order to maintain a dough-like consistency of this preparation. There are two different things you can make out of this dough.

1. You can make small pancakes by flattening the little dough each time on a pre-heated non-stick pan that should be oiled a little. Cook on low heat and turn it around. Make sure that all the vegetables and besan cook well. This preparation can be served with mixed vegetables or with mixed salad.

2. You may make small balls out of this dough and deep-fry them. Remember that according to Ayurvedic recommendation, deep-frying should be avoided. That is why I have added one extra teaspoon of ajwain in this preparation. For deep-frying, put the balls in very hot oil. If the oil is very hot, they cook very rapidly and soak less fat. These courgette balls can be served as such with a mixed vegetable plate. The traditional dish of Northwest India is to cook these balls in the Basic sauce. The balls are called 'koftas' in Hindi. However, 'kofta' is a general word for this kind of balls, which are generally put in the sauce. 'Koftas' can also be from other vegetables or meat. This preparation is delicious but a little heavy. You may serve it with plain rice.

3. If you do not want to deep fry, replace the besan with semolina or powdered dried bread. Add enough semolina or the bread powder to make the dough hard. Make balls from the dough and put them in the boiling water. Cook for about five minutes at high temperature and take them out immediately after. They can be added in Basic sauce or can be served as such with mixed vegetables.

BITTER GOURD OR *KARELA* IN HINDI

Karela is a very important vegetable from the point of view of Ayurveda. As the name says, it is very bitter. It is available at Indian grocery stores abroad. Bitter gourd is a blood purifier; it pacifies the aggravated pitta, throws out excessive heat from the body and is a part of diabetes medication. Its regular use is preventive against diabetes.

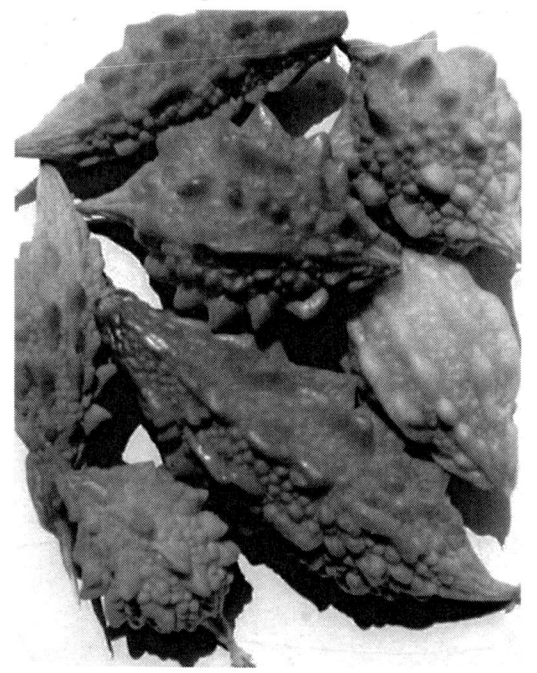

An interesting incident relating to this vegetable happened once in my Ayurvedic workshop in Germany. One of the students who was supposed to do shopping for the cooking class landed up at an Indian grocer shop near Frankfurt railway station. She told the Indian shop owner about the Ayurveda workshop and the cooking class. With the best of his knowledge, the nice shopkeeper gave her the healthiest vegetables from an Ayurvedic point of view. These were Lauki (see picture on page 175) and Karela. I was pleasantly surprised. But when the students tasted a little of the bitter gourd during preparation, they all refused to eat it. They all thought it was awful because it was so bitter. Amazingly, during lunch, the bitter gourd preparation was the first one to vanish. In the final preparation, the bitter gourd dish, which was prepared along with tomatoes, onions and spices, acquired all the rasas, including bitter, which was slightly dominating. Somehow, to the tongue or to the system, the vegetable then gave a very satisfying feeling and people really liked this unknown dish.

BITTER GOURD WITH TOMATOES

Ingredients:

For 3 to 4 portions, you need:

Bitter gourd	½ Kg (about 1 lb.)
Onions	3 medium-sized
Tomatoes	4 medium-sized
Cooking oil	2 tablespoons
Mixture A	1 ½ teaspoon
Turmeric	1 teaspoon
Salt	1/3 teaspoon
Chilli	1 small (optional)

Cut the bitter gourds into small pieces. Put 1 tablespoon of cooking oil in a wok or a pan, heat it and put the vegetable in the hot oil. The cooking oils suggested are sesame, mustard or olive. Stir the vegetable in oil and cook for 5 minutes on a high flame while stirring constantly. Lower the heat and continue cooking while stirring from time to time. Bitter gourd takes very long to cook. You have to cook for about 20 minutes or until they become crisp and brown. Separately, cut the onions in lamellae and fry in one tablespoon of oil until sauté. Add the salt, Mixture A, turmeric and chilli cut into small pieces. Mix everything together and cook for about 2 minutes on low heat. Add tomatoes cut into small pieces, stir well, put the lid on and cook on low fire for about five minutes. Uncover, stir and cook a little more while stirring. Now add the fried bitter gourd into this preparation and cook everything together for about 10 more minutes while stirring from time to time. This cooking time may be less in some cases. If the vegetable is sticking to the surface, stop cooking. No water should be added into this preparation.

Serve with flat bread or any other kind of bread.

Comments: Bitter gourd can be prepared in many different manners. Since many people find bitter not palatable, this recipe seems to be the best. In many Indian homes, to make bitter gourd less bitter, salt is put on the vegetable, which is then left standing for several hours and then squeezed. According to the Ayurvedic principles, it is not a good idea to squeeze out the bitter rasa because, as it is, we generally lack this rasa in our modern way of eating. Secondly, the vegetable absorbs too much salt in this process.

FRIED BITTER GOURD AND STUFFED BITTER GOURD

Bitter gourd can be just fried like you did in the above recipe and then salt and chillies are added. This preparation is served with flat bread and dal (lentils).

Bitter gourds are also prepared in whole by filling them from inside. For this preparation, they are cut open from one side and filled with a preparation of onions and spices. The onions are crushed and not cut, then fried adding the same spices mentioned above. After filling the bitter gourd with this preparation, a cotton thread is turned around it so that it can hold the filling. The filled and tied bitter gourds are fried in a pan with a little fat. They are turned around several times so that they are cooked well on all sides. They should be cooked on medium or low fire so that the filling gets cooked.

Comments: Bitter gourd is a summer vegetable and it is cold in nature. Since nowadays, vegetables are grown under artificial climatic conditions; most vegetables are available around the year. Avoid eating bitter gourd in winter and especially during winter nights.

OKRA

Okra is also called Lady's Finger. It is a common vegetable in Asia and America but rather rare in Europe. It is a very special vegetable, as it becomes very sticky as soon as it comes in contact with water. It is cold in its Ayurvedic nature and is highly kapha. For preparation, it has to be washed and dried properly before cutting. It has to be cooked without any water. I give below two simple methods for its preparation.

Version A

Ingredients:

For 3 portions, you require:

Okra	500 gm (about 1 lb.)
Onions	3 medium-sized
Ginger, chopped	1 tablespoon
Cooking oil	2 tablespoon
Salt	¼ teaspoon
Mixture A	1 teaspoon
Mixture F	½ teaspoon
Turmeric	½ teaspoon

Wash and dry okra and remove the cap-like broader end of the vegetable. Cut horizontally into small pieces. Cut the onions into lamellae. Heat oil in wok or pan and add onions and ginger. Fry until slightly brown (sauté). Add salt and the spices and stir for a minute or two. Add okra, stir and mix well. Cook for about 10-12 minutes while stirring from time to time. Do not put the lid on. The vapours from the vegetables condense and make the okra sticky and slimy. More oil in this preparation than usual is used because it is not possible to cook this vegetable with the lid on.

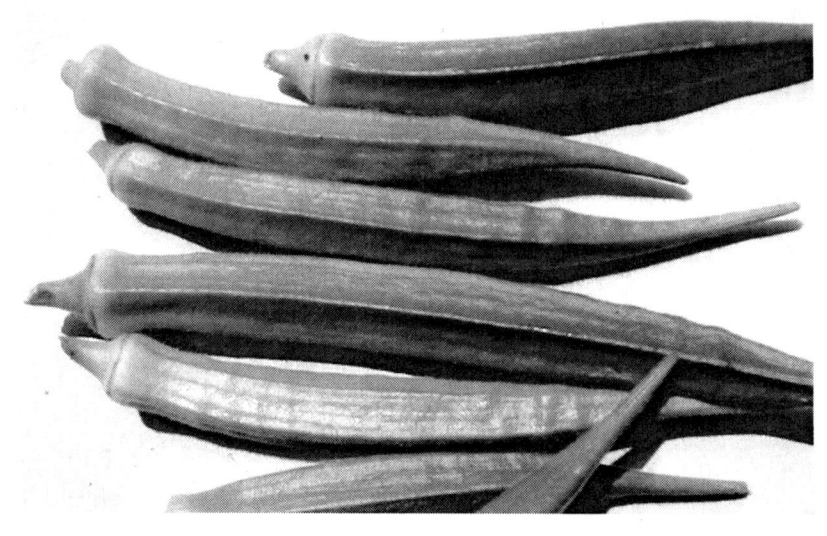

Main Meals

Version B

Ingredients:

For 3 portions you require:

Okra	500 gm (about 1 lb.)
Mixture F	2 teaspoons
Salt	1/3 salt
Cooking oil	1 tablespoon

Wash and dry the vegetable and remove the cap-like ends. Mix the salt with the spice mixture. Give a horizontal cut on each okra on one side and go on filling a pinch of spice mixture into it. Heat the oil in a non-stick pan and put your vegetables in it. Let them cook on medium heat. After a few minutes, turn them delicately. You will need around 15 minutes of cooking time. The okra should be well roasted and turn slightly brown.

Like the bitter gourd, okra also makes a better combination with flat bread or any other kind of bread.

Comments: Okra is kapha inducing and persons with kapha constitution should not have it too often. Because of the kapha qualities of the vegetable, it is cooked with oil and not with ghee. This is also the reason for using the sour spice mixture in both the versions of okra. In Version A, I have also added ginger and on the other hand, in Version B, I have added more of the spicy and sour mixture.

It is a summer vegetable and it is cooling in nature. It is recommended for the summer.

POTATO PREPARATIONS

Potatoes are considered a vegetable in India and are generally cooked with other vegetables. However, in Europe, potatoes are eaten the way rice or bread is eaten in India. For most Indians, it is hard to replace their rice or chapati (freshly made flat bread) with potatoes. Bread, rice and products from other grains are bulk promoting and it is good to replace these preparations with potatoes from time to time. In urban India, over-weight has become a serious problem.

There is a high consumption of potatoes in Northern Europe, and some excellent preparations are made from potatoes. Potatoes are hot in nature and therefore should be prepared with spices or herbs, which are cold in nature, such as

Mixture C or herbs like coriander leaves or dill leaves etc. In France, they make purée from potatoes with a little milk in it. This is a balanced preparation as potatoes are hot and milk is cold. Whole potatoes baked in oven or directly on coal or fire are delicious. They taste the best when cooked in solar oven. Solar oven makes them nice and brown without burning them. These potatoes may be eaten with one of the cheese preparations or cream yoghurt sauce described later in the book. Alternatively, they may be served with mixed vegetables or spinach dishes.

There are many fried preparations of potatoes the world over. The most popular preparation probably is 'Pommes frites' or French fries as the Americans call them. For this preparation, the potatoes are cut finger shaped, salted and deep-fried. This preparation is very unhealthy as firstly, it has too much fat, and secondly the potatoes are hot and so is the oil in which they are fried. If at all, potatoes should be fried in ghee. Put the potatoes in very hot ghee for frying so that they do not soak up too much fat.

For other preparations, in order to avoid taking too much fat with potatoes, boil them first with the skin on. Do not let them become too soft. Peel and cut into small pieces or thin and flat pieces and fry in a non-stick pan with a little ghee. For example, for half kilo potatoes, you need one tablespoon of ghee. Keep stirring and when they are crispy and brown, add ½ teaspoon of freshly ground fennel seeds, a pinch of pepper and some salt. Fry a little after adding the spices. Alternatively, you can simply add some raisins and leave out salt and spices. You may add salt if you cannot eat potatoes without salt.

Swiss and German preparation of Rösti is very tasty but often it is prepared with lot of fat. One can make a Rösti the Ayurvedic way.

RÖSTI

Ingredients:

Potatoes	½ kilo (1 pound)
Ghee	1 to 2 tablespoons
Salt	¼ teaspoon
Pepper	a pinch
Mixture C	½ teaspoon
Cumin	¼ teaspoon
Fresh coriander leaves	1 tablespoon (finely chopped)

Main Meals

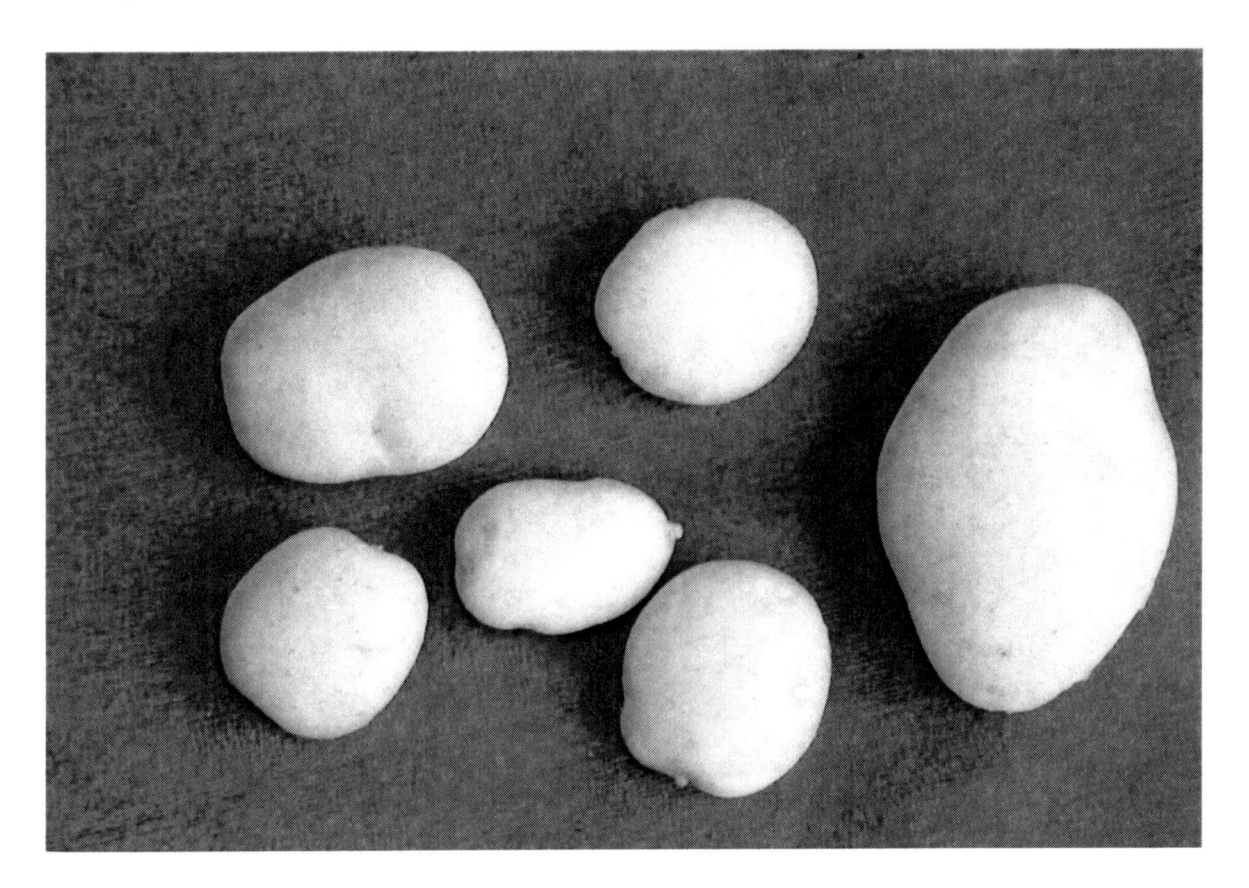

Boil the potatoes with the skin on. Do not boil them too soft. Peel and grate through a thick mesh. Add all the spices except coriander leaves and mix well. Heat ghee in a large sized non-stick pan and spread the spiced potatoes on it. Let them cook on a medium fire. Turn after cooking for about 2-3 minutes. The grated potatoes will soon become like a thick pancake and can be easily turned over like a pancake. After both the sides are golden brown, reduce the heat and cook each side for about 5 more minutes to make it crispy. Serve this with coriander leaves on the top. Rösti can be served with mixed vegetables or with a mixed salad.

Suggestions: You can make various versions of Rösti. For example, fry a finely cut onion before you add the potatoes in the pan. Or mix finely chopped onions and ginger into the grated potatoes. You may make Rösti with Mixture F. Add 1 ½ teaspoon of Mixture F along with Mixture C. In an alternate recipe, you can mix some finely chopped almonds and raisins into the grated potatoes.

You may make Rösti from raw potatoes. Peel and grate the potatoes and mix the spices as described above. Do not make the Rösti as thick as above. Make two Röstis instead of one with the above given quantity. You will have to cook a little longer as compared to the Rösti with pre-cooked potatoes.

BAKED VEGETABLES

Baked vegetables with cheese and cream are delicious but they are rich as compared to the vegetables prepared with the recipes described earlier. Baked vegetables are generally prepared with white sauce made of butter, flour and milk. The pre-cooked vegetables are mixed with this sauce and covered with a layer of cooking cheese. Then they are baked in the oven. There are vegetables like potatoes or sweet potatoes or other root vegetables like beetroot, which can be baked directly in the oven, wrapped in aluminium foil. These baked vegetables can be served with little butter and salt.

There are also different kinds of ovens in the world. The most common ovens these days are electric ones with an electric heater inside. Microwave ovens are used more and more because they are fast and easy to use, but according to Ayurvedic principles, these ovens must be considered detrimental for the food, as they kill its prana or the living element. The traditional Indian ovens are earthen ones and are called *Tandoor*. We have solar ovens in our Himalayan Centre, which cook very slowly and with the rays of the sun. In my recipes below, I will indicate the cooking times for a normal electric oven.

The essential thing to learn about baked vegetables is to create an Ayurvedic balance by using different spices and to make them easily digestible by adding other ingredients. Alternatively, the menus should be made in such a manner that the other courses of the meal are agni enhancing. Always remember the Ayurvedic mantra of eating less of rich and heavy foods. Less quantity of a heavy food makes it lighter to digest and excessive quantity of lighter food makes it heavy to digest.

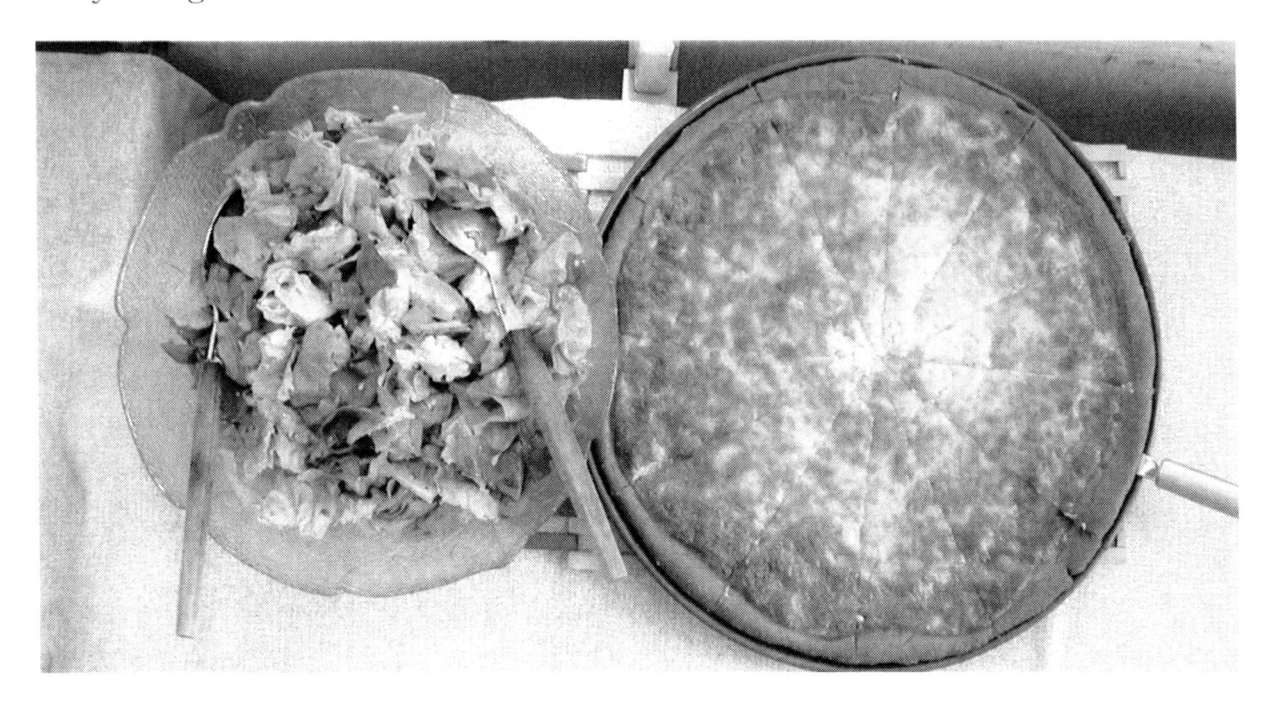

White sauce or Sauce Béchamel

It is quite simple to make this sauce. With due apologies to Monsieur Béchamel, I am going to add few things to his sauce in order to create an equilibrium from Ayurvedic point of view.

Ingredients for a sauce for about half kilo (1 pound) of vegetables:

Wheat flour	2 tablespoon
Ghee or butter	1 tablespoon
Milk	500 ml (2 ½ cup)
Nutmeg (powdered)	¼ of a nut
Salt	a pinch
Mixture H	½ teaspoon
Powdered ginger	¼ teaspoon

Heat the ghee or butter in a pan and add flour. Fry while stirring. When it turns slightly brown after a minute or two on medium fire, slowly add milk into it and keep stirring continuously. This has to be done very carefully so that the flour does not make knots. When all the milk is added, add salt and spices into it and stir for another minute or until the sauce is thick and homogenous.

Preparation of Different Vegetables before Baking

Various vegetables need slightly different preparation. They need to be pre-cooked a little before being baked in the oven with the sauce and cheese. Obviously, the spices are different according to the nature of the vegetables. I give below the preparation for about 500 gm (about 1 pound) of vegetables.

1. **Potatoes:** Potatoes are hot in nature. Therefore, use Mixture C in their preparation. Peel and cut the potatoes into thin slices. Put two tablespoons of water in a pan, add potatoes, cover and cook in vapour on low heat for 10 minutes. The potatoes should not be cooked too much as they are going to be baked later. Add ½ teaspoon of Mixture C and ½ teaspoon of ajwain or thym. Put the potatoes in a buttered baking dish and pour the white sauce over them. Cover everything with a thin layer of grated cooking cheese. You may take Gruyere, Emmenthal or any other cheese of your choice that is meant for baking.
2. **Cauliflower:** Cauliflower makes a delicious baked dish. It is also hot in nature. Excessively big cauliflower grown with artificial fertilisers is mostly hard to digest and vitiates vata. In addition to the above-mentioned spices for the potatoes, add ½ teaspoon of dill seeds and 5 powdered cardamoms. Cook

the cauliflower in vapour like you have done above for potatoes but only for 5 minutes.

3. **Courgette with plain rice:** Courgette or zucchini is a balanced vegetable. Because it is soft, you need not pre-cook it. Prepare the plain rice as has been described earlier. You need about 6 tablespoons of cooked plain rice. To the white sauce, add a teaspoon of thyme and a tablespoon of finely chopped fresh basil leaves. In a buttered dish, add a layer of courgette cut in thin roundels, then a layer of white sauce and then a layer of rice. Add more layers of white sauce, courgette and rice. Cover the preparation with grated cheese before putting it in the oven.

Baking: Baking time with medium heat is 15 to 20 minutes. When the cheese is light brown, take the dish out of the oven.

Suggestions: I have given you above three standard recipes, which are easily adapted to other baked vegetables. Instead of rice, one can use pasta and add vegetables like aubergine, tomatoes and mushrooms. Wherever you use tomatoes, do not use white sauce, as the sour taste of the tomatoes is antagonist to the milk of the white sauce.

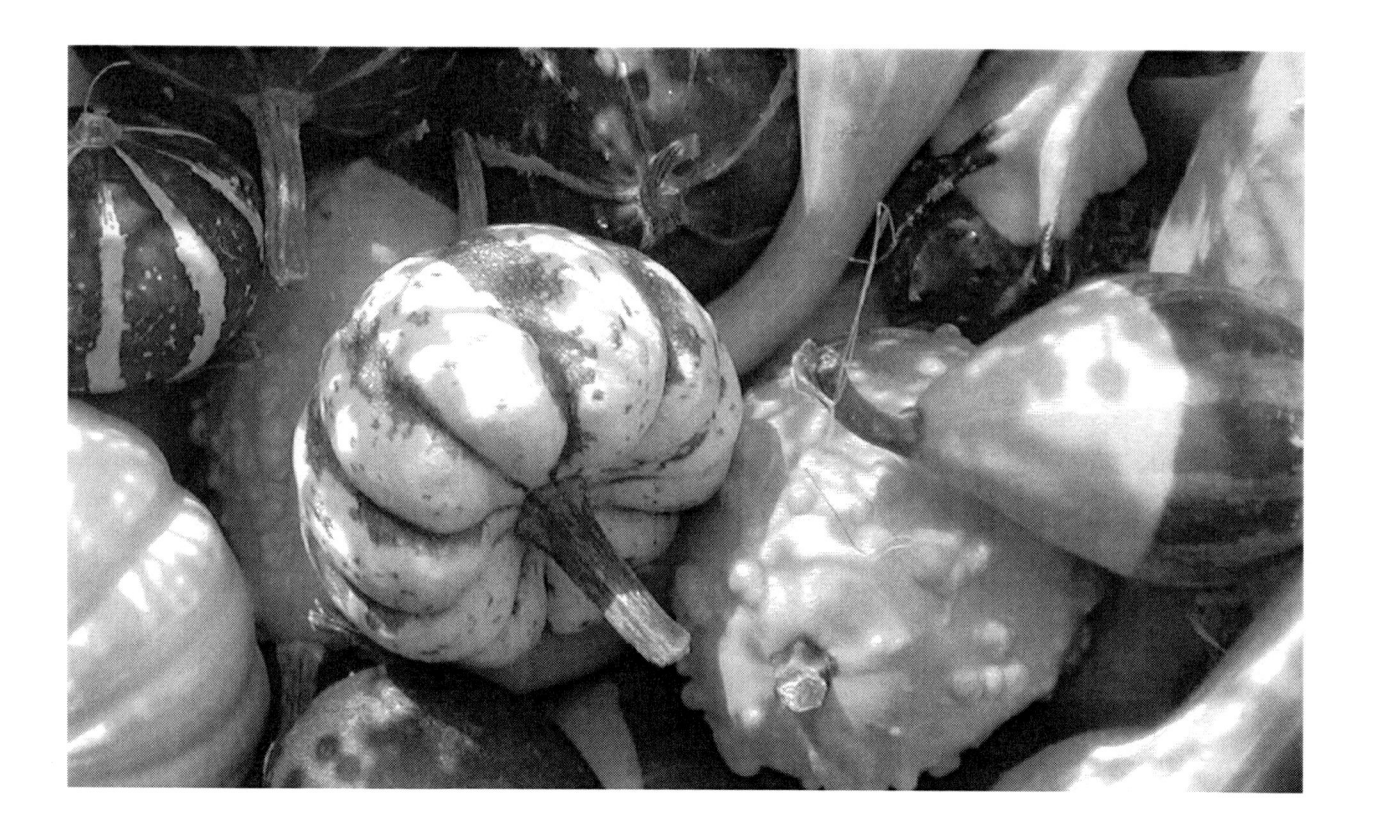

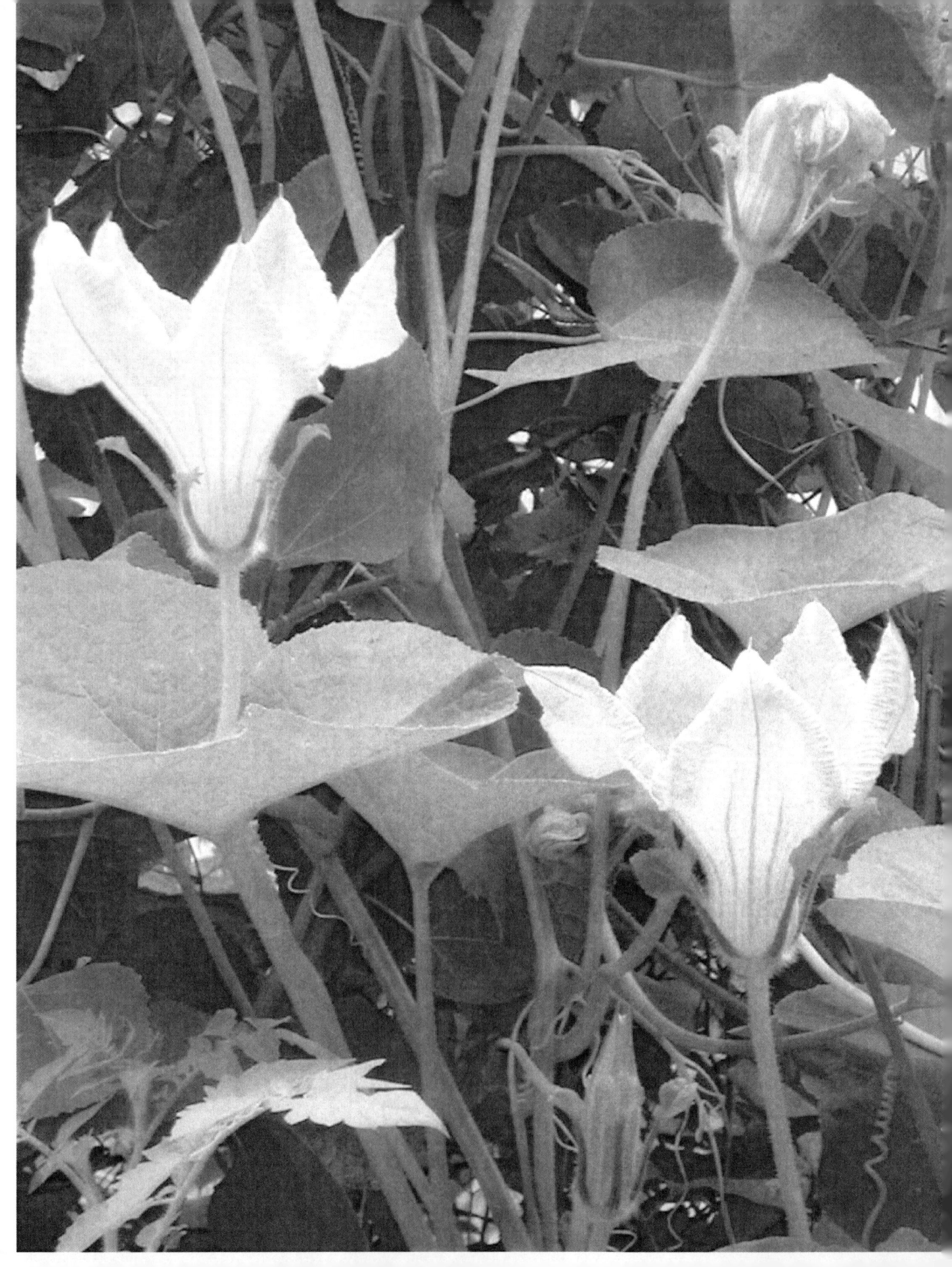

CHEESE

There are large varieties of processed cheeses in the world, specially in Europe. France, Switzerland, Holland and Italy are famous for their cheeses. Basically, cheese is the solid parts of the milk as described above for making paneer or cheese from milk and from yoghurt by eliminating the fluid of the milk that is called whey. Whey is rich in lactose, minerals and vitamins and is a good drink especially for those who have weak digestion or during convalescence periods after an ailment. In the solid part, principally the proteins and fats of the milk are retained. Humans have made cheese since antiquity from the milk of various animals. The importance of cheese is also for milk preservation, as the milk cannot be kept very long despite modern technology. Besides, the milk is very bulky and is relatively difficult to transport from one place to the other. In the former times, when there was no electricity, the cheese was preserved in dried form.

The various kinds of cheese differ according to the type and treatment of the milk, presence of fat contents, heating and pasteurising process and the addition of enzymes. In general, cheese is kapha-pitta enhancing but the degree of that depends upon the quality of milk. Cow milk or cheese promotes these energies less, and is more balanced whereas cheese made from water buffalo is heavier and more kapha promoting. Goat milk and cheese is lighter than that of cow and is more balanced. Sheep milk and cheese on the contrary is very hot in its Ayurvedic qualities.

Cheese should not be taken in excess and meat and cheese together should be avoided, because they are both very high-protein diets. From the Ayurvedic point of view, meet and cheese are both rich and heavy. We observe also that in most Western countries, where both meat and cheese are consumed in large quantities, the major part of the malnutrition stems from the excessive consumption of the highly protein and fat rich diet. Remember that out of all the cheeses, goat cheese is light and balanced. In fact, in Ayurveda, goat milk and mother's milk are also used for several remedies.

In the previous Section, I have given two methods to make paneer and a kind of fresh cheese from yoghurt. I will now give some recipes for these to make cheese with various herbs and spices.

Cheese

CHEESE FROM YOGHURT

Hang the full cream yoghurt, preferably home made, in cheesecloth (see page 79) to drain out water. When most of the water is drained out, mix the solids with various herbs and spices, as given in the recipes below. Mix the ingredients and the cheese well, put it in a small dish or a cup and fill it to the brim by pressing the cheese a little bit. Turn the cup upside down, put on a cheese plate and lift the cup. You get a nicely shaped cheese on your cheese plate. Serve with some fresh vegetables like pieces of paprika, cucumber, beetroot, basil leaves or other herbs.

Here are the ingredients for about 150 gm (¾ cup) of cheese.

A. Cumin, pepper and cardamom

Cumin	1 teaspoon
Pepper	a pinch
Cardamom	4
Salt	a pinch

Heat a pan and put a spoon of cumin into it. Roast a little while stirring on medium fire for less than a minute to make the cumin seeds crisp. The seeds should not turn dark. Remove the pods of cardamom and crush their seeds and cumin seeds to have a sandy consistency. Add to the cheese these along with salt and pepper and mix well. Make a round piece and serve with herbs and salads as described above.

B. Garlic and herb cheese

Garlic (crushed)	5 cloves
Salt	a pinch
Dill leaves chopped	1 tablespoon
Tender fennel leaves (chopped)	1 tablespoon

Mix all the ingredients together along with the cheese and do the same as above for making a mound of this cheese.

C. Paprika and mint cheese

Grated paprika	2 tablespoons
Mint leaves (chopped fine)	1 tablespoon
Mixture F	½ teaspoon

Mix all the ingredients together along with the cheese and do the rest as described above.

D. Mixed herb cheese

Various kinds of herbs (chopped)   3 tablespoons
Salt   ¼ teaspoon

Take a variety of herbs, especially tender leaves of garlic, parsley, basil, coriander leaves and so on and chop them very fine. Mix them with cheese along with salt and serve and decorate in a similar manner as described above.

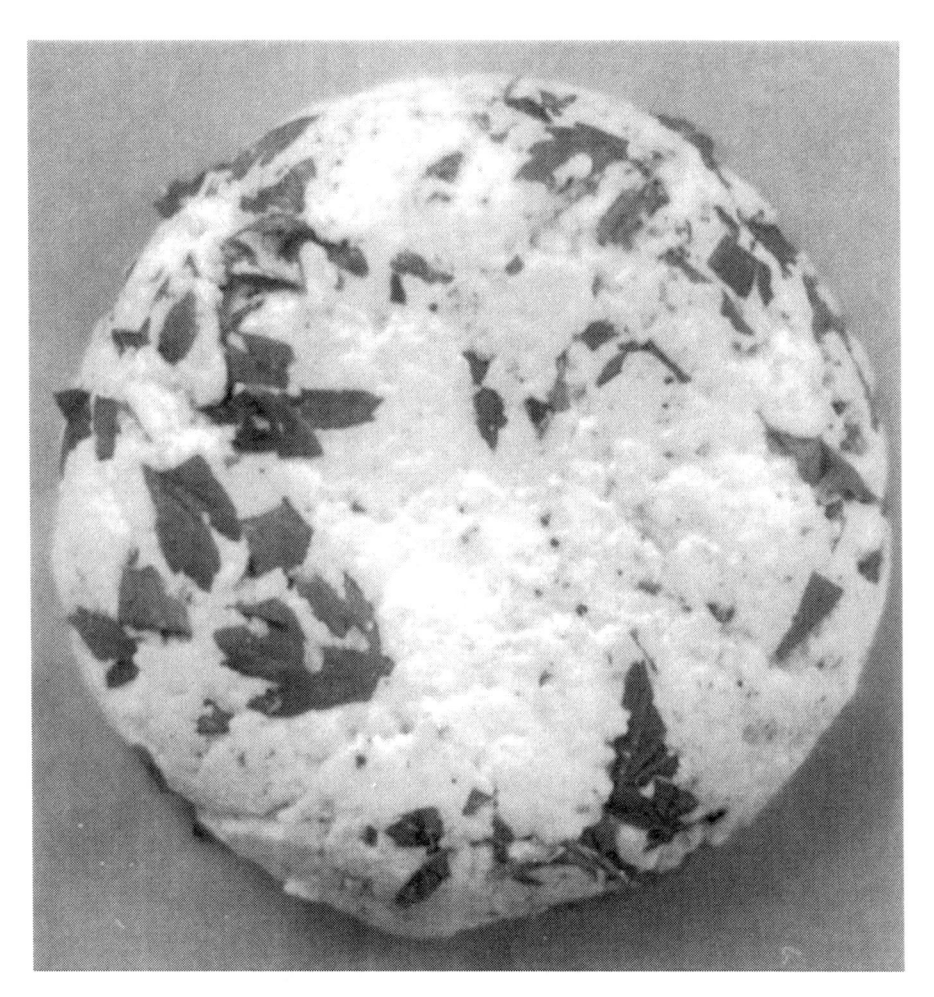

PANEER-CREAM CHEESE

Make paneer, hang it in a cheesecloth in order to drain out the whey. Mix it half-and-half with fresh cream. Mix well to get a homogenous mixture. With this, you can make any of the recipes described above or any other combination of herbs and spices of your choice.

YOGHURT-CREAM CHEESE

Four parts of the cheese obtained after draining out the water from yoghurt is mixed with one part (25%) of fresh cream. Mix well and add herbs and spices as in the above recipes.

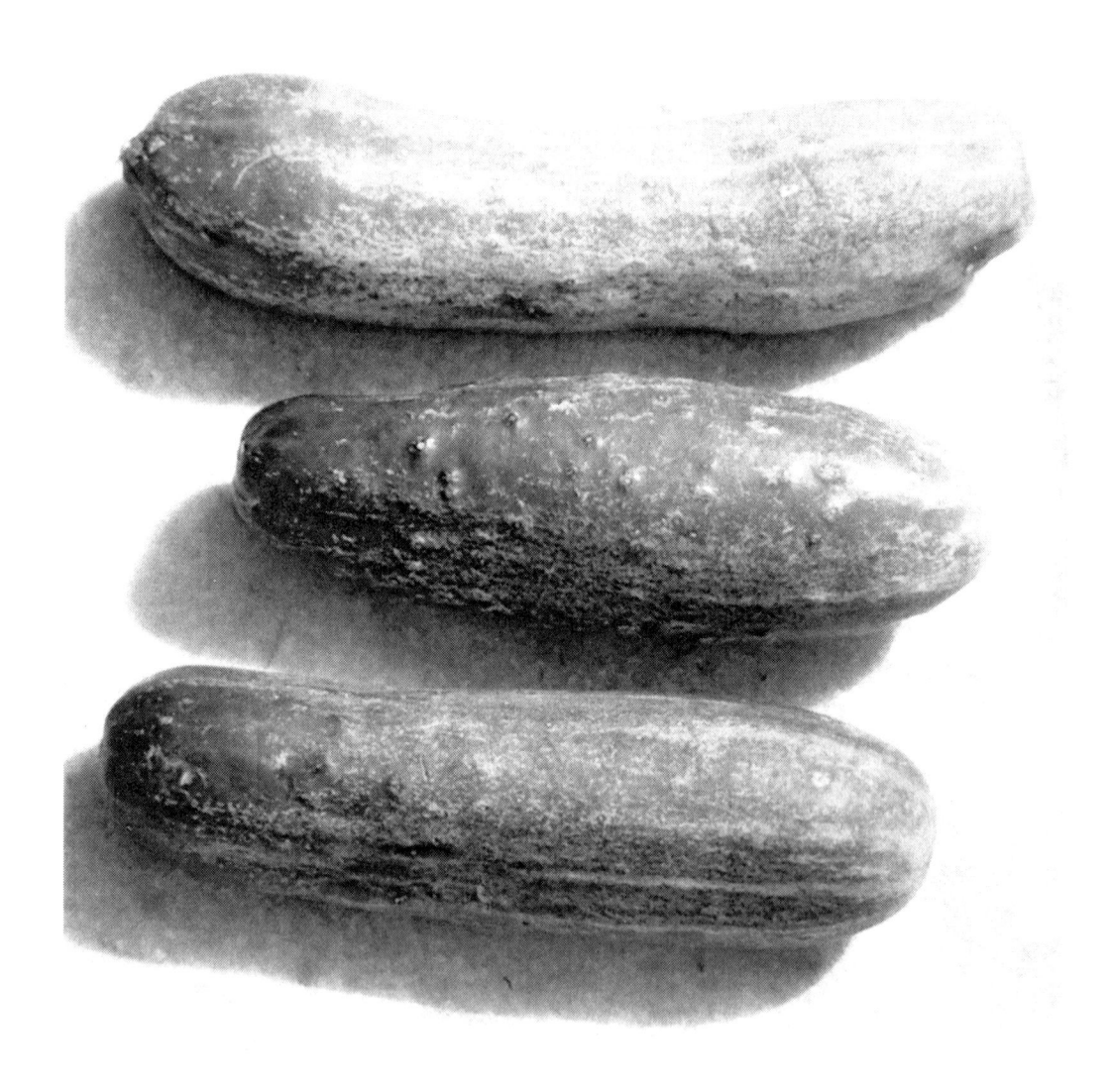

SALADS

Salads generally accompany the main meals in Ayurvedic tradition. Since main meals do have some fat in one form or another, salads are used for enhancing agni (digestive fire). Unlike in the West where sometimes people replace a meal with a huge salad, Ayurveda will not recommend that. It is advised not to eat raw products exclusively. Salad as side-dish is generally prepared with rock salt and fresh lemon juice or with yoghurt in the form of rayatas. Rayatas are whipped yoghurt mixed with different ingredients. The recipes for rayatas will be given later with the side-dish recipes. I will give below some recipes for salads with lemon juice dressing as well as with European classical dressing with wine-vinegar.

SPRING ONION SALAD

Ingredients:

For 2-3 portions, you require:

Spring onions	200gm (½ lb.)
Paprika	1 medium-sized
Tomato	1 medium-sized
Coriander leaves or other herbs chopped	2 tablespoons
Rock salt	¼ teaspoon
Pepper	a pinch
Lemon juice	1½ tablespoon

Cut the spring onions very fine and do not use the lower green part, as it is too fibrous for being eaten raw. However, you may keep it for soup. Cut tomatoes and paprika into very fine pieces. Mix everything including green herbs and add salt and pepper. Add lemon juice and mix. Salt and lemon juice should be added just before serving.

Salads

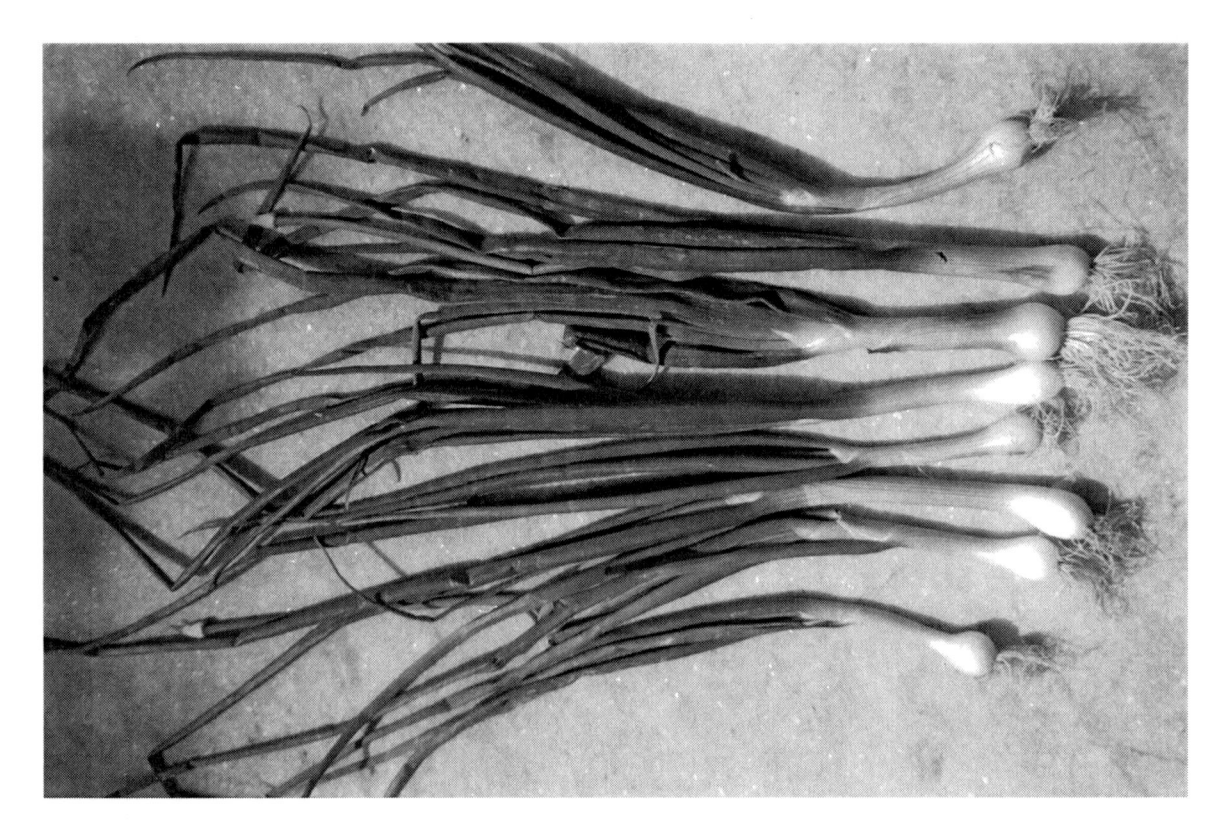

Suggestions: You can add cucumber in this salad or replace paprika with it. The spring onion taste should stay predominant in this salad. You can prepare any other salad in this simple way but remember that these salads are eaten with the main dish.

SALADS WITH SAUCE

In the West, most salads are made with various kinds of sauces, some of which are creamy and heavy to digest. Different salad sauces are also sold readymade in bottles, obviously with some preservatives. I recommend making a simple sauce just before use. The salad sauce recipes with cream or milk are not recommended as sour with cream and milk is antagonist.

Choice of vinegar and oil: It is important to choose a good vinegar. In India, we have sugar cane, jamun (a fruit) and apple vinegar. Italian Balsamico vinegar is very good and is available practically everywhere.

To make a balanced salad sauce, add two tablespoons of vinegar in a salad bowl. Add ¼ teaspoon of salt, ¼ teaspoon of Mixture H, and some finely cut onions and garlic. Stir and leave for about 15 minutes. This neutralises the strong smell of onions and garlic. Add three tablespoons of olive or sesames oil and stir well. Finally, add a teaspoon of honey or jaggery or raw sugar and stir well. Your sauce is ready. Add it into your salad and mix well. The amount of sauce varies according to the quality of the salad. Leafy salads need less sauce as compared to salads with rice or potatoes. Decide that according to taste and make sure that your salad is not too sour. The reason to add honey or sugar is also to create a balance of sour and salty rasas.

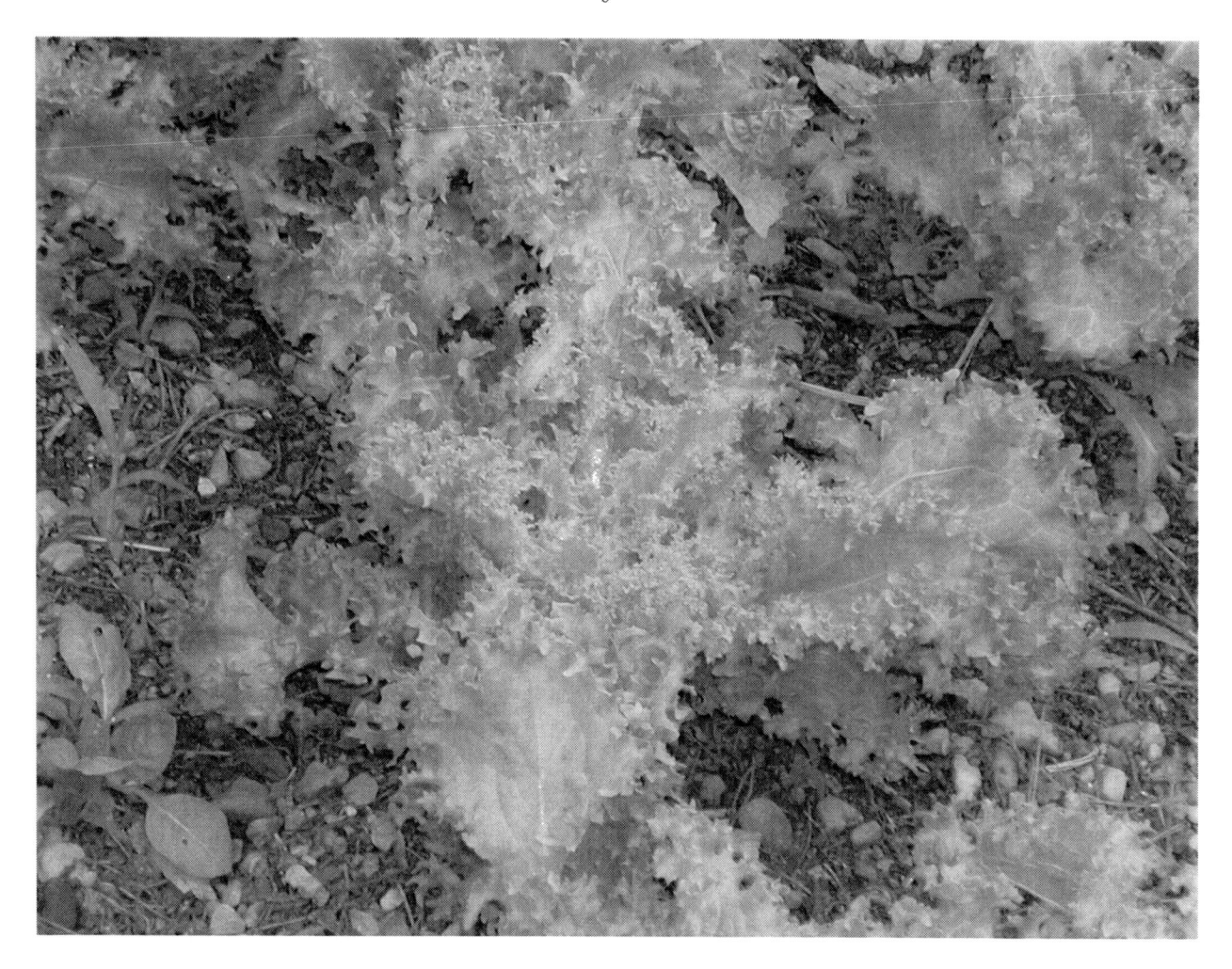

RICE SALAD

One can add various vegetables and spices to the rice, which makes this salad all-rasa containing healthy food.

The quantity of the salad for one person depends upon whether the salad is eaten as a small side-dish or almost an entire meal after soup. I give below the ingredients for big portions.

Salads

Ingredients:

For 2-3 portions, you require:

Basmati rice	150 gm or ¾ cup
Cucumber	1 small sized or half from a big one
Paprika	1 medium-sized
Tomatoes	2 medium-sized
Carrots (grated)	2 medium-sized
Apple (sweet)	1
Lettuce leaves or some other green salad	Few leaves
Mixed green herbs	4-5 tablespoons finally chopped
Spring onions or	2
Small onion	1
Garlic	4-5 cloves
Vinegar	5 tablespoon
Olive or sesame oil	6 tablespoons
Salt	½ teaspoon
Mixture H	1 teaspoon
Raw sugar	1 teaspoon

Pour vinegar in a big salad bowl and add finely chopped onions, garlic, salt and spice mixture. Stir and leave for about 15 minutes. Add sugar and oil and stir vigorously. Separately, boil the rice in double the quantity of water as explained earlier. Let the rice cool down. Cut vegetables into small pieces and add them with the rice into the sauce. Stir gently to mix everything together.

MIXED SALAD

Mixed salad is made in a similar manner as rice salad. In this recipe, the rice is replaced by mushrooms, beetroot or any other ingredients of your choice to go with the vegetables described above. Remember always to put some sweet fruit like the apple in the above recipe. You can also add some dried raisins, almonds or sesame seeds.

CARROT SALAD

Ingredients:

For 2 or 3 portions, you need:

Carrots	5-6 medium-sized
Onions	1 medium-sized
Vinegar	3 tablespoons
Olive oil	5 tablespoons
Salt	¼ teaspoon
Mixture H	½ teaspoon
Sesames seeds	2 teaspoons
Raw sugar	½ teaspoon

Prepare salad sauce as described above. In this recipe, sesame seeds are replaced with garlic. Carrots should not be grated too fine otherwise they become like a purée. Unlike the green salads which should be added into the sauce just before serving, this salad needs to be kept in the sauce for at least about ½ an hour before serving.

BEETROOT SALAD

Beetroot should be cooked before making the salad. Then peal and cut into small pieces. Add the sauce as described above.

For a mixed salad, add boiled potatoes and paprika. This makes a very colourful salad. Make the sauce as has been described above.

TOMATO SALAD

Sauce for tomato salad is made with only garlic and not onions. Remember to soak the garlic in vinegar as described above. Add a teaspoon of honey and also fresh coriander and basil leaves.

In fact, this preparation is a fine way of consuming garlic as due to vinegar and sour of the tomatoes, the garlic odour is suppressed.

Salads

AVOCADOS WITH SPECIAL SAUCE

Ingredients:

For four portions, you require:

Ripe avocados	2
Paprika	½
Tomato	1 medium-sized
Garlic	2 cloves
Vinegar	3 tablespoon
Olive oil	4 tablespoons
Salt	¼ teaspoon
Mixture H	½ teaspoon
Mustard paste	¼ teaspoon
Honey	1 teaspoon
Chopped dill leaves or Coriander leaves	1 teaspoon

Cut the avocados into halves and remove the seeds. Make the sauce as described above and add finely chopped paprika, tomato and green herbs. Mix the sauce well with all these ingredients. Fill into the avocados halves and serve the extra sauce on the table. Avocados should be cut and filled with the sauce just before serving otherwise they get black.

ENDIVE SALAD WITH NUTS

This is a fine preparation from France. You may not get the cheese mentioned here in some countries. In that case, just add some paneer.

Ingredients:

For 2 or 3 portions you need:

Endives	4
Rockford cheese	50 gm
Walnuts	6
Vinegar	2 tablespoons
Olive oil	3 tablespoons
Salt	¼ teaspoon
Mixture H	½ teaspoon

The sauce for this salad does not contain onions or garlic. Olive or sesame oil is also not used because of the delicate flavour of Endives and the Rockford cheese. Make the sauce and add into it small pieces of walnuts and cheese. Endives should be cut into fine pieces. Mix everything together delicately.

GREEN SALADS

There are many kinds of green salads in the world. Salads like cress, rocket salad (arugula) and dandelion are good for the liver and for purifying blood. One should eat a variety of green salads. Any green salad should be very well washed, especially if it is not from your own garden. After washing, the salad should be dried. One can do that by putting the salad in a napkin. These days there are also small machines available for drying salads. Wet salad will ruin the preparation by diluting the sauce. The recipe of the sauce is as described above. Green salad requires less sauce than the other salads, therefore be very careful with the amount of sauce.

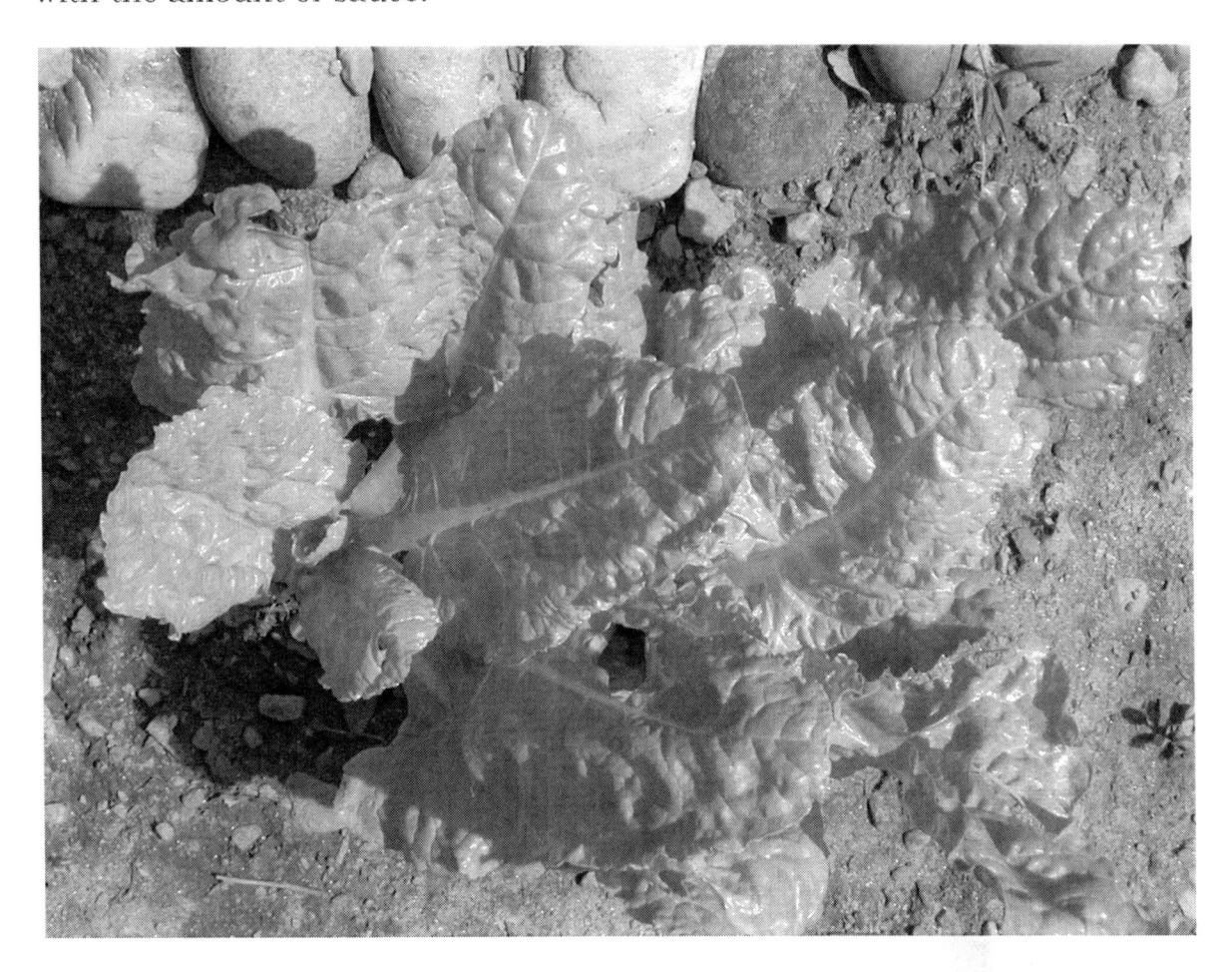

Note: Persons with weak digestive system or suffering from liver ailments should not eat green salads. Instead, they should eat simple and cooked food with cumin and ajwain until they are cured.

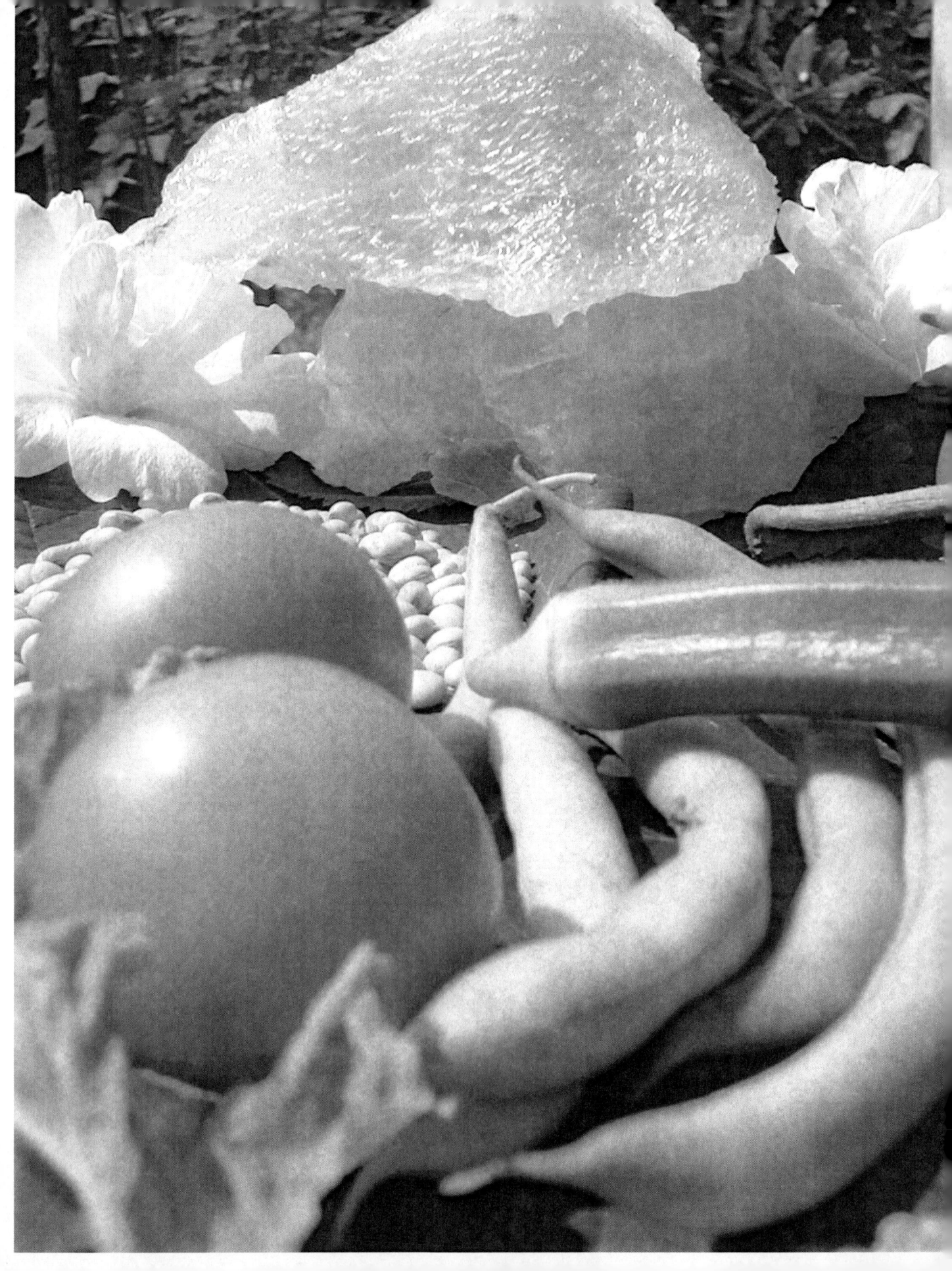

BREADS

GERMINATED WHEAT BREAD

Breads are made from various kinds of flours from diverse grains all over the world. But this specific bread is from germinated wheat and it is highly strength promoting. Besides Ayurveda, germinated wheat and its extract are recommended in many other alternative systems of medicine for healing and strength promoting. Since it can sometimes be difficult to take certain things as medicine, I developed ways to take germinated wheat in the form of delicious food. Earlier in this book, I have also described a recipe for breakfast with germinated wheat.

Ingredients for 3 or 4 flat breads like the pancakes:

Wheat grains	250 gm
Salt (optional)	¼ teaspoon
Ajwain	½ teaspoon
Kalonji	¼ teaspoon
Ghee or cooking oil	2 teaspoons

Germinate the wheat by soaking it in water as has been described earlier. The grains should be just at the beginning of germination. Crush the germinated wheat in wet grinder. Add a few tablespoons of water if it is too dry for grinding. Take out the crushed wheat and add salt and spices into it. You may leave out salt if you are eating the bread with some vegetable preparations which are already salted. If you like to eat the bread with butter and jam, you can add salt.

Mix the spices and the crushed grains well. Heat a non-stick pan smeared with a little ghee. When it is very hot, put 2 to 3 tablespoons of your dough (it is something between dough and batter in consistency) on it and spread it with a wooden flat spoon. After about half a minute, reduce the heat and let the bread cook slowly. Put the wooden spoon under the sides of the bread to make sure it is not sticking. After about a minute, turn the bread over and add a little more ghee on the pan. Let it cook on medium fire until both sides of the bread are light brown. Normally, if you are patient, you will have to turn the bread over only one time. The important factor in making this bread is that the dough should be spread properly on the pan to make a thin bread. Thick bread takes very long to cook and sometimes remains uncooked in the middle.

Breads

GERMINATED WHEAT BREAD WITH VEGETABLES

Use the same recipe but add finally chopped vegetables like onions, ginger, tomatoes and paprika. You can add also grated carrots or simply some green herbs. Follow the instructions given below for the maize flour breads.

MAIZE BREAD

This bread is very simple and quick to make. You should have the right flour, not too fine or sandy in consistency. I will give below three different recipes of maize bread.

Plain bread

Ingredients for 2-3 breads:

Maize flour	150 gm (½ to ¾ cup)
Salt (optional)	¼ teaspoon
Ajwain	½ teaspoon
Kalonji	¼ teaspoon
Water	about 100 ml (½ cup)
Ghee or cooking oil	2 tablespoons

Add the entire ingredients together and stir properly. If the dough is too dry, add a little more water. It should not be too fluid.

Heat a non-stick pan after smearing it with some ghee. When the pan is hot, take a handful of the dough and flatten it on the pan with a flat wooden spoon as you did for the previous recipe. You can also do that with your hand but in that case use a crepe pan (or dosa pan in India) and be very careful not to touch the hot pan. Expert cooks can do that easily but the novice will find a wooden spoon very helpful. Reduce the fire after a little while. Carefully turn the bread after about a minute. Apply a tiny bit of ghee or oil on the other side. Make sure that the bread is cooked well from both sides. If your bread is thick, cook a little longer on low fire.

Maize bread with vegetables

For making vegetable maize flour bread, add the following in addition to the above ingredients:

Grated carrot	1 medium-sized
Finely chopped paprika	1 small or half from a big one
Finely chopped tomato	1 medium-sized

Finely chopped green herbs	1 tablespoon
Finely chopped onions	2 tablespoons
Finely chopped ginger	1 tablespoon
Mixture A	1 tablespoon
Chopped green chilli (optional)	1

Mix all ingredients well and cook the bread in a similar manner as described above.

Maize flour bread with Methi (Fenugreek leaves)

Replace the mixed vegetables in the above bread with about 100 gm (¼ pound) of finely chopped fenugreek leaves. Make the bread in a similar manner as above.

BESAN (CHICKPEA FLOUR) BREAD

Besan is a high protein diet. It is highly recommended for children and those suffering from kapha vitiation. The first two preparations given for the maize bread can be also made with besan. However, in this case make a batter, not dough. The bread is made like a crepe and should be thin.

MIXED FLOUR BREAD

This bread is made by mixing four different kinds of flours in equal quantities: wheat, maize, chickpea (besan) and Finger millet. Mix the flours and use the same recipes as described above for maize bread. Finger millet alone also makes very good bread. It is strength promoting and brings equilibrium of the three energies of the body.

GREEN BREAD

I call this green bread because the dough for this bread is made with flour and puréed green vegetables and the bread looks green. Cook vegetables like spinach, arugula or dandelion or any other vegetable or mixture of vegetables of your choice. You may also include tender leaves of radish, beetroot or turnips if you have a garden.

After cooking the vegetables, make a purée. Prepare the dough with this purée. Take different kinds of flours or simply with Finger millet or maize flour. Add a little ajwain and salt. Make the bread on the pan as explained above.

Breads

CHAPATI, ROTI AND PARANTHAS

Chapati is the simplest form of flat bread with just whole-wheat flour and water; it is baked on a pan without any fat. Chapati is always made fresh and eaten hot. The same dough is used for chapati, roti and parantha. It is made by adding water little by little into the flour and kneading constantly. After kneading a lot, the dough becomes elastic and does not remain sticky. The dough should be kept for about 15 minutes before making chapatis or paranthas.

Take nearly one tablespoon of dough between your palms and make a ball from it. Flatten it first by pressing it on the sides with your fingers and then with a rolling pin.

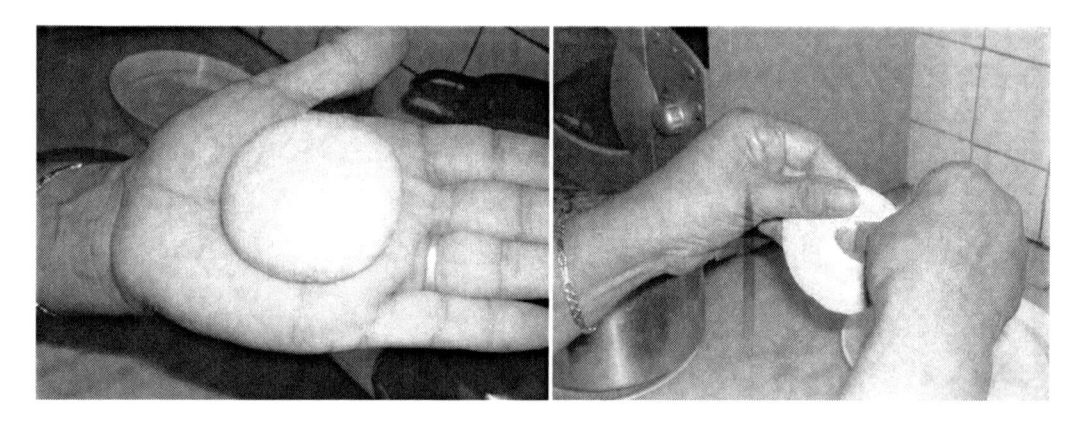

Use some flour for preventing it from sticking on the surface while rolling. Roll it as thin as possible. Pick it up very carefully and put it on a pre-heated pan. Turn it over after a few seconds. Turn it over once again after about 20-30 seconds and press the surface gently with a cotton napkin. By doing so, chapati will puff up. It is ready. You can smear little bit of ghee on the surface after removing it from the pan.

Ayurvedic Food Culture and Recipes

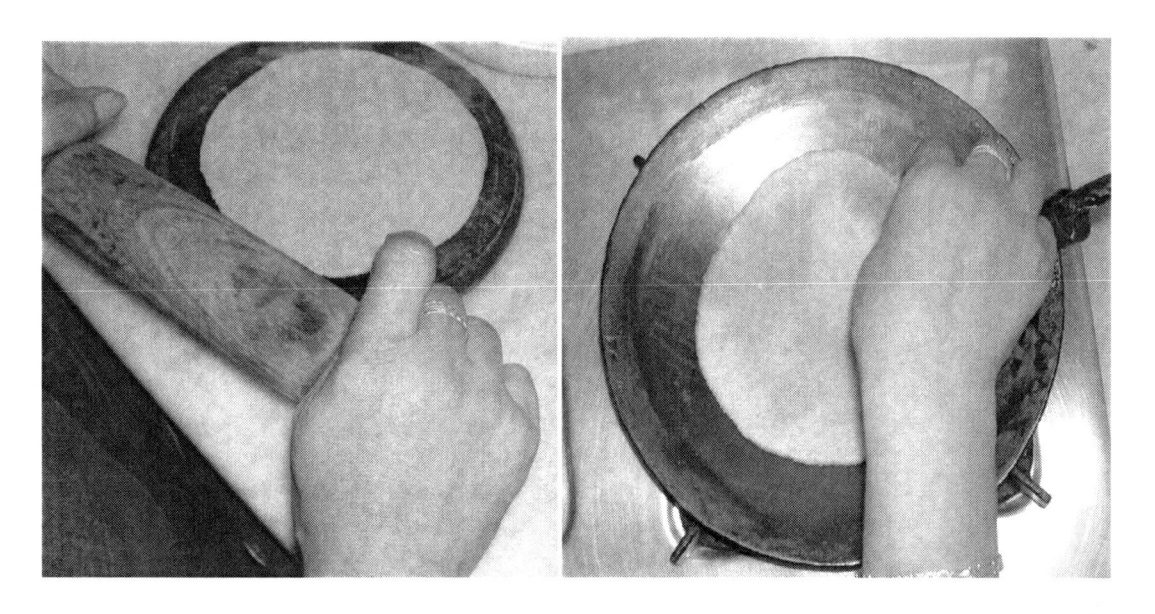

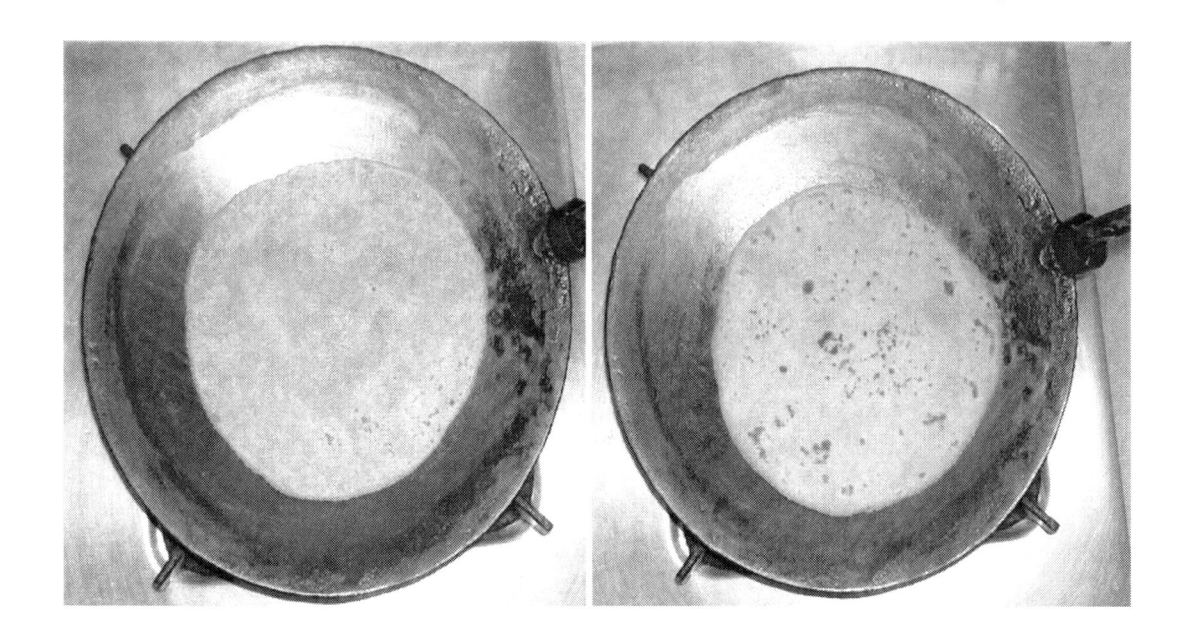

Breads

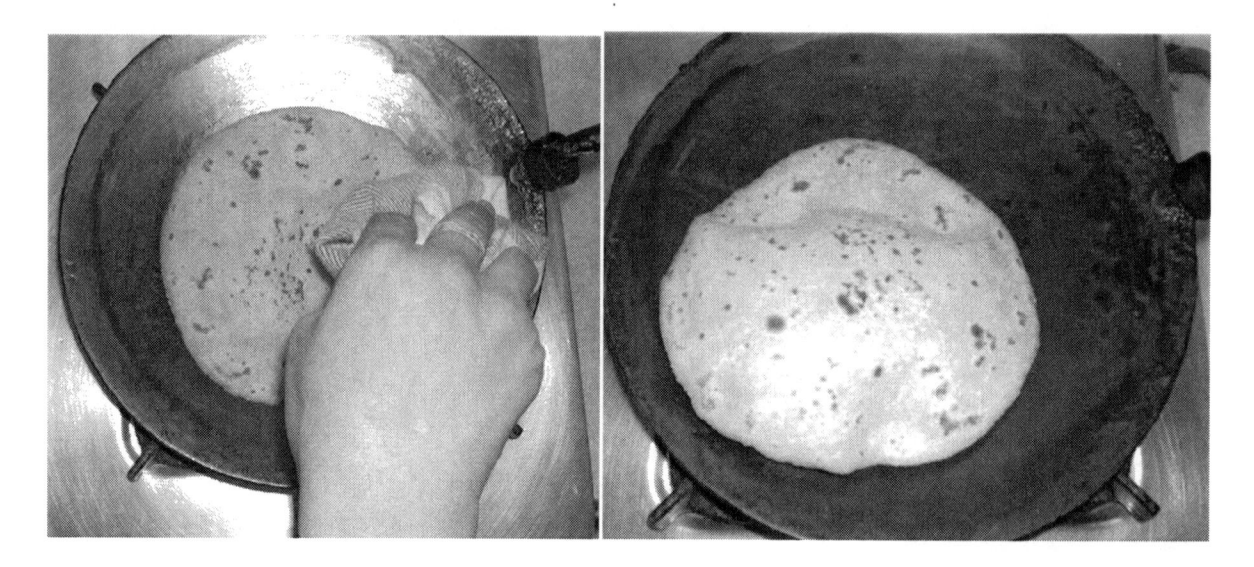

Comments: You can add some ajwain seeds in chapati dough especially during winter months.

Chapatis are generally eaten with different vegetable preparations or dals for the main meal. You can also eat them with butter, jam and marmalade for breakfast.

Roti is thicker than chapati. When roti is baked in a tandoor (traditional earthen oven with firewood), it tastes very delicious. There are also electric tandoors available now, but I will write a very simple technique for making tandoori roti on a normal heating plate or gas stove.

Take double the amount of dough than for chapati. Make a ball in your palms and wet this ball in water. Put it in your hands and clap until flat. In case you find it difficult to do that, use a rolling pin and smear some water on it so that it does not stick on the surface.

Put the roti (flattened dough) on a very hot iron pan. After few seconds, turn the pan upside down so that the roti is facing the hot plate. Keep heat on very high and hold the pan over the hot plate until the roti begins to detach itself from the pan. At that point, quickly turn the pan around again. Cook for another minute from both sides. Smear a little ghee on the roti and eat when still warm, otherwise it gets hard.

Serve chapati or roti with various vegetables and dal dishes. Shown below is a traditional thali or a trey of food with chapati and vegetable dishes.

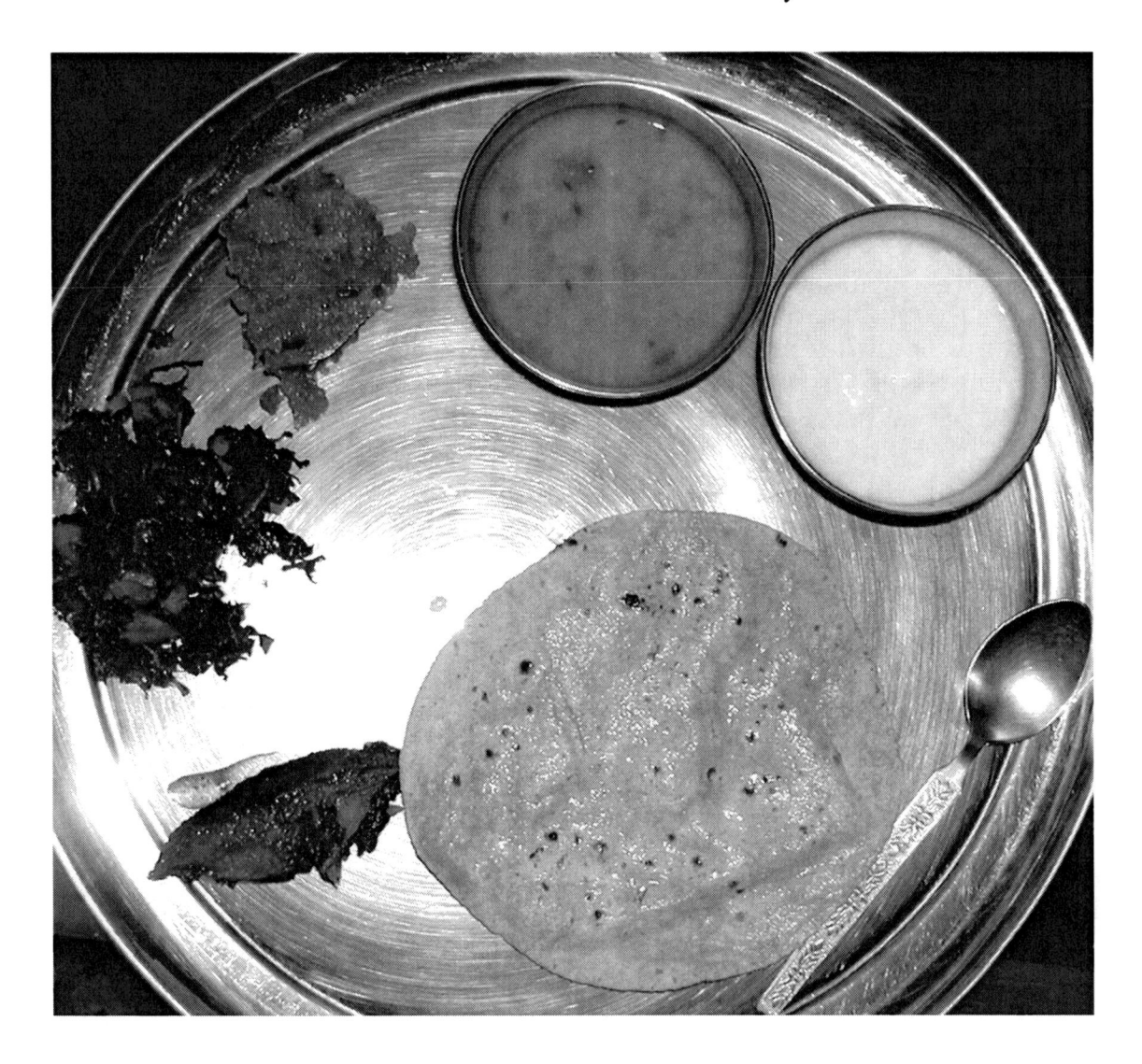

Paranthas: There are several kinds of paranthas:

a. **Simple parantha with ghee inside**
b. **Parantha with salt and spices**
c. **Parantha stuffed with various vegetables**
d. **Besan parantha**

For the first three kinds of paranthas, chapati dough is used. For Besan-parantha, the dough is made with wheat flour and besan as described below.

Simple Parantha: Take twice the amount of dough you took for a chapati (nearly two tablespoons), form a ball and flatten it with a rolling pin. Smear a little ghee on the top and fold like an envelope into a pocket. Flatten this pocket of dough and put it on a pre-heated pan. Turn over to bake from the other side. Turn it over again after about 20 seconds and smear a little ghee on its surface.

Breads

Turn over once more and smear ghee also on the other surface. After adding ghee, the parantha should not be cooked too long. It is not good to burn the fat.

Spicy Prantha: Roll dough as above and put a pinch of mixture F and some salt along with the ghee. Fold and continue as above.

Stuffed parantha: To make this parantha, you require more skill than for the above two. Instead of ghee and spices, add some vegetable stuffing and close it as shown in the following sequence of pictures. Flatten carefully so that the stuffing does not come out. Fry the parantha as described above.
I give below the sequence of pictures for making stuffed pranthas.

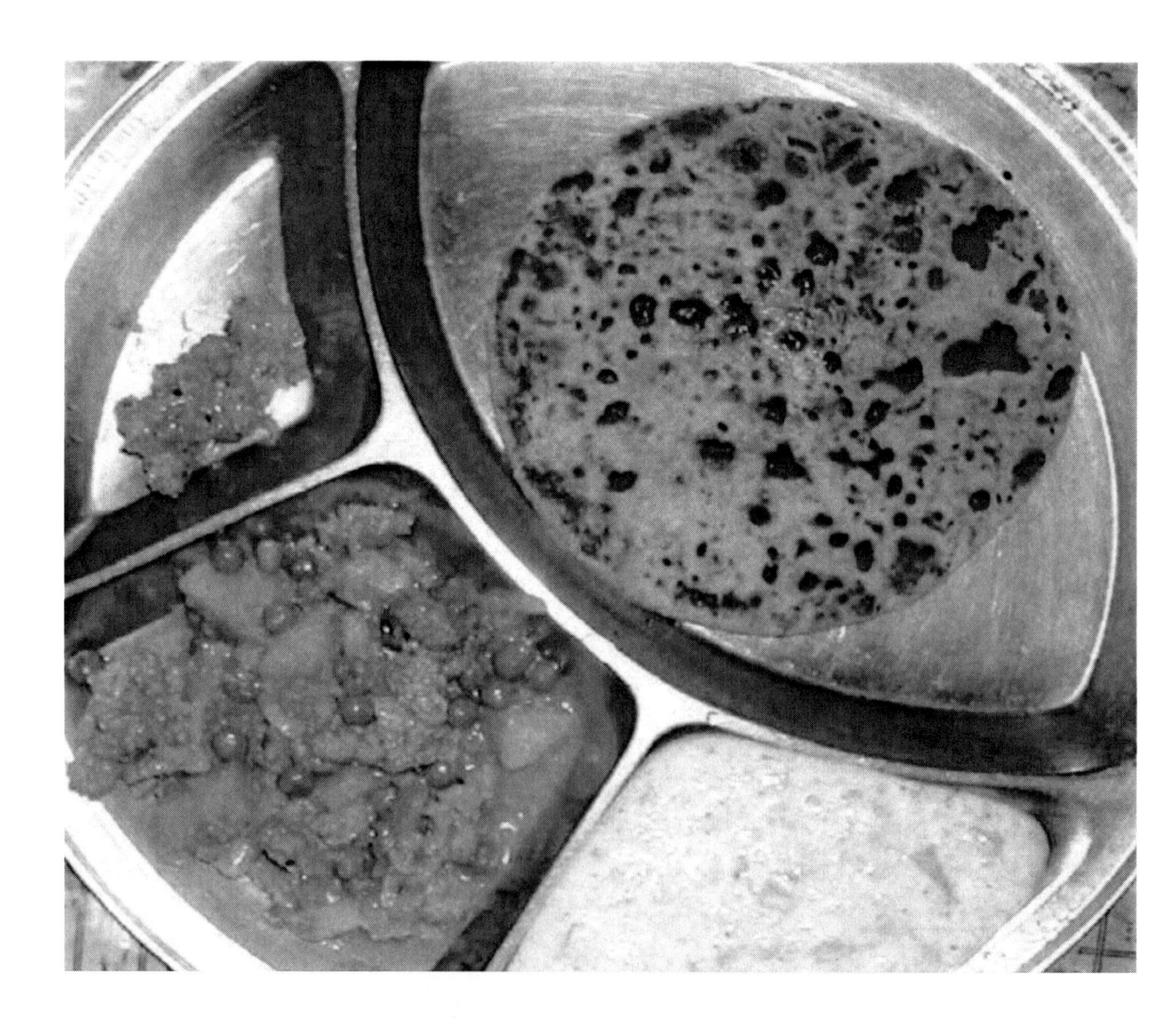

1. Take the dough and make it in the form of cavity.

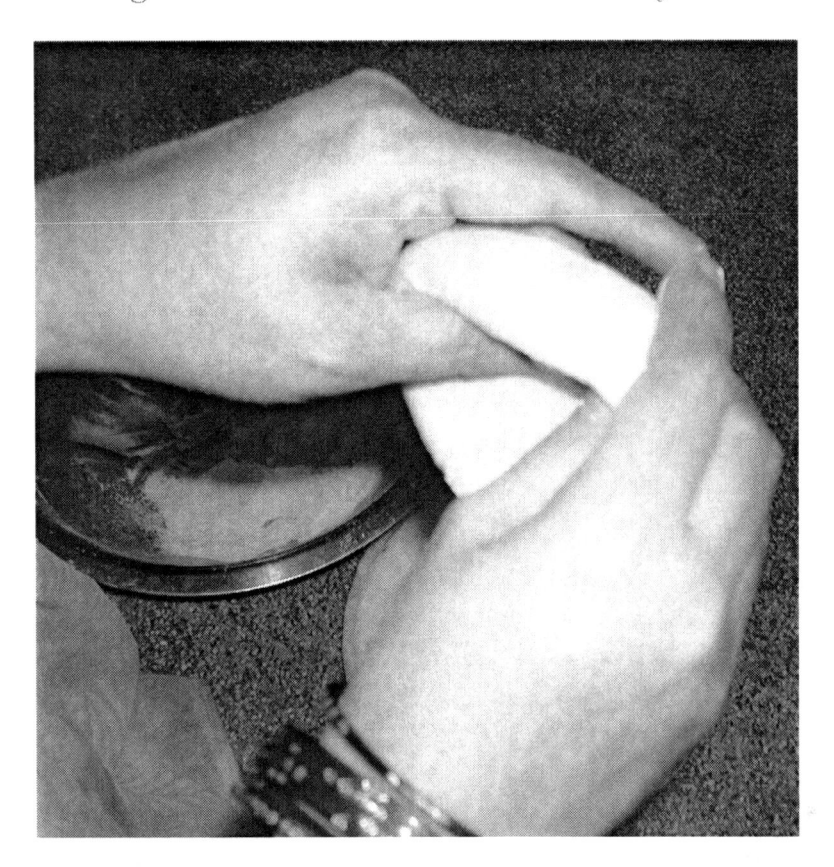

2. Fill the cavity with the parantha stuffing.

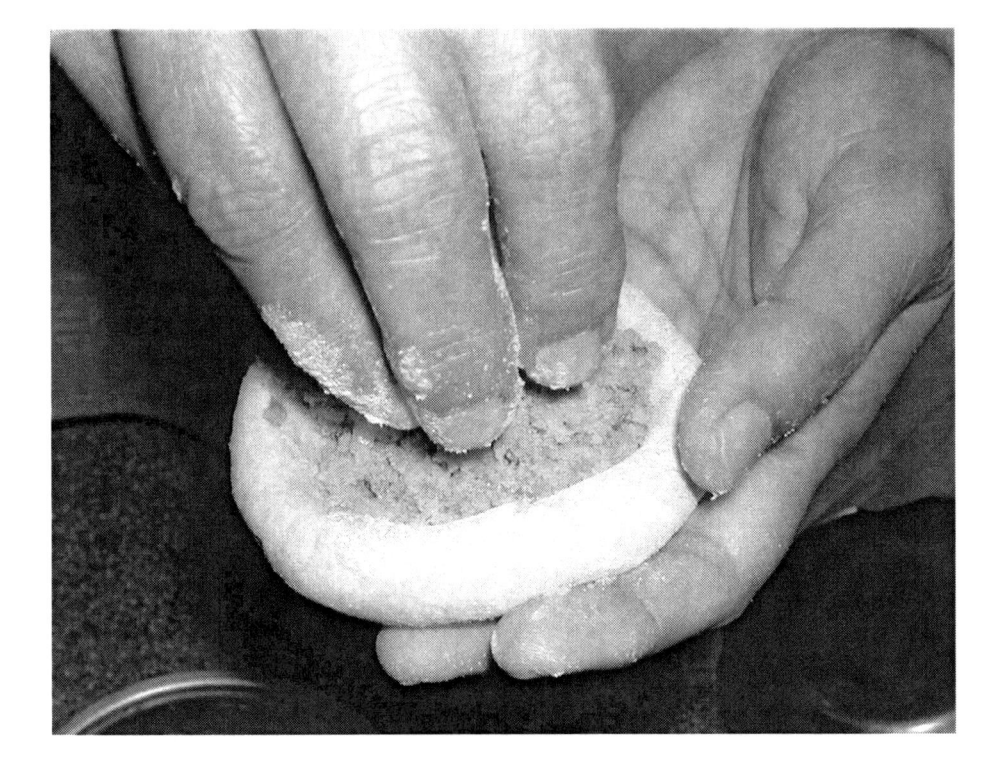

Breads

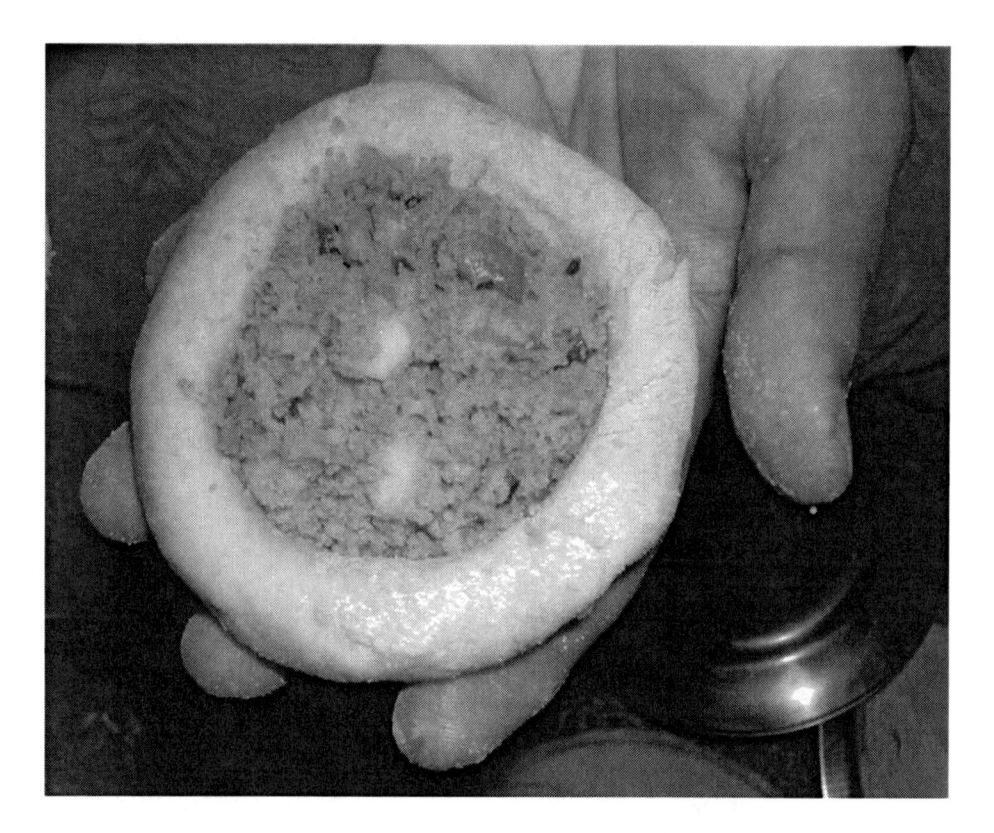

3. Close the stuffing inside the dough

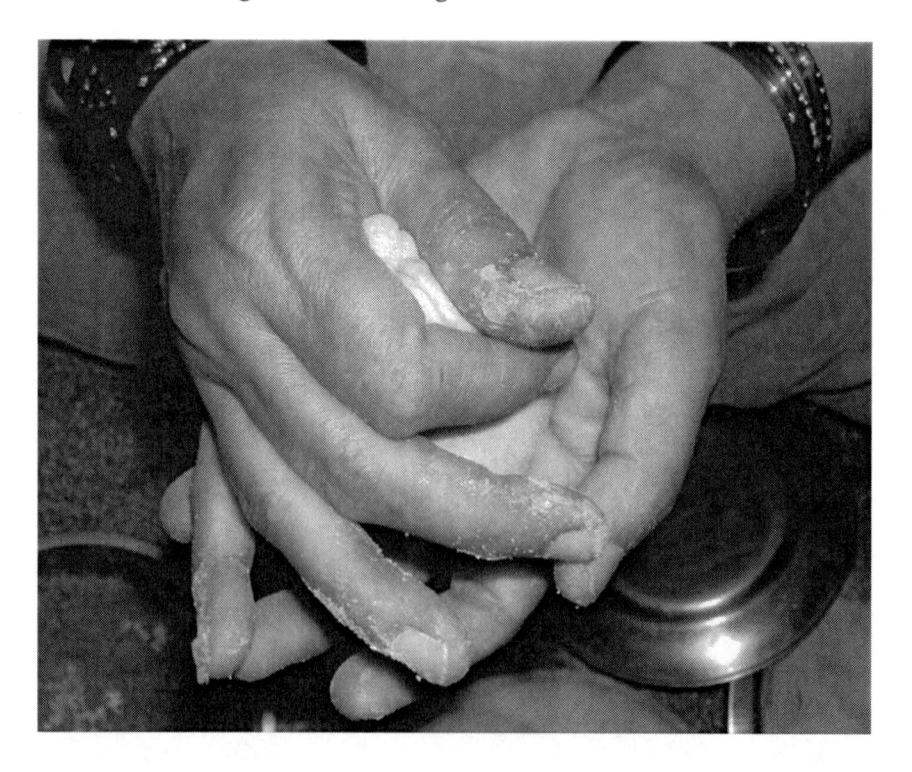

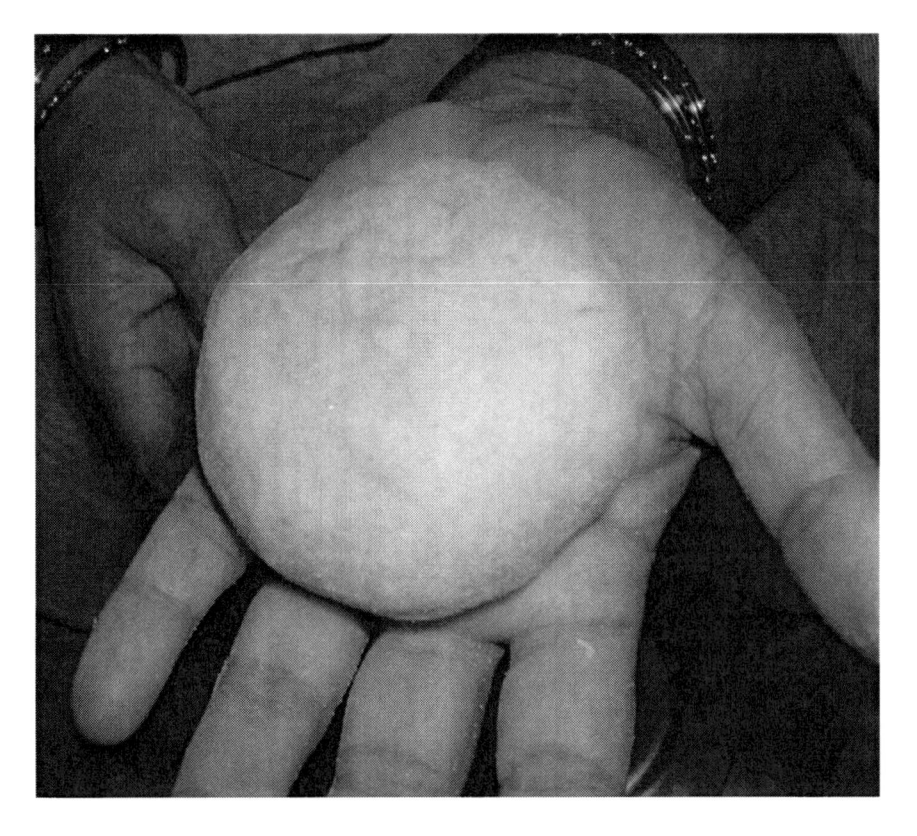

4. Flattened the filled dough carefully and bake it on a hot pan with little ghee.

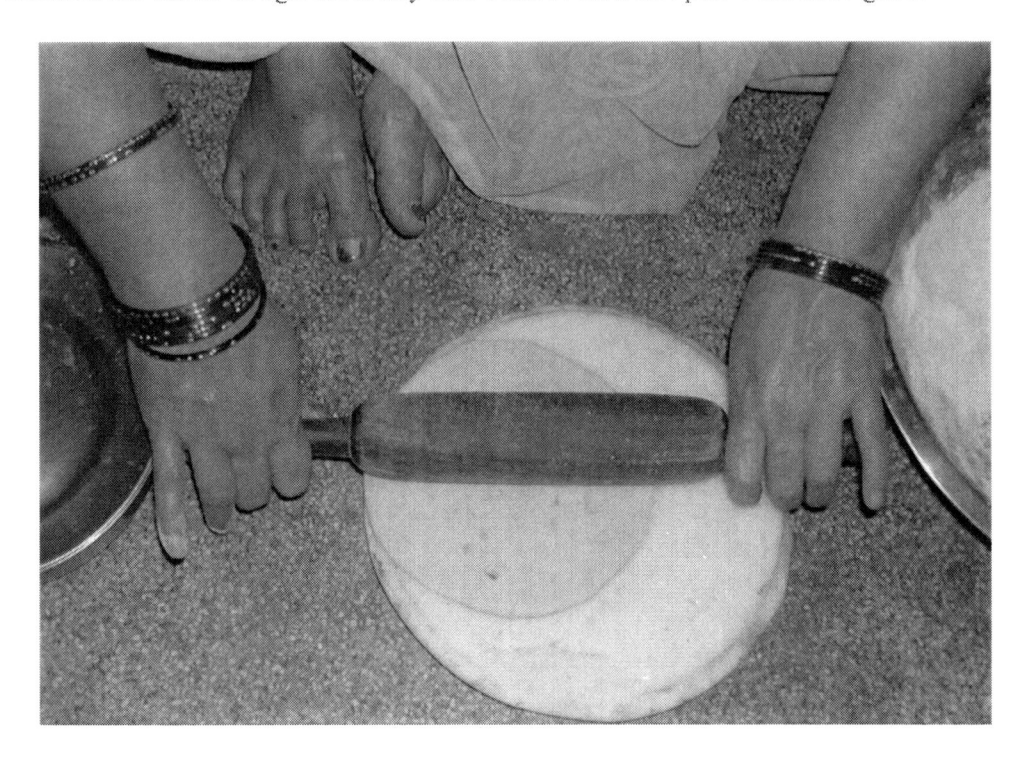

Breads

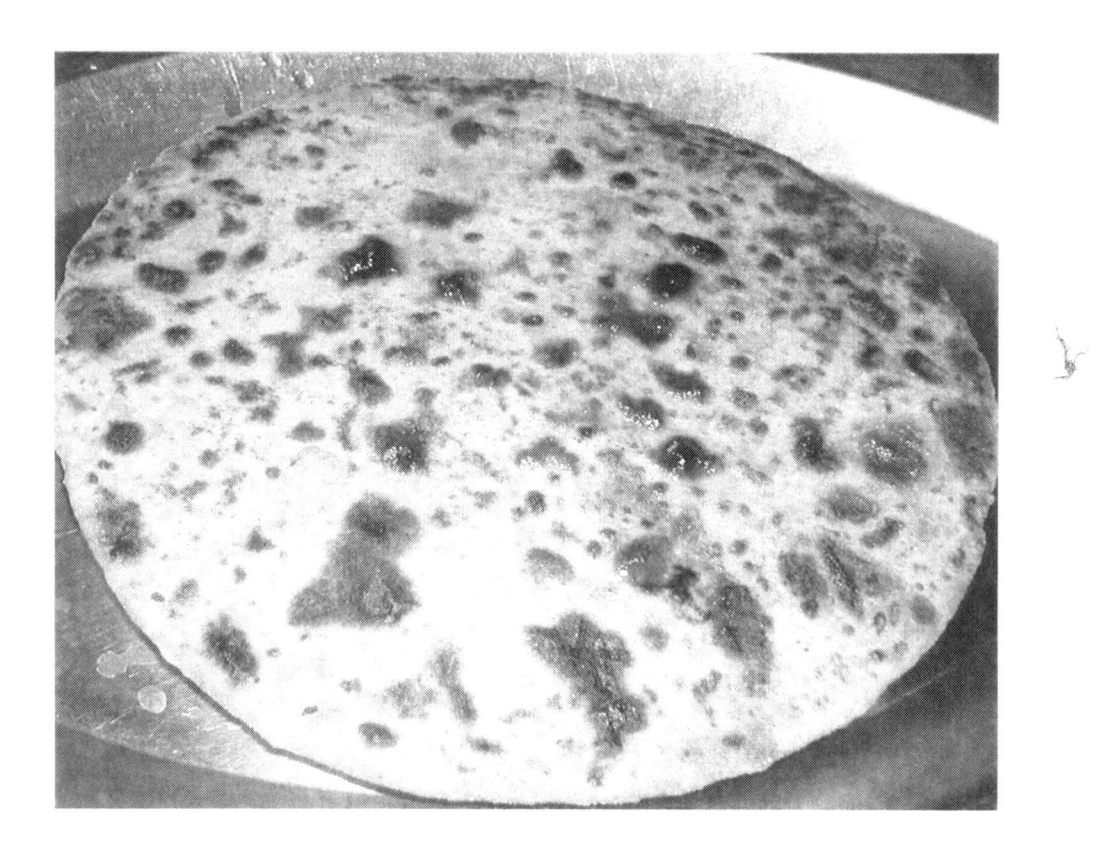

The stuffing can be prepared with various vegetables. I give some ideas below.

1. **Potato filling:** Boil 4-5 medium-sized potatoes with skin. Peel and add one finely chopped onion and one tablespoon each of finely chopped ginger and parsley or coriander. Add ¼ teaspoon of salt, 1 teaspoon of mixture A and 1 teaspoon of mixture F. You can add one finely chopped green chilli if you like it hot. Mix everything together by mashing the potatoes with your hands. Do not do that with a blender, as the filling should not be puréed. This filling will be enough for about 5 paranthas.

2. **Cauliflower filling:** Grate one medium-sized cauliflower and add other ingredients in the same quantity as described above for the potato filling. Mix everything together.

3. **Radish filling:** Grate 2-3 big radishes and mix with them only salt, herbs and spices. Leave out ginger and onions.

Besan-parantha: Take 100 gm (½ cup) of besan and 300gm (1½ cup) of wheat flour and add finely chopped one medium sized onion, one tablespoon of fresh ginger and one green chilli (optional). Add ½ teaspoon each of ajwain and salt and 1 teaspoon each of mixture A and F. Mix everything together and make dough by adding water as for chapati. Wait for about 15 minutes before making paranthas. Take double the amount of dough as for chapati, form a ball in your palms, sprinkle some wheat flour on it and flatten it with a rolling pin. Put the parantha on the pre-heated pan and fry the same way as has been described above.

Suggestion: You can also make tandoori parantha from the dough for besan parantha. For this, add a little ghee like for the normal parantha and fold into a pocket. Flatten it by smearing a little water on it. Bake the same way as for tandoori roti described above.

Note: Normally, a chapati pan or pan for cooking all these varieties of breads is made of wrought iron and is called tava. But you can take any other iron pan with a smooth surface. For making chapati, do not use a non-stick pan as you have to heat the pan without fat, which is not recommended for non-stick pans.

DOSA

Dosa is a thin and fine bread from Southern India. It is made of Urd dal and rice. You need to soak the ingredients two days in advance. Quick dosa mixtures are available but as you know that will give you dosas without prana.

Ingredients for 10-15 dosas:

Rice (white, of thick variety)	400 gm (2 cups)
Urd dal	200 gm (1 cup)
Salt	½ teaspoon

Soak dal and rice separately over night after washing them a few times. The next day, drain out the water, grind them separately in a wet grinder to make purée of rough consistency and mix them together. Leave over night so that the mixture gets slightly fermented. Add a little salt into this batter.

Heat a non-stick pan with a little ghee or oil. Spread two tablespoons of the batter on the pan and make sure that the layer is very thin. Turn over after a little while. Dosa cooks very quickly and is a very healthy food. The Urd dal, which is hot in nature, is balanced with rice, which is cold in its Ayurvedic nature.

Dosas can be eaten plane or filled with vegetables.

Fillings for Dosa

Dosa can be filled with diverse vegetable preparations. Besides mixed vegetables, green vegetables like broccoli, spinach, arugula (rucola) etc. make excellent fillings. For a good filling, the vegetables should be cut very fine. Put a little of

Breads

Mixtures B and F along with salt and turmeric in some hot ghee or oil. According to taste, add finely chopped green chilli. Stir-fry the vegetables in these spices. Put two tablespoons of filling in the middle of a dosa and fold it over from both sides.

SOME FILLED BREAD PREPARATIONS

There are many food preparations in various parts of the world where vegetables and salads are used as toppings for some kinds of dough preparations. The most popular of such foods are pizzas, which are originally Italian but are sold all over the world. However, in most restaurants these days the pizzas are not prepared with fresh vegetables. I am giving below two recipes for filled breads, which are very refreshing and nice.

FLAT BREAD OR CHAPATI WITH SALAD AND YOGHURT

Ingredients for one portion:

Chapati or flat bread	1
Lettuce or some other green salad	few leaves
Tomato	1 medium-sized
Paprika or cucumber (chopped)	1 tablespoon
Carrot (grated)	1 tablespoon
Salad sauce	1 tablespoon
Yoghurt	2 tablespoons
Salt and pepper	1 pinch together
Garlic	2 cloves
Olive or sesame oil	1 teaspoon

Make sure that your salad ingredients are not cold. Keep the vegetables at room temperature a few hours before preparation. Chop all the vegetables into small pieces and make a salad with a salad sauce as described earlier. Separately, make a sauce from yoghurt with salt, pepper, a teaspoon of oil and finely chopped garlic. Mix well everything together.

Put the salad in the middle of a hot chapati or flat bread and pour the yoghurt sauce on the top of it. Fold the chapati over from two sides.

This preparation should not be served for dinner, as there is yoghurt in it. You can replace yoghurt with paneer mixed with herbs and garlic.

FLAT BREAD OR CHAPATI WITH HOT VEGETABLES AND YOGHURT SAUCE

For this recipe, add the mixed vegetable filling along with the yoghurt sauce. You may use the same recipe for mixed vegetable as has been described for dosa filling or you may take one of the previously described recipes.

If you are serving this preparation for dinner, replace the yoghurt sauce with carrot salad or paneer mixed with herbs and garlic.

BAKED BREAD WITH VEGETABLES

In the two recipes described above, the bread was prepared separately. Here the vegetables are enclosed in the flattened dough and baked. However, pre-cooking of the vegetables is essential. The vegetables are stir-fried so that they remain crisp.

This recipe can be made with whole-wheat chapati flour. But it tastes better with white flour. Most white flours available in the West have 85% of the wheat constituents. I suggest a mid-way, which is to pass the chapati flour through a fine strainer and take out a part of the wheat husk. You can try out different kinds of flour according to your taste.

Ingredients for 4 breads:

For dough:

Wheat flour	300 gm (1 ½ cup)
Salt	a pinch
Ajwain	½ teaspoon
Ghee or butter	2 tablespoon

Mix together all the ingredients for dough. Make the dough with minimum amount of water and knead it well.

Split the dough into four parts and flatten each piece with a rolling pin just as for chapatis. Fill the stir-fried vegetables in the middle and fold in from two ends by joining them on the top. It should look like a little boat. Bake at a high temperature for about 20 minutes.

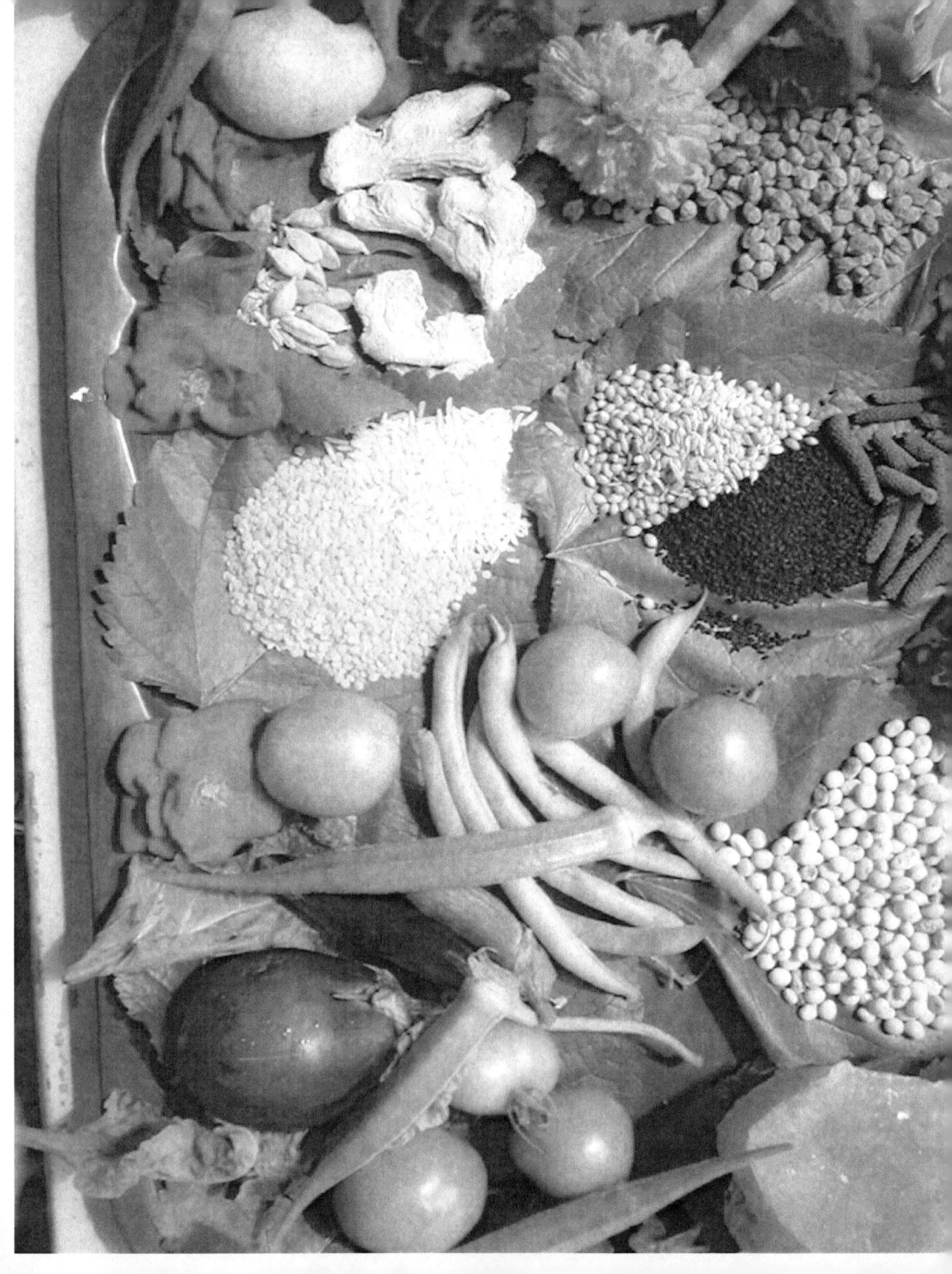

BEANS AND LENTILS

Beans and lentils are staple food in some parts of the world and an important source of protein. They are used more in the southern parts of the globe, and there are numerous recipes especially in African countries and South America. With the recent wave of health consciousness and vegetarian diets, beans and lentils are also becoming popular in the affluent countries of the Northern Hemisphere. However, they take long to cook and are heavy to digest. Thus, it is very important to cook them well and to use appropriate spices or other ingredients for a balanced preparation. A quicker way to cook beans and lentils is in the pressure cooker. But cooking under high pressure is too drastic and destroys the living element (prana) of the food. Cooking on slow fire for a long time is recommended. For those who eat them often, I suggest that they should buy a slow electric cooker. Solar cooking is another alternative, but unfortunately solar cookers are not easily available in some parts of the world.

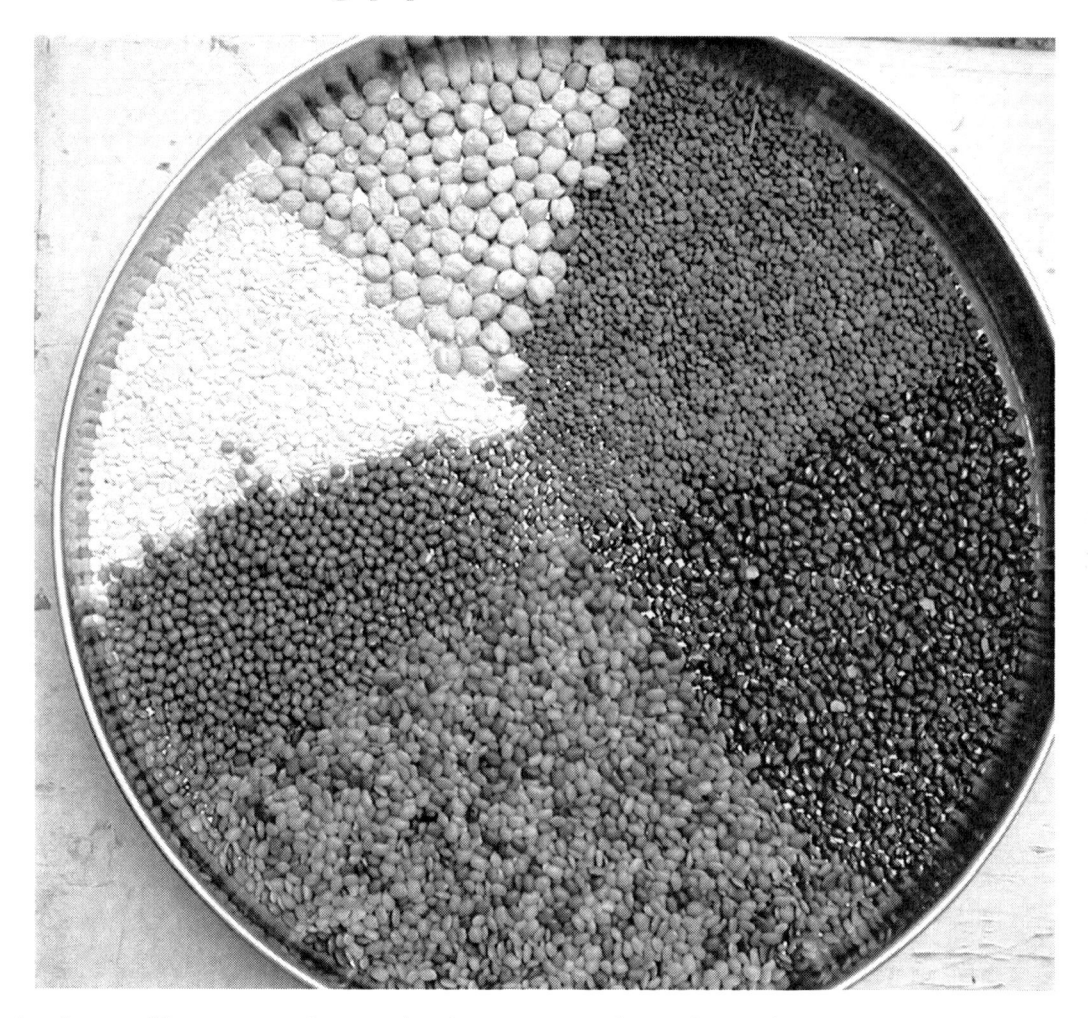

CHICKPEA PREPARATIONS

Chickpeas are available all over the world. As said earlier, the darker and smaller variety of chickpeas, called also black gram, is healthier than the big and white chickpeas. Although both the varieties are called chickpeas, but they taste different. Therefore I have included separate recipes for each of them.

White chickpeas

This is the most common type of chickpeas. There are two kinds available; one is slightly smaller than the other is. Buy the smaller variety.

Version A

Chickpeas with tamarind

Ingredients:

For 3-4 portions, you need:

Chickpeas	200 gm (1 cup)
Salt	¾ teaspoon
Mixture B	1 teaspoon
Mixture A	1 teaspoon
Turmeric	1 teaspoon
Onions	3 medium-sized
Ginger (chopped)	2 tablespoons
Garlic	4 cloves
Cooking oil	2 tablespoons
Dried fruits of tamarind	100 gm (¼ pound)
Jaggery or raw sugar	1 tablespoon
Green chilli	1 small (optional)
Cucumber, paprika, tomato	Few pieces of each

Soak the chickpeas in water for about 24 hours to germinate them as described earlier. Take a pot large enough to remain at least half-empty after putting 1 litre (5 cups) of water into it. Boil the water and add turmeric, Mixture B and only half the salt into it. Add germinated chickpeas after draining out the water in which they were soaking and bring to boil. Reduce the heat, put the lid on and cook for an hour. Add more water if needed. Make sure that the chickpeas are soft enough. They should be cooked well otherwise they will vitiate vata. Depending upon the quality of water, you may have to cook longer than one hour. Always add boiling water and never cold water into a cooking dish.

Remember that in this recipe, we want the chickpeas almost without water in the end.

Soak the tamarind fruits for about 15 minutes in hot water and squeeze them through a strainer to take out their juice. Soak and strain again until you have removed all the juice from the fruits.

Grate or mash the onions and fry in the oil along with the ginger. Add finely chopped green chilli into it if you like to have the preparation slightly hot. When the onions are sauté, add mixture A and rest of the salt. Stir-fry for another 2-3 minutes. Add tamarind juice and stir. Cook for few minutes and add the previously cooked chickpeas. Stir everything together and cook uncovered on the low heat for about 15 minutes or longer if your preparation has too much fluid. Taste and add a little more salt if needed to have equilibrium with the sour of the tamarind. Add raw sugar or jaggery and in the end add the finely chopped garlic.

Serve this dish decorated with some cucumber, paprika and tomato pieces on the top.

Version B

Chickpea preparation without fat

In this preparation, there is no oil, onions, fresh ginger or garlic. Cook the chickpeas as described above but add a teaspoon of powdered dry ginger. After the chickpeas are cooked, add in them Mixutre A, tamarind juice and sugar. Add one teaspoon of paprika powder for colour and the other half of the salt. Cook them until a little sauce is left in them. Mash some chickpeas between two wooden spoons to make the sauce thicker. Compared to the above recipe, this preparation is fluid. Decorate this dish with chopped green herbs like chive, mint, coriander and basil.

Suggestions: The above two dishes are best served with flat bread or tandoori roti or parantha. I suggest that you serve Version A with roti whereas Version B, which is without fat, with parantha.

Version C

Chickpea purée

This is a purée made from germinated and boiled chickpeas along with some oil and spices. This can be used as topping on the bread or can be eaten with some

Beans and Lentils

salad. One can also make little rounds of this purée and fry them in non-stick pan.

Ingredients:

Chickpeas	100gm
Olive or sesames oil	2 tablespoons
Lemon juice	2 tablespoons
Ginger powder	1 tablespoon
Mixture E	1 teaspoon
Salt	½ teaspoon
Garlic	3-4 cloves
Green herbs (chopped)	3 tablespoons
Green chilli (optional)	1

Germinate and boil chickpeas as described above. Put all the ingredients in a wet grinder and make a purée. This purée can be kept in the refrigerator for a few days.

Suggestions: You may make diverse versions of this recipe. For example, you may add vegetables like tomatoes, paprika, onions etc. to get diverse flavours.

Black gram or dark chickpeas

I have already mentioned this type of chickpeas in the breakfast recipes. This variety takes shorter time to cook than the white chickpeas. Soak these in water for 24 hours in order to germinate them.

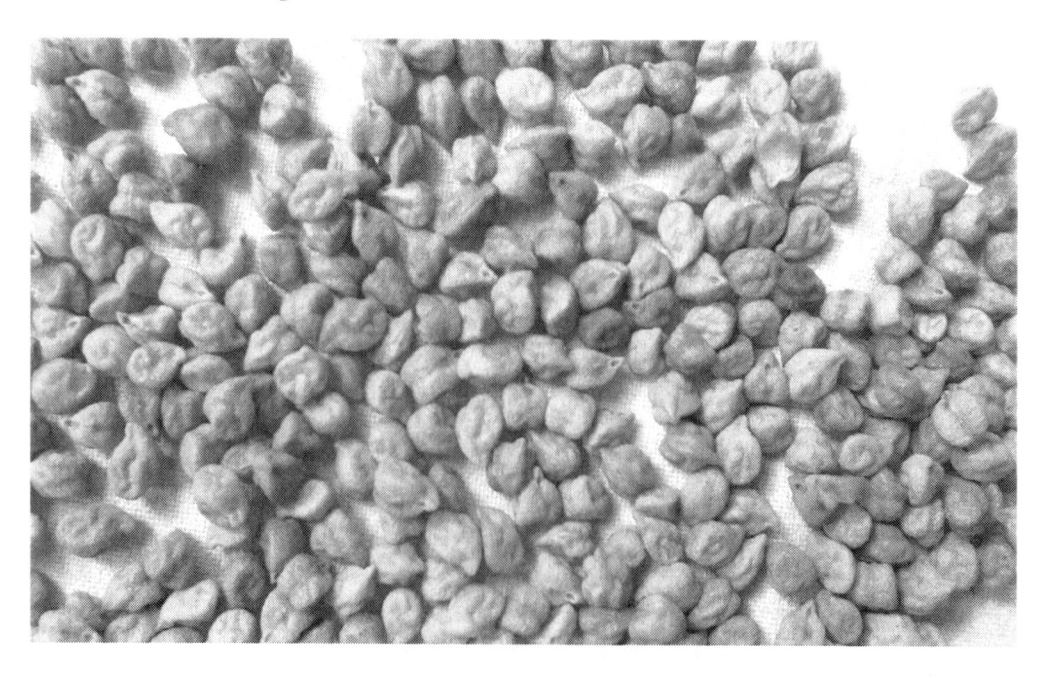

Version A

Ingredients:

For two portions, you require:

Chickpeas	100gm (½ cup)
Salt	1/3 teaspoon
Mixture F	½ teaspoon
Cumin	½ teaspoon
Ajwain	¼ teaspoon
Cooking oil	1 tablespoon
Lemon juice	1 teaspoon

Heat oil in a pan and add salt and spices. After few seconds, add the germinated chickpeas after draining out the water in which they were soaking. Stir-fry for about 2 minutes and then reduce the heat and put the lid on. Cook them for about 15 minutes and stir from time to time. If the chickpeas stick on the bottom, add one or two tablespoons of water. Make sure that they are cooked soft. If needed, cook a little longer. After taking them off the heat, add lemon juice and stir well to mix the juice.

Version B

For this recipe, boil the germinated chickpeas in salted water from ½ hour to 45 minutes. Make sure that they are well cooked. Prepare the basic sauce as described earlier (Page 150) and add it into the cooked chickpeas. Add extra water to the dish so that the chickpeas are in a soupy basic sauce. Add the mixture of ginger, garlic and herbs in the end as described for the basic sauce.

Version C

You can make a purée as described above for the white chickpeas.

Suggestions: Boiled black gram can be used to replace green peas in the rice. They can be also added in various salads. Chickpea purée can be used as filling in dosas or other bread recipes, which are described above.

KIDNEY BEANS AND OTHER SIMILAR KINDS OF BEANS

There is one basic recipe for all those beans which do not germinate as chickpeas or mung beans. It is essential to soften them by soaking them in water over-night. All these beans require cooking for a very long time. They are cold, heavy to digest and vata promoting. Therefore, they should always be

Beans and Lentils

cooked with spices, ginger and garlic. They should not be eaten too often and not for dinner.

Pay attention that your beans are cooked very well. That means if you press them with the back of the spoon against the wall of the pot while holding the pot with one hand, they should be mashed. If the beans are not well cooked, they vitiate vata. Always cook the beans with a teaspoon of Mixture B to have equilibrium. Normally the beans take about two hours to cook. That is twice the time than the chickpeas.

Prepare the beans with following two recipes:

1. Use the recipe described for Version A of the Chickpeas. That is with onions, ginger etc. and by adding tamarind juice in the sauce.

2. The second recipe for these beans is to prepare them with the basic sauce as has been also described above for black gram.

Remember in both cases that the beans should be cooked in the sauce for another hour. Add water if necessary. In the end, crush some beans to make the sauce thicker.

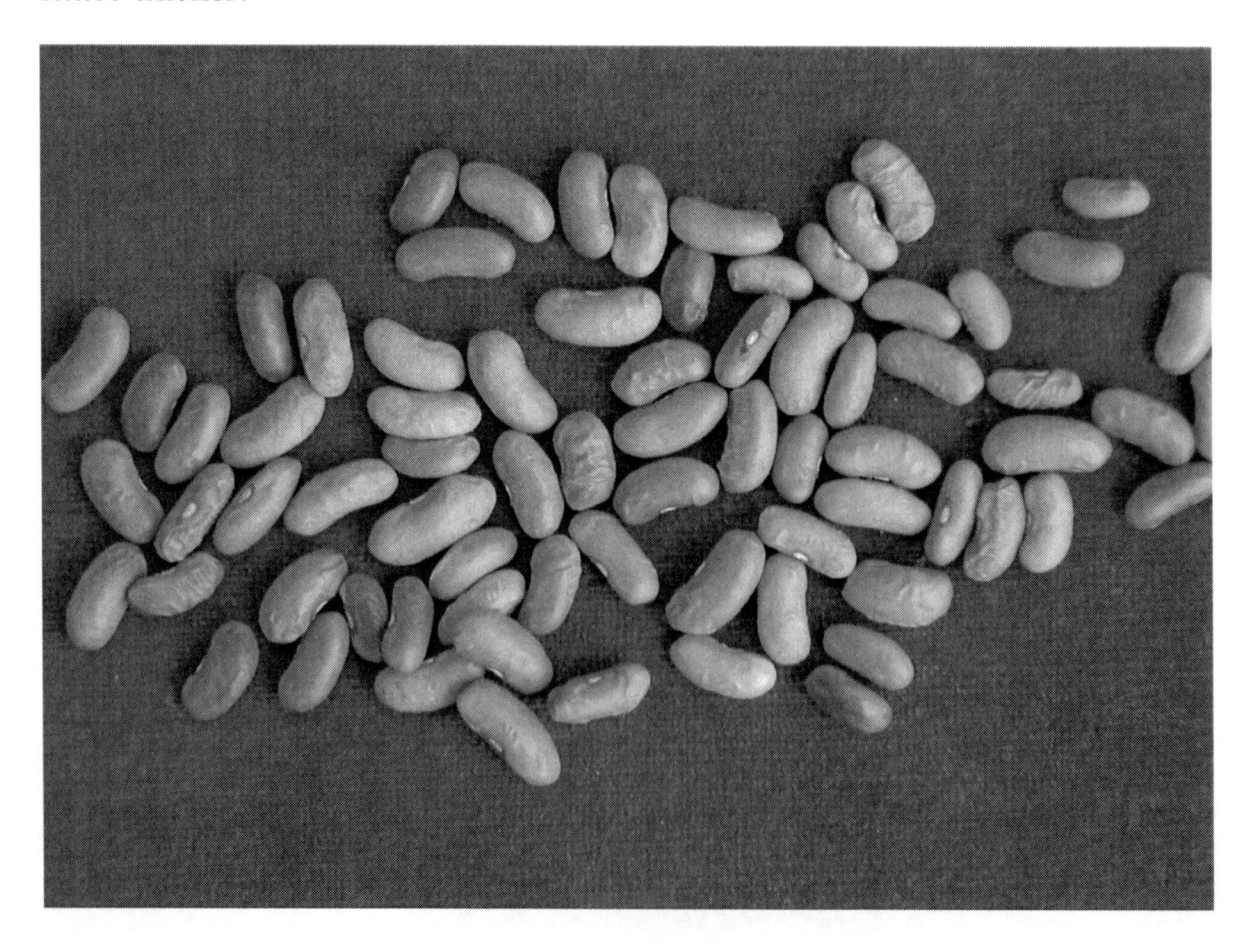

SOYA BEANS

Soya beans in sauce

Soya beans are different than the above-described beans as they are hot in their Ayurvedic nature. They are not vata promoting, but on the contrary, they cure vitiated vata and kapha and enhance pitta. You can prepare them like the other beans but altering the recipes a little as suggested below:

1. Add a spoon of Mixture C instead of B.
2. Add ghee instead of cooking oil.
3. Do not add garlic.

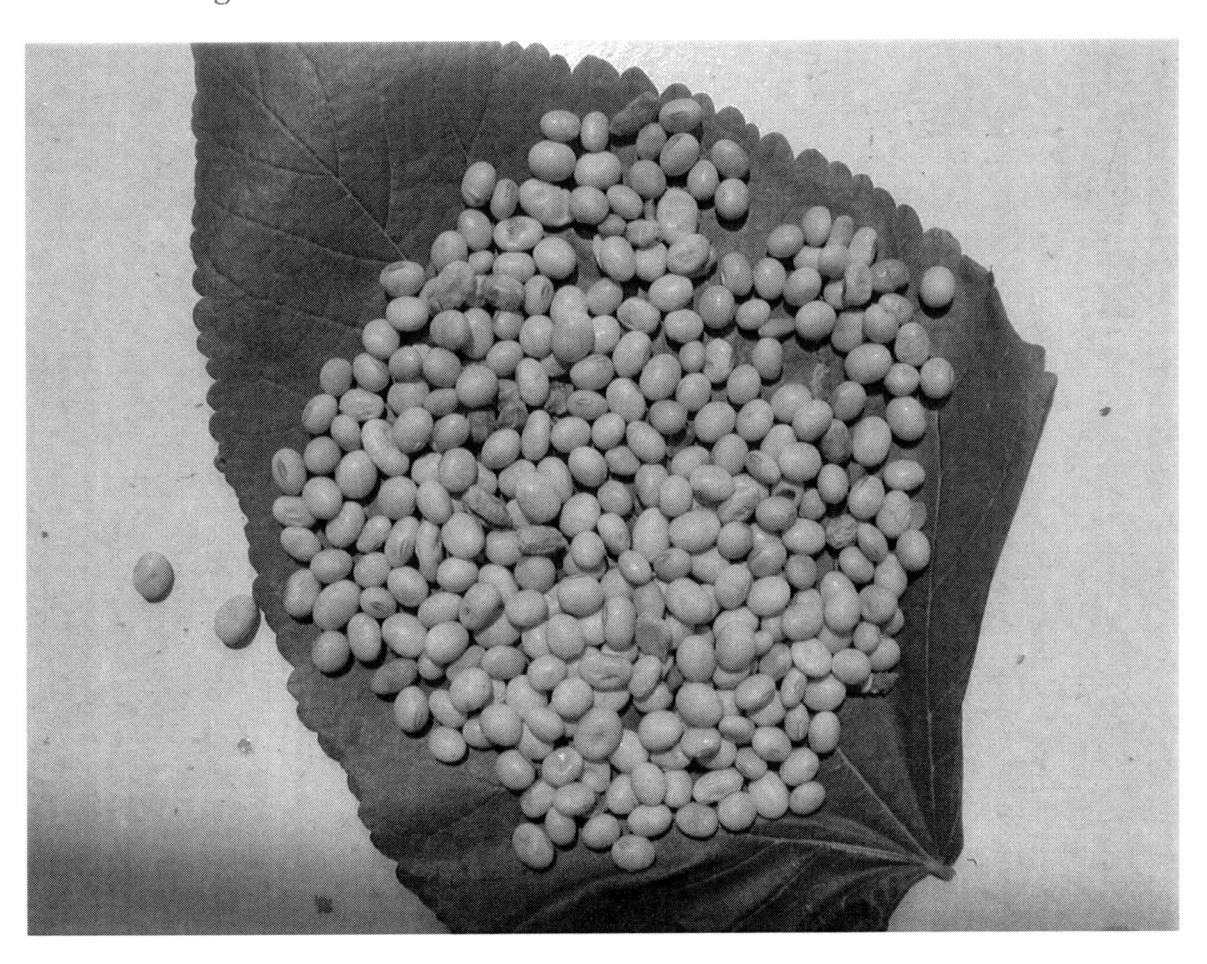

Fried Soya beans

Soya beans can also be prepared like nuts and eaten as snack. Soak the Soya beans in water for about 24 hours and take off their husk by crushing them in your palms. Soak them in a little water with a teaspoon of salt and let them stay

Beans and Lentils

for few hours. Drain out the water and let the beans dry. Roast them in a non-stick pan by adding a little ghee. Stir-fry them and in the end add a little of Mixture F if you want them spicy.

MUNG BEAN PREPARATION

Mung beans are very healthy and bring the energies in equilibrium. They are lighter and easier to digest than all other beans and lentils. The best preparation from a health point of view is to soak in water for 24 hours and let them germinate.

Ingredients:

For 3-4 portions, you require:

Mung beans	200 gm (1 cup)
Salt	½ teaspoon
Mixture B	1 teaspoon
Turmeric	1 teaspoon
Chopped fresh ginger	2 tablespoons
Green chilli	1 (optional)

Put germinated beans in about a litre (5 cups) of boiling water and add salt, Mixture B, turmeric, and, if you like, add also the chilli. Bring to boil, reduce heat, cover the pot and let the beans cook for an hour or until they become soupy. Go more by appearance because the cooking time depends upon the quality of the Mung beans and that of water.

Suggestions for garnishing:

1. If to be eaten as a soup, add Mixture H and butter or ghee; or

2. Add Mixture H, ghee or butter and a little lemon juice; or

3. Fry two finely chopped onions, in two tablespoons of ghee. When sauté, add a teaspoon of cumin, ½ teaspoon of ajwain and 1½ teaspoon of mixture F. Cook for a minute and add this to the cooked mung beans. Cook for another 3-4 minutes. Garnish with two tablespoons full of finely chopped fresh herbs; or

4. Prepare basic sauce described earlier and cook the mung beans in it for another five minutes.

MUNG DAL PREPARATION

As already mentioned, mung dal is split mung beans with the husk removed. It has small yellow grains. The advantage is that this dal can be cooked fairly fast. Soaking for 5 to 10 minutes is enough. The other method is the same as for the mung beans. You can prepare this dal in one of the ways described above for mung beans.

URD DAL PREPARATION

Urd dal is very highly pitta and kapha and is hard to digest. Since it is an aphrodisiac and also makes a delicious preparation, I will give one recipe for it. In my previous books, I have given several recipes related to enhancing sexual capabilities with this dal but most of them are sweet preparations. This is a recipe for a main meal to be eaten with flat bread, tandoori roti or chapati.

Ingredients

For 3-4 portions, you require:

Urd dal	200 gm (1 cup)
Fennel	1 teaspoon
Salt	1/3 teaspoon
Turmeric	1 teaspoon
Ginger (chopped)	2 tablespoons
Green chilli	½ to 1 (optional)
Ghee	2 tablespoons
Onions	2 medium-sized
Mixture A	1 teaspoon
Cumin	½ teaspoon
Mixture C and F	½ teaspoon each
Tomatoes	3 medium sized
Garlic	4 cloves
Coriander and dill leaves	2 tablespoons (chopped)

Measure the dal, wash it and soak for about 15 minutes. Bring to boil double the quantity of water, add fennel, salt, turmeric, ginger, green chilli and the dal after draining out the water in which it was soaking. Cover and cook on low heat for about 15 minutes. It should be cooked like rice; that means all the water is soaked into the grains and no fluid is left.

Separately, cut the onions into lamellae and fry them in ghee. After they are sauté, add Mixtures A, C and F and cumin. Stir a little and add tomatoes chopped into small pieces. Stir, cover and let them cook until they are soft and well cooked. Add the dal and mix it with the sauce. Cook another 2-3 minutes. In the end, add finely chopped garlic and decorate the dish with chopped herbs.

Suggestions:

1. You can add a little lemon juice along with the garlic in the end.

2. Since this dish is heavy to digest, do not eat too much of it. Preferably, make this preparation for lunch or if for dinner, have an early dinner.

Note: All the lentils, beans and dals etc. are heavy to digest and it is written in the ancient texts that they should be prepared with spices, ghee and something sour. Urd dal is excessively pitta and kapha promoting and therefore a special care is taken. The preparation tastes very good but be careful not to eat it too much.

Please note that eating urd dal enhances stool. It is good for those suffering from constipation.

KHICHARI

Khichari is a prepararion of rice and mung dal together. A large number of Indians eat rice and dal along with some vegetable preparations for lunch. Khichari is a replacement of a big meal and is quick and easy to prepare because both dal and rice are cooked in one pot. In Ayurvedic texts, khichari is described as a light and easy to digest meal. It is given to people who have a weak digestion or are convalescent. It is also recommended after pancha karma treatments. It is a good food for dieting after you have been having too many big meals.

Basically khichari is two portions of rice and one portion of mung dal and cooked together like a dal as described above. There are many versions of khichari with different garnishing and consistencies.

Version A

This is a soupy preparation and garnished in a simple way for those with weak digestion.

Ingredients:

For 2-3 portions you need:

Rice	100 gm (½ cup)
Mung dal	50 gm (¼ cup)
Turmeric	½ teaspoon
Salt	½ teaspoon
Ghee	2 tablespoons
Onion	1 medium-sized
Cumin	½ teaspoon
Fennel	¼ teaspoon
Ajwain	½ teaspoon
Ginger (chopped)	1 tablespoon
Lemon juice	1 tablespoon (optional)

Wash mung dal and rice and soak them in water for 15 minutes. Boil about a litre of water (5 cups) in a pot of at least two-litre capacity and add turmeric and salt. Add dal and rice after draining out the water in which they were soaking. Bring to boil, put the lid on and cook for an hour on low fire.

Separately, fry the onions and ginger in ghee and when they are sauté, add fennel, cumin and ajwain. Stir-fry for a few minutes and add to the soupy khichari. Cook for another 2-3 minutes. Add lemon juice before serving.

Version B

You can garnish the cooked khichari with the usual basic sauce prepared with onions, tomatoes, ginger etc. already explained (page 150). Alternatively, you can add 2-3 tomatoes after frying the onions as described in Version A. However, for persons with weak digestion or suffering from ailments, the above preparation is better.

Version C

The above two versions are soupy, whereas this version of Khichari is like rice. Take the same ingredients as in version A. Do not cook dal and rice in water but stir fry them in onions and spices instead. Add thrice the volume of water than the grains. Add boiling water after having stir-fried dal and rice for about two minutes in onions and spices. Cover and cook on low fire with the lid on. It is just like cooking basmati rice.

In case you wish to make this version with tomatoes, then cook dal and rice in thrice the quantity of water along with turmeric and salt. Briefly cook together

Beans and Lentils

with the Basic sauce or simply with onions and tomatoes. Remember that in sour medium, dal does not cook well. If the dal is not well cooked, it vitiates vata.

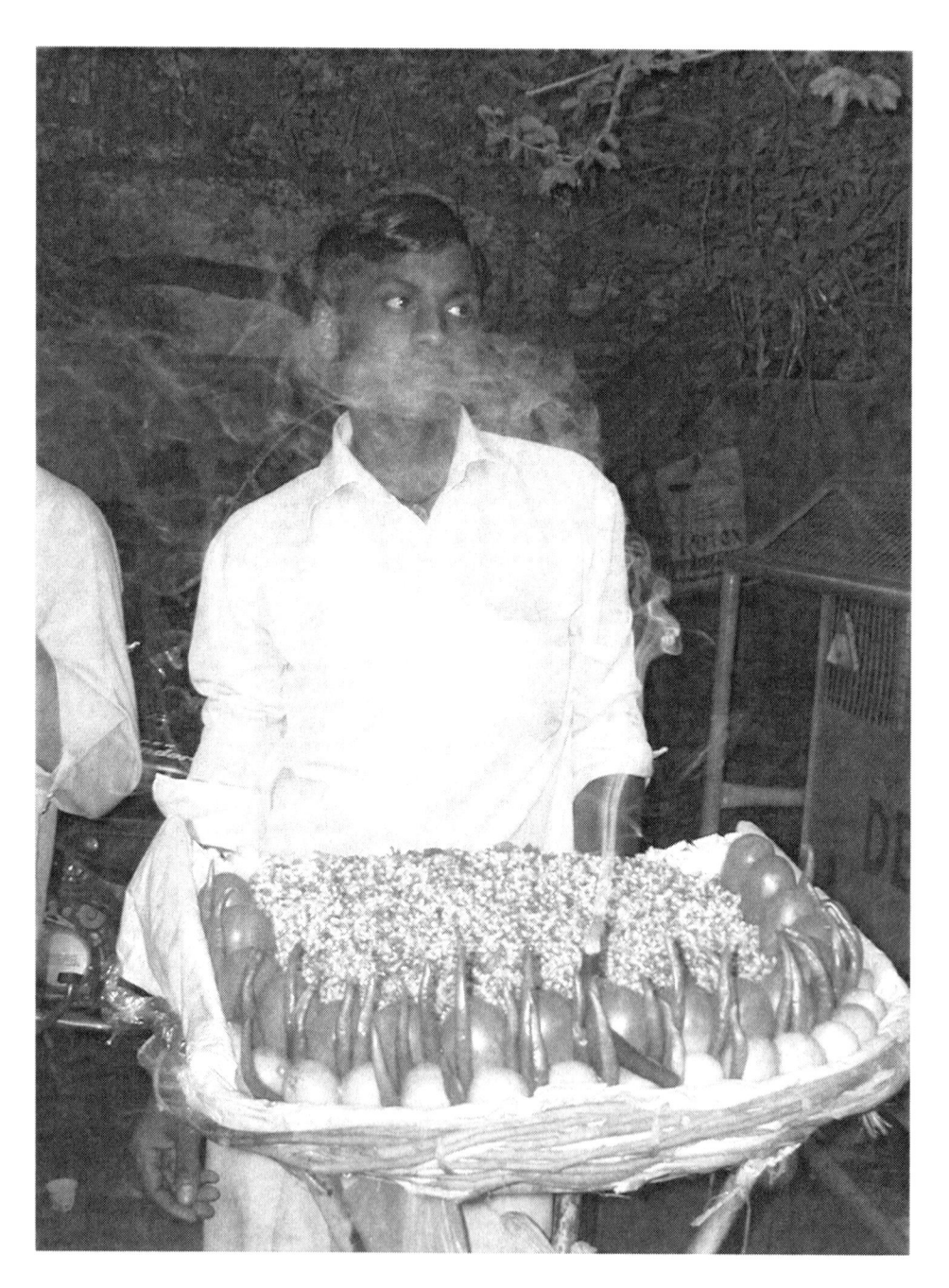

A baked beans vendor in Delhi

SMALL MEALS

There is an increasing need for the lighter and smaller meals, as our modern day lifestyle requires very little physical labour. I have given some recipes below but there are many others which can be used from the cheese and breads sections of the book. Filled breads with salads and vegetables very well make the small meals.

CURD-RICE

It is a southern Indian preparation and makes a very fine small meal for summer mornings. According to Ayurveda, yoghurt is nectar when eaten in the morning, good at noon and poison at night.

Ingredients for 2-3 persons:

Rice	100 gm (½ cup)
Yoghurt	400 gm (2 cups)
Sesame oil	2 tablespoons
Cumin	1 teaspoon
Mustard seeds	1 teaspoon
Salt	½ teaspoon or according to taste
Fresh coriander leaves (chopped)	1 tablespoon
Ajwain	½ teaspoon
Grated coconut	2 tablespoon
Pomegranate fruit	1

Wash and soak the rice and cook it in water as has been described earlier in the book. Put it on the side and let it cool. Heat oil in a pot and when it is very hot, add cumin and mustard seeds in it, reduce the fire and fry for about 20 seconds. Put off the heat and add grated coconut, salt, ajwain and coriander leaves immediately and stir. Mix all this with the rice. Separately, whip the yoghurt and prepare the pomegranate seeds. Add these two ingredients to the rice. Make sure that the rice is at room temperature. As I wrote in the beginning of this Section, yoghurt, when heated becomes hard to digest.

SEMOLINA WITH VEGETABLES (UPAMA)

It is a quick and easy to prepare small meal, it tastes very good and is light to digest.

Ingredients for 2-3 persons:

Semolina	100 gm (½ cup)
Chopped ginger	1 tablespoon
Paprika	2 medium sized
Carrots	2 medium sized
Green peas (tender)	3 tablespoons (optional)
Tomatoes	2 medium sized
Fresh ginger (chopped)	1 tablespoon
Green herbs (chopped)	1 tablespoon
Salt	½ to ¾ teaspoon
Cumin	1 teaspoon
Mustard seeds	½ teaspoon
Mixture F	1 teaspoon
Cooking oil	1 tablespoon

Cut paprika and tomatoes into small pieces but keep them separately. Grate the carrots. Heat the oil in a pot and add cumin and mustard seeds. Reduce the heat and add salt and rest of the spices including ginger. Fry for 20 seconds and add paprika, carrots and peas, and stir-fry. After about 5 minutes, add tomatoes and stir-fry another 5 minutes. Add semolina and stir everything together for about a minute. Add gradually thrice the quantity of water than semolina. You should always measure semolina to know about the exact quantity of water you will require. Keep stirring and bring it to boil. Reduce the fire very low and stir from time to time. Semolina will very quickly soak all the water and it is ready.

Note: You may use different vegetables of your choice. Use only tender green peas and not the over-ripped ones. You may add onions but if you are preparing this dish for breakfast, leave out the onions.

IDALY

Ingredients for 3-4 persons:

Urd dal	100 gm (½ cup)
Rice	200 gm

Wash and soak dal and rice separately over-night. Grind them in a wet grinder and then mix them together. Do not grind them too fine and add minimum water so that your batter is not fluid. It should be something between dough and batter. Leave the batter for another night at room temperature and next day you can use this batter for making idalies.

Idalies are cooked in vapour and you need to buy either a complete pot with treys or simply these treys. It is cheaper to buy only the treys and you can keep them in a tightly closed pot that can withhold the vapours. Many people make them in pressure cooker. The treys have a stand, small round moulds and holes for vapours. Smear the moulds with a little oil and put the dough in them after having prepared it with spices or vegetables as described below. The cooking time is 15 minutes.

Different versions of idalies:

Version A

Idalies can be made by simply adding a pinch of salt in the batter. In that case, you need some other accompaniment with them. For a small meal, you can have them with a preparation of mixed vegetables. You can have them simply with coconut chutney. In Southern India, they eat them with sambar (a preparation from arhar dal along with vegetables.

Version B

This is made by adding vegetables in the batter. In the above quantity of batter, add the following:

Carrots (grated)	2 medium sized
Paprika (finely chopped)	2 medium sized
Ginger (finely chopped)	2 tablespoons
Green herbs (finely chopped)	1 tablespoon
Cumin	1 teaspoon
Mixture F	2 teaspoons
Salt	½ teaspoon

Mix all these ingredients with batter and make the idalies as has been described above. You can serve them either with coconut chutney or roast them with very little oil or ghee on a non-stick pain. The reason to do this is that some amount of fat is essential with this meal. Otherwise it is hard to digest and body is unable to assimilate certain essential components from the vegetables.

Version C

You can make different variations. Add tender green peas instead of paprika. You can also make another version by adding tomatoes and mushrooms.

Small Meals

Version D

Chop some mixed green vegetables and stir-fry them with a little oil. Cook until tender and make sure that most water from them evaporates. Mix these into the idaly batter and make green idalies.

Uttapam (a vegetable pancake)

Uttapam is made with the same batter as idaly. The diiference is that uttapam is made on a pan with a liitle oil. It is made with different vegetables in it. Use the mixed vegetable recipe as in Version B for the idalies. Take a non-stick pan so that you are able to use minimum amount of oil. Use either sesame oil or ghee. Smear the non-stick pan with oil and when it is hot, flatten the batter with mixed vegetables on it. Reduce the heat after about 20 seconds so that it can cook slowly. After about a minute, turn it over and add a little oil once more. Make sure that both the sides are cooked golden brown.
Uttapam can be served with coconut chatani.

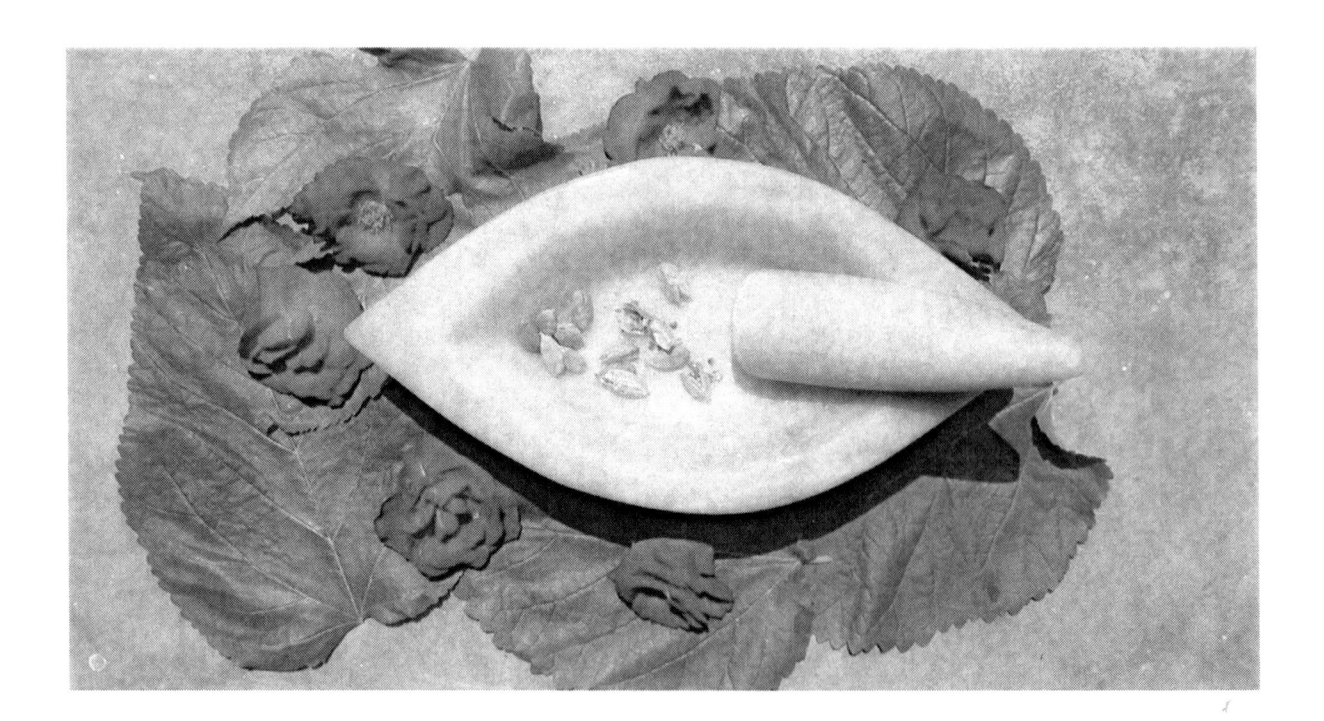

SIDE-DISHES

In this category you will find different preparations for yoghurt, chutneys from different herbs or fruits, pickles from fruits or vegetables and so on. The purpose of side dishes is to enhance the rasas in some main dishes or to pacify some of their extreme rasas.

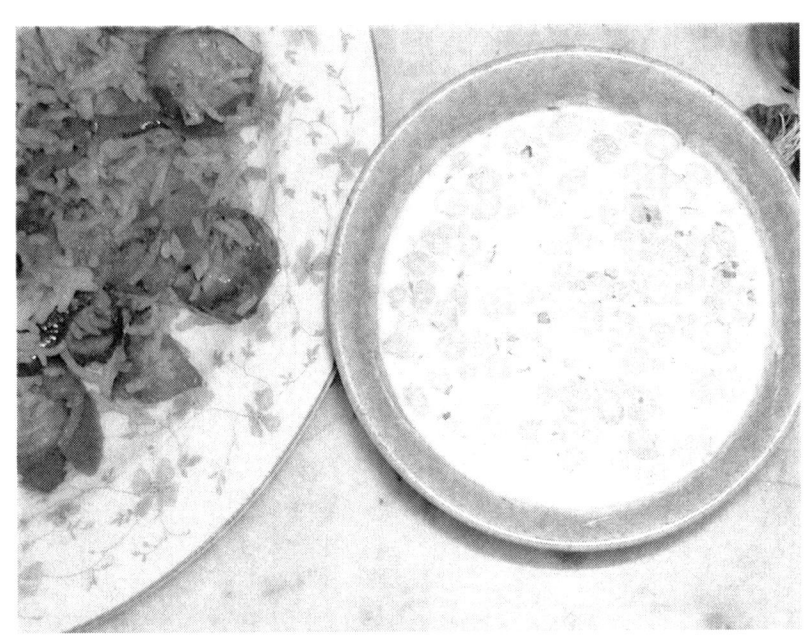

I recall a French young man's comment on Indian Food when I invited him over long ago in the seventies. Today, people in the West eat more spices but those days, the only spice in countryside in France was pepper and that too was used in molecular quantities. The young man from Cognac commented that the rayata in the meal we offered him worked as a fire extinguisher. It was a profound statement from the point of view of Ayurvedic pharmacology that came so naturally from him. So is the whole wisdom of Ayurveda, which is based upon cosmic phenomena.

Technically speaking, salads also come in this category but I have described them in a separate section. The reason for this is that the modern day human beings have very little physical work and they need lighter meals. The soups and salads make very good combinations and light meals. Salads have acquired more importance and are needed to simplify main courses.

RAYATAS

Rayatas are principally made of yoghurt (called curd in India) along with some vegetables or fruits and spices for flavouring. Sometimes nuts are also added. Rayatas are very simple to make and are an excellent side-dish for lunch. However, as said earlier, the yoghurt should not be eaten at night and thus, the rayatas should not be served for dinner.

Side-Dishes

Banana rayata

Ingredients:

For two portions you need:

Yoghurt	200 gm (1 cup)
Bananas	2 medium-sized
Salt	a pinch
Mixture H	½ teaspoon

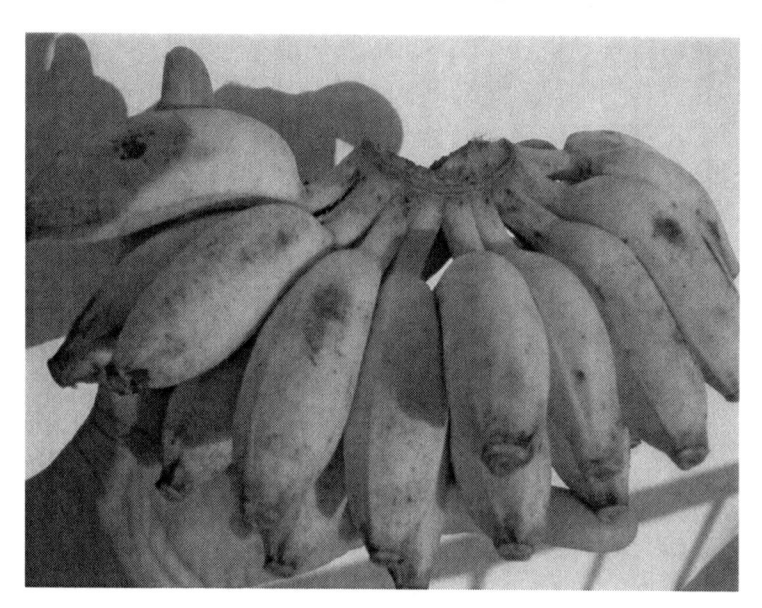

Whip the yoghurt after adding salt. Cut bananas into roundels and put into it. Stir with a spoon to mix well. Spread Mixture H on the top of the dish. Mix it just before serving.

Cucumber rayata

Version A

In this rayata, replace the banana with small pieces of cucumber. Take cucumber and yoghurt in equal parts. Add Mixture H and in addition some finely chopped fresh mint leaves.

Version B

Add some crushed peanuts to the above-described cucumber rayata. For 200 gm (1 cup) of yoghurt, add 50 gm (¼ cup) of crushed peanuts.

Ginger, onion and tomato rayata

Take yoghurt, whip it and add salt and Mixture H, as for the banana rayata. Add one small finely chopped onion, one medium-sized tomato and one tablespoon of fresh ginger pieces.

Courgette rayata

This rayata is made by adding grated courgette or lauki (big variety of a kind of courgette from India, see page 176) in yoghurt. The grated vegetable is cooked for about 10 minutes with the lid on. Keep the heat low and vegetable will cook in its own vapours. If there is too much water after cooking, drain it out by squeezing the vegetable a little. Add this vegetable in the yoghurt after it cools down. Whip it a little with a spoon. Add the spices as has been described for banana rayata.

CHUTNEYS

"Chutney" is the traditional British spelling which does not accurately reflect the actual pronunciation in Hindi. The proper pronunciation is more like "Chattani" where both 'a`s' are short (almost like "e") and the 'i' is long.

Chutneys are generally predominant in sour, hot and sweet rasas. They promote digestion by enhancing digestive fire.

Mango chutney

Mango chutney is famous all over the world. It is made from raw mangoes, principally from a variety called "pickle mangoes". Normally, the mangoes sold in Europe tend to be sour, and one can make this recipe from these. The mangoes for the chutney should be hard enough so that one can grate them. If you are unable to grate, chop them into small pieces.

Ingredients for 1 Kg (2 pounds) of fruit pulp:

Hard and raw mangoes or	2 kg (5 pounds)
Grated fruit pulp	1 kg (2 ½ cup)
Sugar	700 gm (3 ½ cup)
Cumin	1 ½ teaspoon
Salt	1 ½ teaspoon
Mixture A	2 tablespoons
Pepper	1 teaspoon
Dried dates	100 gm (½ cup)
Dried raisins	50 gm (¼ cup)

Side-Dishes

Nuts from pumpkin seeds	100 gm
Vinegar	2 tablespoons

Peel the mangoes and either grate them or chop the pulp into very small pieces. Remove the seeds. Add sugar in the proportion of 0.7 to 1. It is not possible to give you the exact weight of pulp obtained from 2 Kg of mangoes. Therefore, go by the weight of the sugar in proportion to the pulp.

Cook the pulp along with the sugar, salt, cumin and pepper on low heat and covered for about half an hour until it becomes thick like syrup. Stir from time to time.

Chop the dates, add together with the other dried fruits towards the end and cook for another five minutes. Let the preparation cool down, add the vinegar and stir well.

The chutney looks like a jam. Store in clean and dry bottles. The chutney will keep for several months in the refrigerator.

Mint chutney

Ingredients:

Fresh mint leaves:	200 gm (½ pound)
Onions	2 medium-sized
Salt	½ teaspoon
Mixture A	1 teaspoon
Green chilli	1 (optional)
Lemon juice	2 tablespoon
Or tamarind syrup	3 tablespoon
Raw sugar or jaggery	2 teaspoon

Wash the mint leaves well. Cut onions into small pieces. Put all the ingredients in a wet grinder and crush them fine. Mint chutney can be preserved in the refrigerator for 3-4 days.

Suggestions: You can also prepare chutney from coriander leaves in the same way. Coriander chutney has a more subtle flavour than the mint chutney.

Mixed herb chutney

You can mix different sorts of fresh herbs and to make chutney with the above recipe. Coriander leaves, dill leaves, parsley, chive etc. can be all mixed together to make chutney.

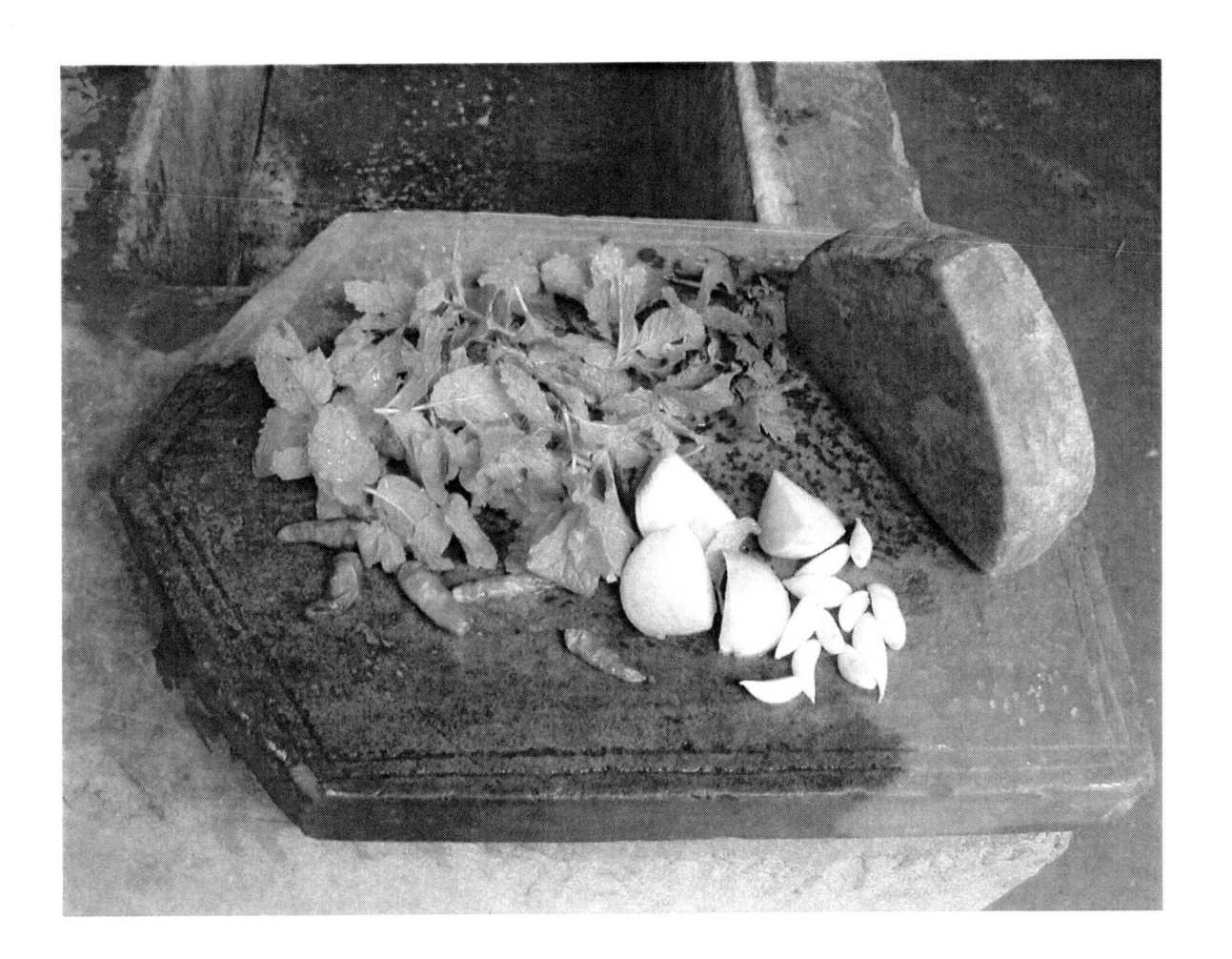

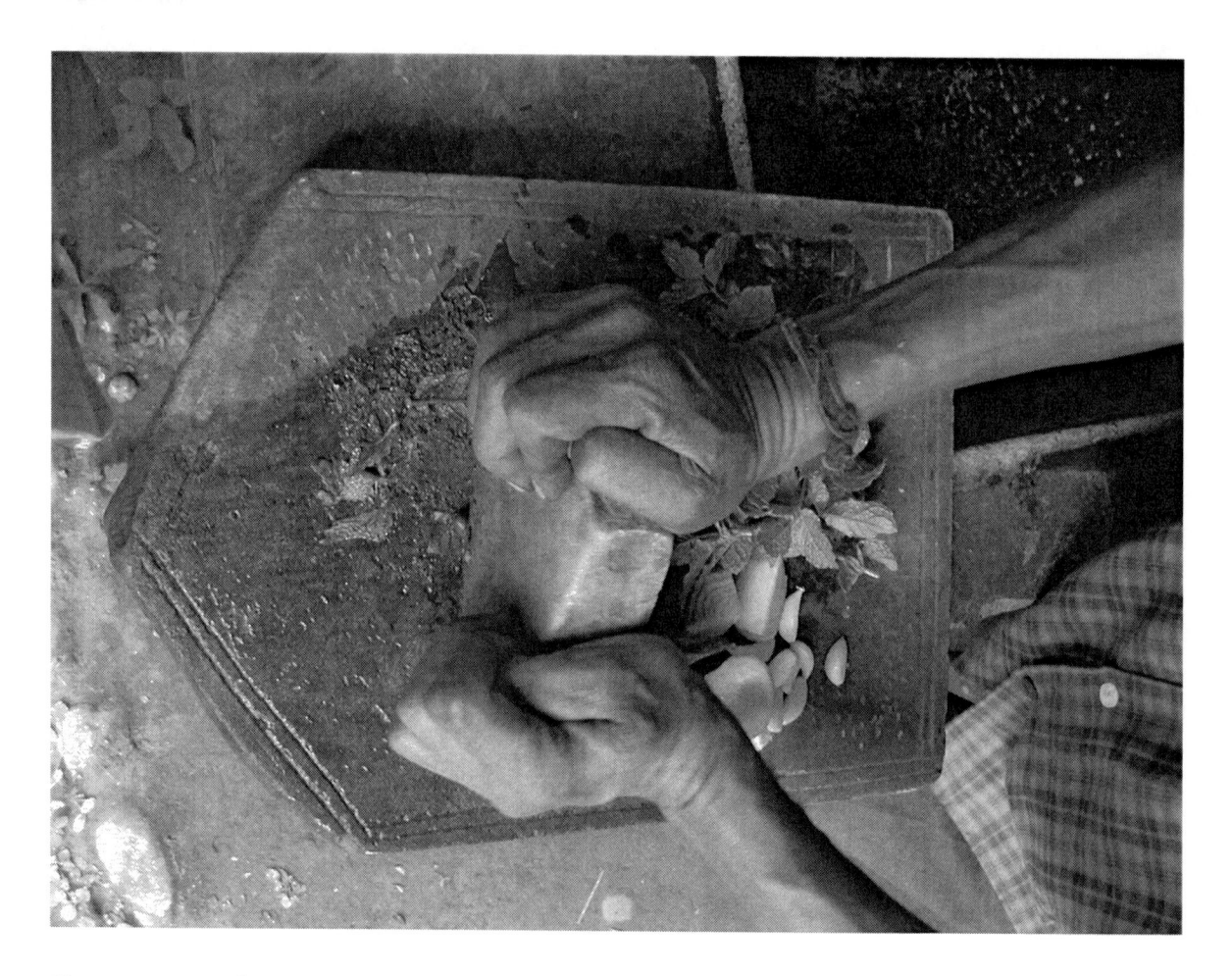

Coconut chutney

This is a delicious and very refreshing chutney made of fresh coconut. If you do not have fresh coconut, take very finely grated dried coconut, which is also available abroad.

Ingredients:

Grated coconut   5 tablespoons
Chopped onion   1 medium-sized
Chopped ginger   3 tablespoons
Lemon juice   4 tablespoons
Salt   1 teaspoon
Cooking oil   1 teaspoon
Mustard seeds   1 teaspoon
Urd dal   2 teaspoons
Green chilli   1

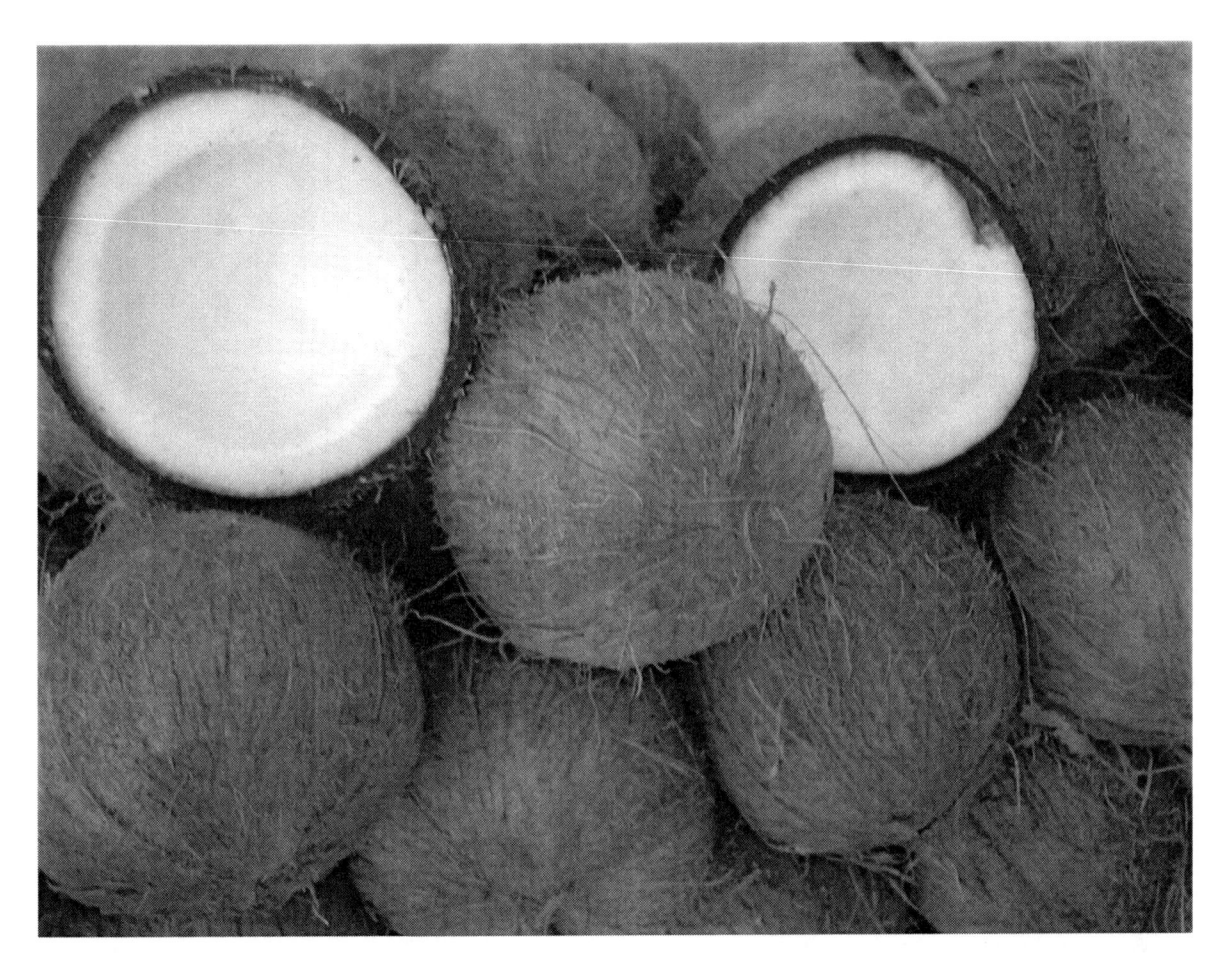

Mix coconut, onion, ginger, green chilli, salt and lemon juice in the blender and make a purée. Add 5-10 tablespoons of water to get the appropriate consistency. Dried coconut needs more water than the fresh. Separately, heat the cooking oil. When the oil is very hot and fuming, add into it the mustard seeds and immediately after add dal. Stir and cook for a minute and then add the contents of the blender into it. Cook for another minute while stirring. Put off the heat and let the chutney cool down. It is served at room temperature.

PICKLES

Pickles are basically a way of preserving vegetables with salt, spices and some sour substances like vinegar or lemon juice. It is good to know some methods of preservation which were used in ancient times and were without the harmful preservatives used in the modern food technology.

Side-Dishes

Ginger pickle

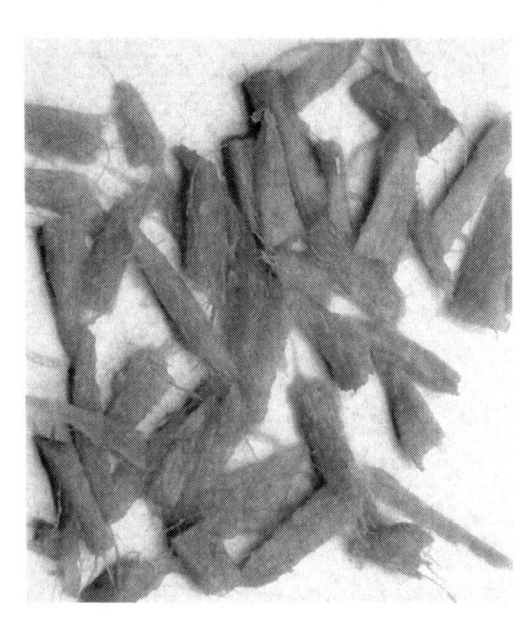

It is the simplest pickle and the preservation time is about a week. It is of great medicinal value and therefore it is important to describe it here. It is beneficial for those who have lack of appetite or slow and partial digestion.

Ingredients:

Ginger	200 gm (½ pound)
Lemon juice	50 ml (¼ cup)
Rock salt	1 tablespoon

Peel and cut the ginger into thin and elongated pieces. Put them in a glass bottle. Put salt and lemon juice, close the bottle tightly and shake it so that all the ingredients mix well together. Leave it like this over-night. The ginger pieces will turn pink. The pickle is ready.

Lemon pickle

This is another pickle that has great medicinal value. After a heavy meal, in case of indigestion or a feeling of heaviness, this pickle is very beneficial. It is also a good cure for mountain sickness and other symptoms arising due to height, like dry throat and restlessness.

Ingredients:

Lemons	½ kilo (1 pound)
Mixture E	2 tablespoon
Ajwain	50 gm (¼ cup)
Salt	2 tablespoon
Sugar	300 gm (1 ½ cup)
Vinegar	300 ml (1 ½ cup)

Take small, organically grown lemons with thin peels. Soak them in water for a few hours and then dry them, if possible in the sun. Cut into four pieces each and put in a clean and dry glass jar that can be closed tightly. Add mixture E and salt and shake the jar after closing it or stir with a wooden spoon. Mix half the sugar into half the quantity of vinegar, pour into the jar and mix again. Close the lid properly and keep in a sunny place. Shake from time to time. It will take several months for the pickle to 'ripe'. After about a month, dissolve the other half of the sugar into the rest of the vinegar and add into the jar. Shake well again. After about 3 months, one can eat this pickle but it is still hard. If you see during this time that the lemons have absorbed all the fluid and look 'dry', add some more vinegar and sugar as you did before.

This pickle practically keeps forever. It will dry up after some time but its medicinal value remains intact. In fact, if it dries out completely, one can grind it and use that powder to promote appetite and to cure indigestion.

Mixed vegetable pickle

This recipe is generally made with carrots, turnips and cauliflower. However, if you wish, you can use only two or even one of the vegetables.

Ingredients:

Chopped vegetables	1 Kg (2 pounds)
Onions	4 medium-sized
Garlic	1 medium-sized
Cooking oil	5 tablespoons
Salt	1 tablespoon
Mixture A	2 tablespoons
Red chilli powder	1 teaspoon (optional)
Vinegar	200 ml (1 cup)
Jaggery or raw sugar	300 gm (1 ½ cup)

Wash, peel and cut the vegetables. Cut the turnips into roundels, cauliflower in small pieces and carrots in finger-shaped pieces and so forth. Boil two litres of water in a big pot and put all the vegetables into the boiling water. Boil only for 1 to 2 minutes and put everything in a big strainer to take the water out. Spread the vegetables on a towel so that they can dry or put them in sun for half an hour if possible.

Side-Dishes

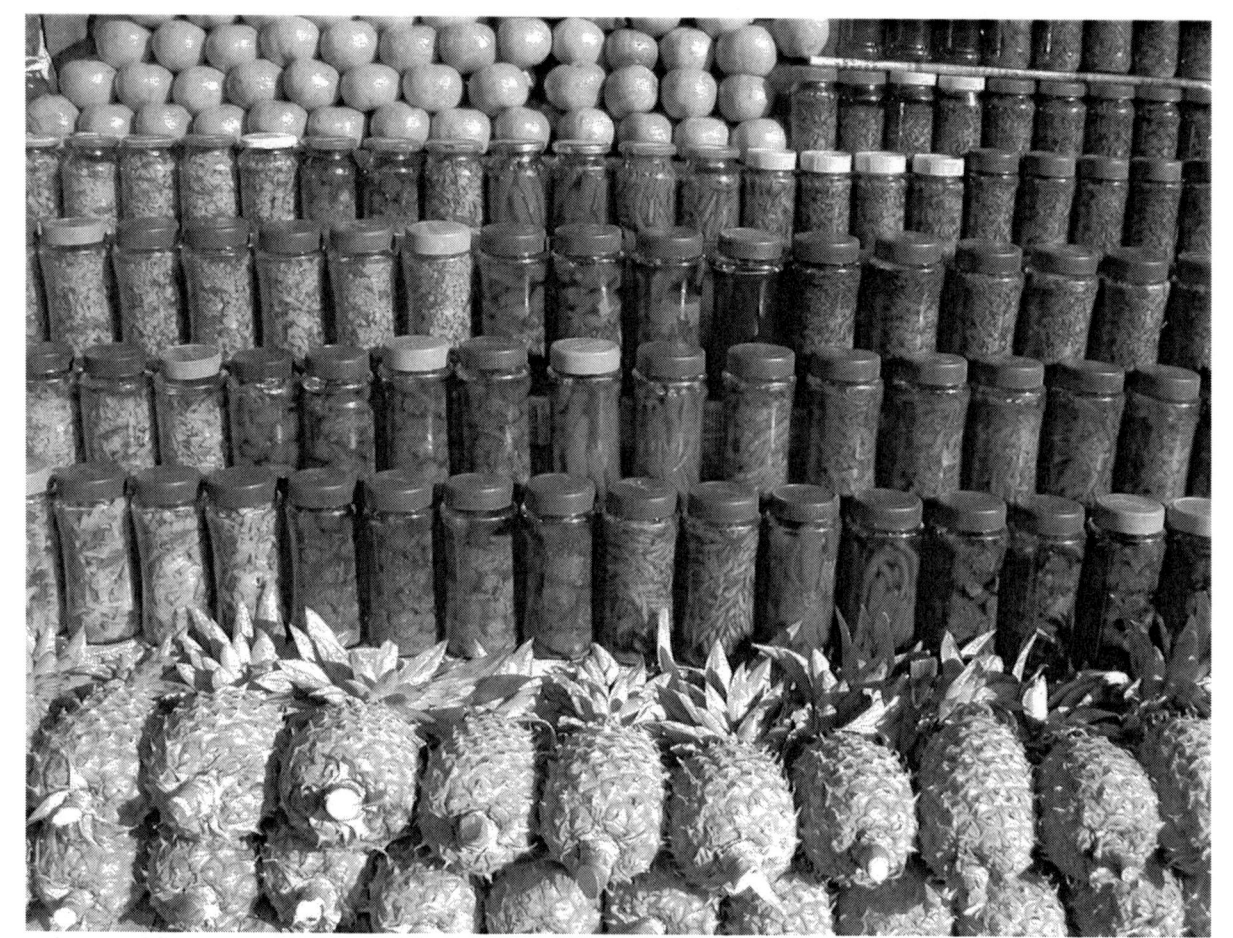

A shop of local pickles and fruits in Meghalaya (east of India). East is particularly famous for bamboo pickles.

Crush or mash the onions and the garlic separately. Fry the onions in the oil and when they are sauté, add the spices and the salt. Fry a little and add vegetables. Make sure your vegetables are completely dry by that time. Stir-fry the vegetables for about 5 minutes and add the crushed garlic towards the end. Let the vegetables cool down. Dissolve jaggery into vinegar and add in the fried vegetables. Mix well and put in a clean and dried glass jar that can be closed tightly. Put the jar in a sunny place and mix the contents from time to time by shaking the jar. This pickle is ready in a week's time. You may have to add a little vinegar later. This pickle can be preserved for several months without refrigeration but you have to be very careful not to open the pickle jar again and again. Rather fill the pickle into smaller bottle for everyday use. In humid climates, it may get fungus.

DESSERTS

According to the Ayurvedic principles, one should finish main meals with something sweet. However, heavy desserts made of flour, rice or other grains are not recommended. Light desserts made of fruits, paneer or nuts with jaggery are recommended in small quantities. If you wish to have a dessert made of rice or wheat, make sure that you do not have the grains (rice, wheat, millet etc.) in the main meal. Keep the main meal light to leave space for a copious dessert. Remember always the principle that the stomach should not be more than two thirds full.

MIXED FRUIT DESSERT

There are several ways of making mixed fruit salad. **Fruit-cream** is made by adding a little cream and sugar to the fruits. Take care that you do not add any sour fruit in this, as milk and cream are antagonist to sour.

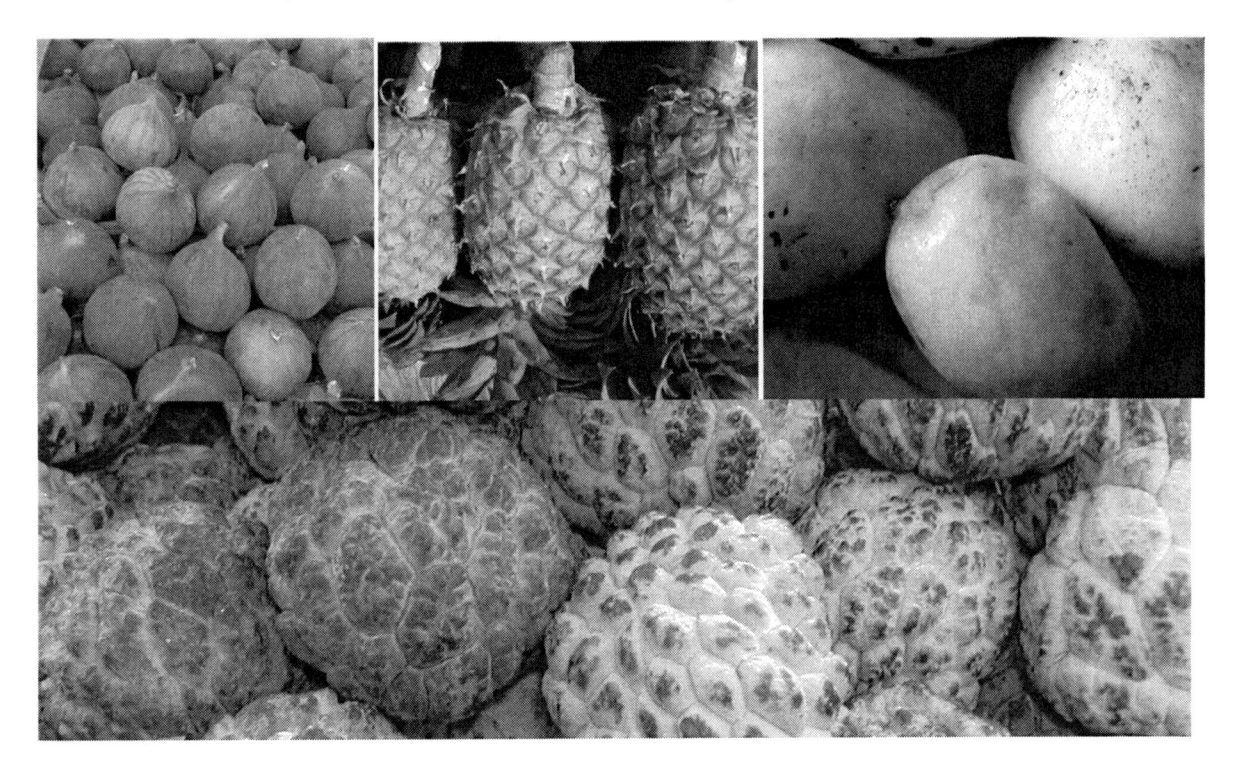

In **mixed-fruit dessert**, one can also add some dry fruits like raisins, almonds, grated coconut and so on. If the fruits are sour and not sweet enough, add a teaspoon or two of honey. A little bit of almond alcohol (Amaretto) gives nice flavour to this kind of fruit dessert.

Desserts

Another idea is to make a **mixed-fruit** dessert with **Mixture F and lemon**. This dessert is particularly good after a heavy meal as sour of the lemon and mixture F help digestion. For four bowls of mixed fruits, you need to add a teaspoon of Mixture F and two tablespoons of lemon juice. Adjust these quantities according to your taste.

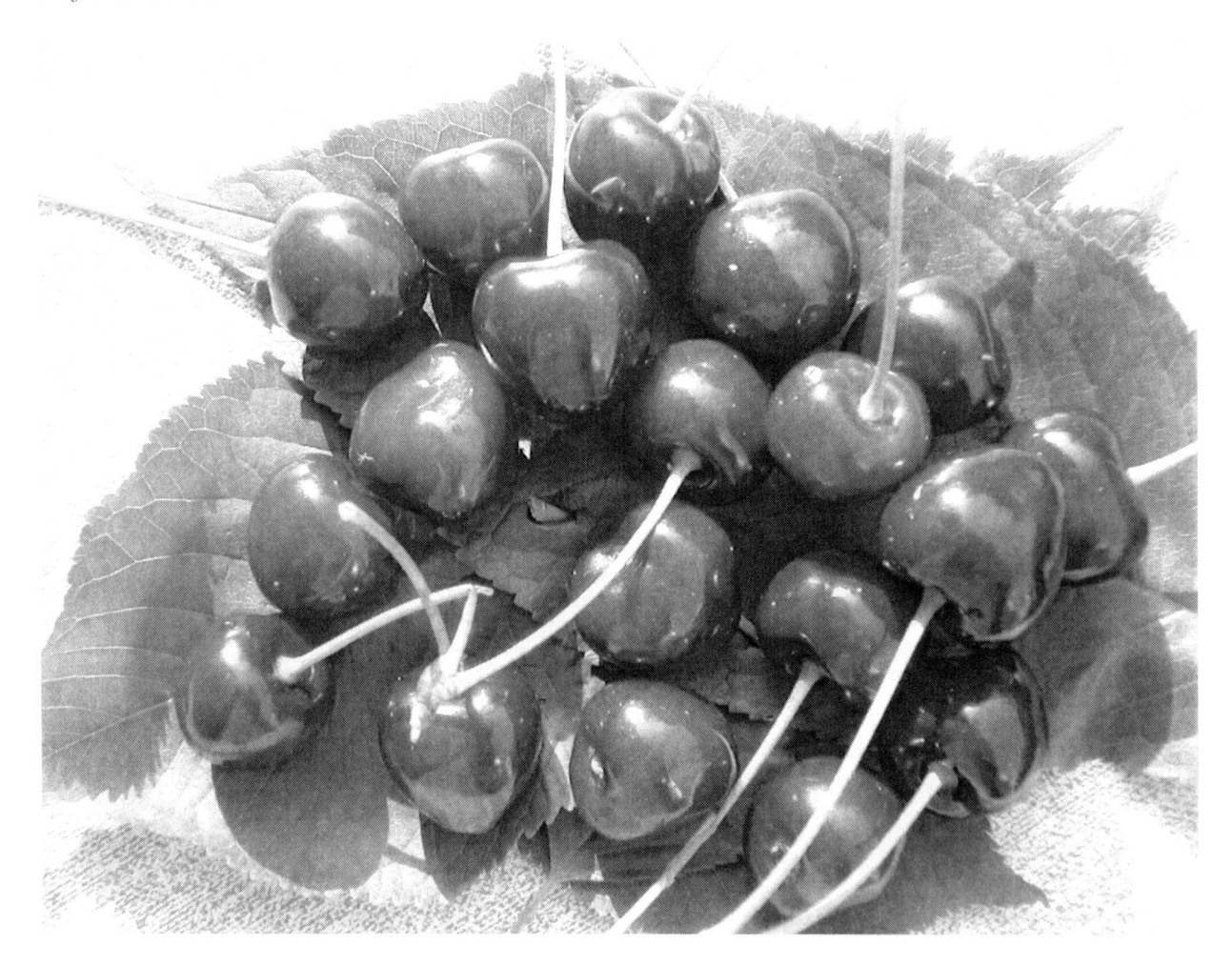

STRAWBERRY AND BASIL DESSERT

This is a simple dessert recipe for strawberry season. Most people add cream and sugar to the strawberries, which make them a rather rich dessert. But this recipe promotes digestion and is refreshing.

Ingredients:

For 3-4 portions you need:

Sweet strawberries	250 gm (½ pound)
Red wine vinegar*	1 teaspoon
Honey	1 tablespoon
Basil leaves (finely chopped)	1 tablespoon
Pepper	a pinch

Cut each strawberry into 4 pieces. Put a teaspoon of vinegar and a tablespoon of honey over the fruit. Let the fruit stay for about 15 minutes. Add chopped basil leaves and some black pepper. Mix all the ingredients well. Decorate the dessert with some basil leaves when you serve.

SUJI (SEMOLINA) HALWA

Semolina halwa is another version of the semolina recipe described for breakfast. It is very quick and simple to prepare.

Ingredients:

For 3-4 portions you need:

Semolina	100 gm (½ cup)
Sugar	50 gm (¼ cup)
Ghee	2 tablespoon
Cardamom	3
Almonds cut into small pieces	2 tablespoons
Pistachio nuts (finely chopped)	1 tablespoon

Fry semolina in ghee for about 2-3 minutes. Separately, heat about 200 ml (1 cup) water and add sugar and crushed cardamoms without the pods and let this cook for 7-8 minutes. Add this into the fried semolina and keep stirring. Add almonds while you are stirring the halwa. Cooking time after the addition of the syrup is about 2-3 minutes. Put some pistachio nuts on the top and serve hot.

---

* The quality of the vinegar is very important in this dessert. In Europe, you can use Balsamico, which is an exclusive Italian vinegar. But you can also take any very good quality red wine vinegar or dark sugar-cane vinegar. In India, Jamun vinegar should be used for this purpose.

Desserts

CARROT HALWA

This is similar to the recipe given in the breakfast section. For dessert, our halwa is slightly different; it is richer and takes longer to cook.

Ingredients:

For 3-4 portions you require:

Carrots	5-6 medium-sized
Milk	1 litre (5 cups)
Sugar	100 gm (half cup)
Cardamom	5
Almonds (chopped)	2 tablespoons
Cashew nuts (chopped)	50 gm (2 ounces)
Raisins (sweet)	2 tablespoons

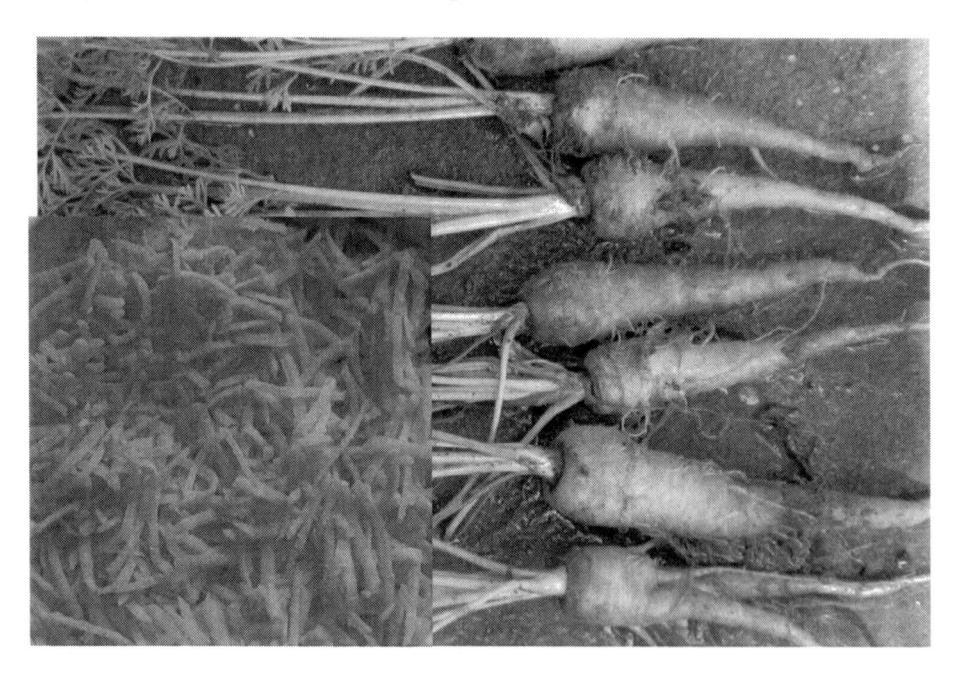

Peel and grate the carrots. Cook them with few tablespoons of water and cardamom. Cardamoms should be taken out from the pods and crushed. Cover and cook on low heat for about half an hour and keep stirring from time to time. If the carrots are sticking to the surface, add a little more water.

Separately, boil milk in a wok and let it simmer on low heat. Stir from time to time. Cook until the milk is reduced to one fourth of its original volume. Put the cooked carrots in the reduced milk and add sugar. Keep cooking while stirring until most of the water is evaporated and the preparation becomes a little solid. Add raisins and almonds and cook for another five minutes. Serve hot or let it cool down so that it can be cut into pieces. Decorate with cashew nuts. To reduce the preparation time, you may use cream instead of milk.

SAFFRON KHIR

Like halwa, kheer is a general term denoting a preparation of grains cooked with milk and sugar and later nuts are added into it. When only the word kheer is used, it generally refers to a preparation with rice.

Ingredients:

For 5-6 portions, you require:

Basmati rice	100 gm (½ cup)
Milk	1 litre (5 cups)
Sugar	100 gm (½ cup)
Saffron	250 mg (a pinch)
Almonds	50 gm (2 ounces)
Raisins (sweet)	30 gm (1 ounce)

Wash and soak the basmati rice and cook it in 2½ times their volume of water. When the rice is cooked, put it in a wok and cook in half the milk. Keep the heat very low. Stir from time to time and when the preparation is thick, add rest of the milk and sugar. Stir well and continue to cook. This kind of khir needs to cook for several hours. By the end, the rice becomes almost homogeneous with milk. Add saffron, chopped almonds and raisins and cook for another 5 minutes. Stir well so that the saffron dissolves completely. Khir can be served hot or cold.

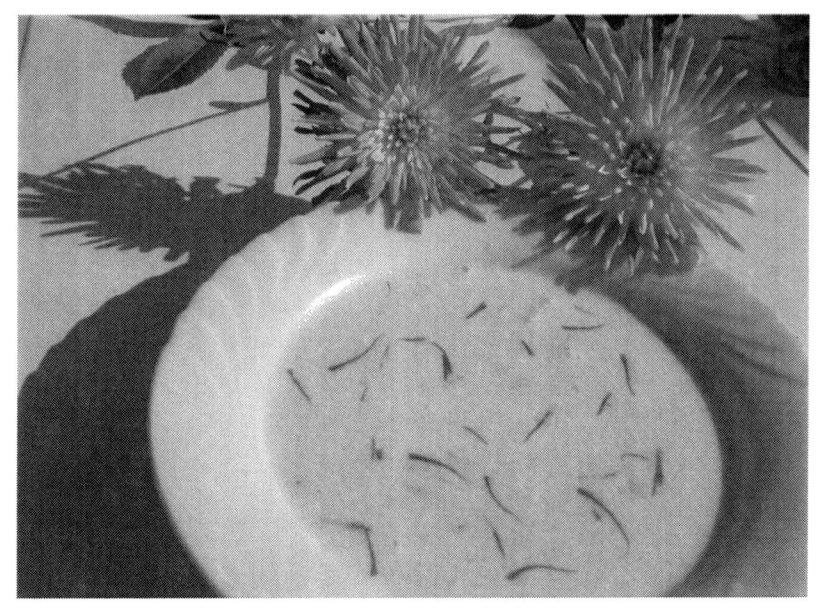

Desserts

SUJI (SEMOLINA) KHIR

Semolina khir is very quick to prepare and it is light. You can make it with saffron as above or with cardamom.

Ingredients:

For 3-4 portions, you require:

Semolina	50 gm (¼ cup)
Ghee	1 tablespoon
Milk	500 ml (2 ½ cup)
Sugar	4-5 tablespoons
Cardamom	4
Almonds	50 gm (2 ounces)
Raisins	25 gm (1 ounce)

Heat ghee in a pan or wok and fry semolina. When the semolina is slightly brown, add about 100 ml (½ cup) water, bring it to boil and add crushed cardamoms. Before the semolina has soaked up all the water, add milk and sugar and stir. Cook on low fire for another 5 minutes and add almonds and raisin. Cook another 2-3 minutes and serve hot.
Note: Wherever the ghee is used for cooking, the preparation is generally served hot. It may also be served at room temperature. It is advised not to drink anything cold with preparations containing ghee. If you wish to drink something along with a dessert that includes ghee, the accompanying drink should be hot.

PHIRANI

Phirani is made from the wheat extract that is taken out from the germinated wheat as described earlier in the breakfast section.

Ingredients:

For 2-3 portions, you require:

Wheat extract	200 ml (1 cup)
Ghee	1 tablespoon
Cardamom	4
Sugar	3 tablespoons
Almonds (chopped)	2 tablespoons
Pistachio nuts (chopped)	1 tablespoon
Cashew nuts (chopped)	1 tablespoon

Stir-fry the wheat extract in heated ghee for about 10 minutes and add the crushed cardamoms without pods. Although the wheat extract is liquid, one needs to stir it because it is not homogeneous. Its solid contents tend to settle down at the bottom and burn. Add sugar and almonds and cook for another 2-3 minutes while stirring. Phirani can be served hot or at room temperature. Decorate with pistachio nuts and cashew nuts before serving.

CHENA MITHAI

This dessert is made from paneer. Chena is another name for paneer and mithai means sweet dish.

Ingredients:

For 3-4 portions, you require:

Paneer	from 1 Litre (5 cups) milk
Ghee	1 tablespoon
Sugar	4 tablespoons
Almonds (chopped)	5 tablespoons
Saffron	250 mg (a pinch)

Take out the whey from the paneer and crush the paneer between two flat wooden spoons or between your palms. Palms do a better job than the wooden spoons. Heat the ghee in a pot and stir-fry this paneer for about 5 minutes on low heat. Add sugar and fry for another 5 minutes on medium fire. Add almonds and saffron and continue cooking for 2-3 minutes more.

Put the contents on a plate and make them flat and round. When it cools down, it can be cut into small pieces. Serve at room temperature.

Desserts

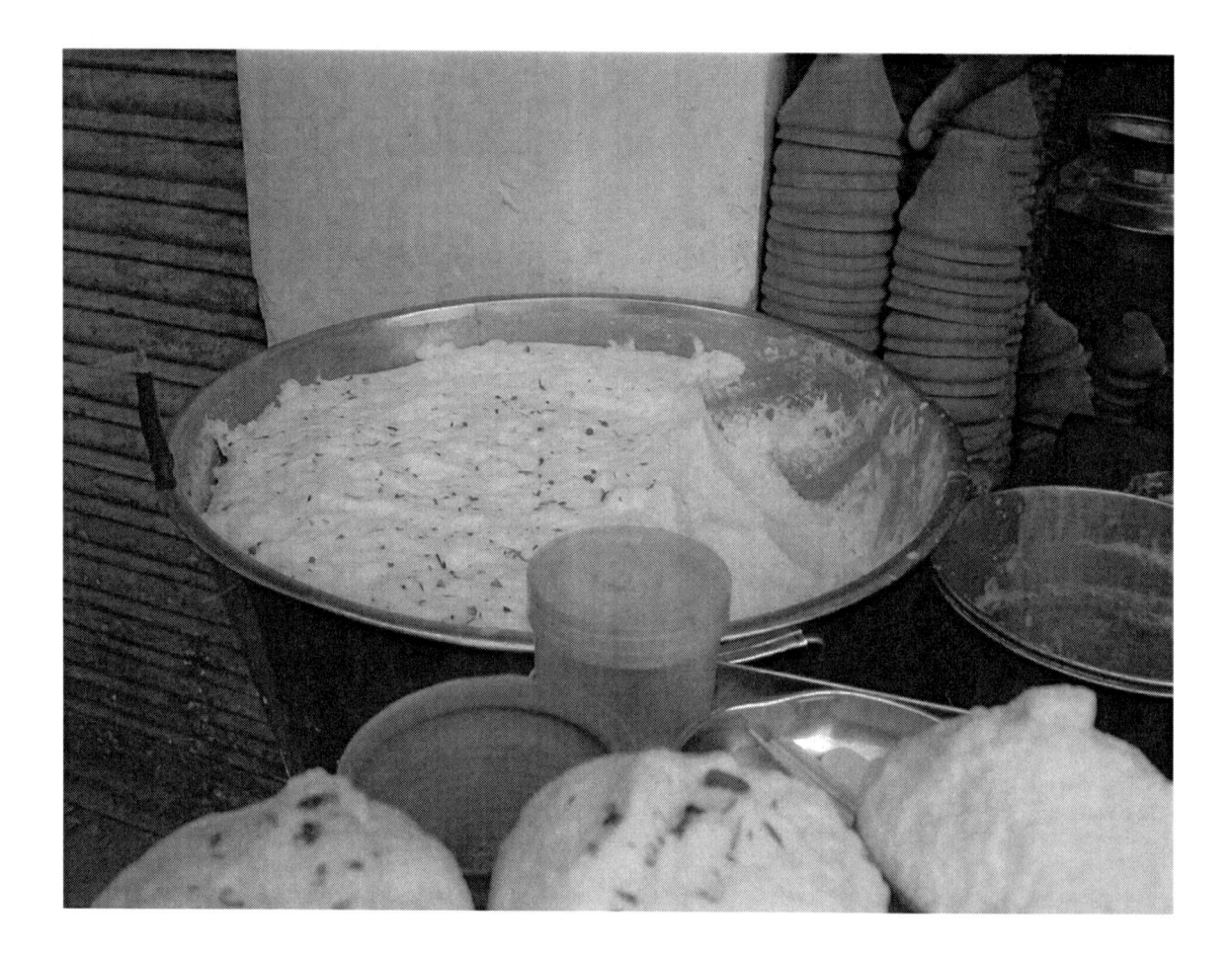

CHOCOLATE

Chocolate is loved the world over. It is stimulating due to the presence of theobromine and caffeine. There are so many delicious preparations of the chocolate specially in Switzerland, Belgium and France. It makes a very good dessert when taken in a reasonable quantity. Chocolate is made of cacao beans and to balance its bitter taste sugar is added. You can end your meal with a moderate quantity of chocolate of your liking. I suggest about 35 gm maximum for one time dessert.

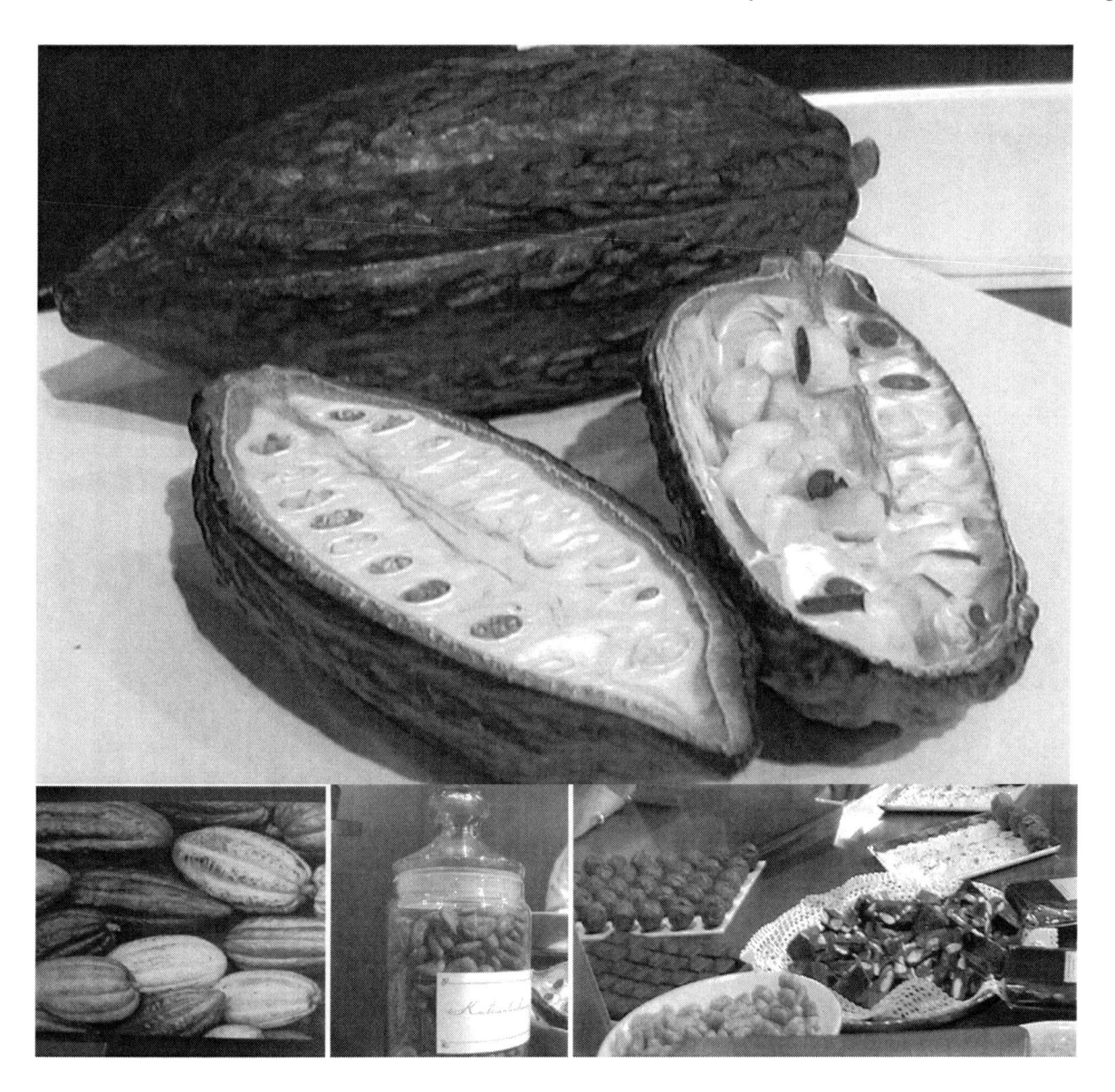

Ayurvedic Food Culture and Recipes

Desserts

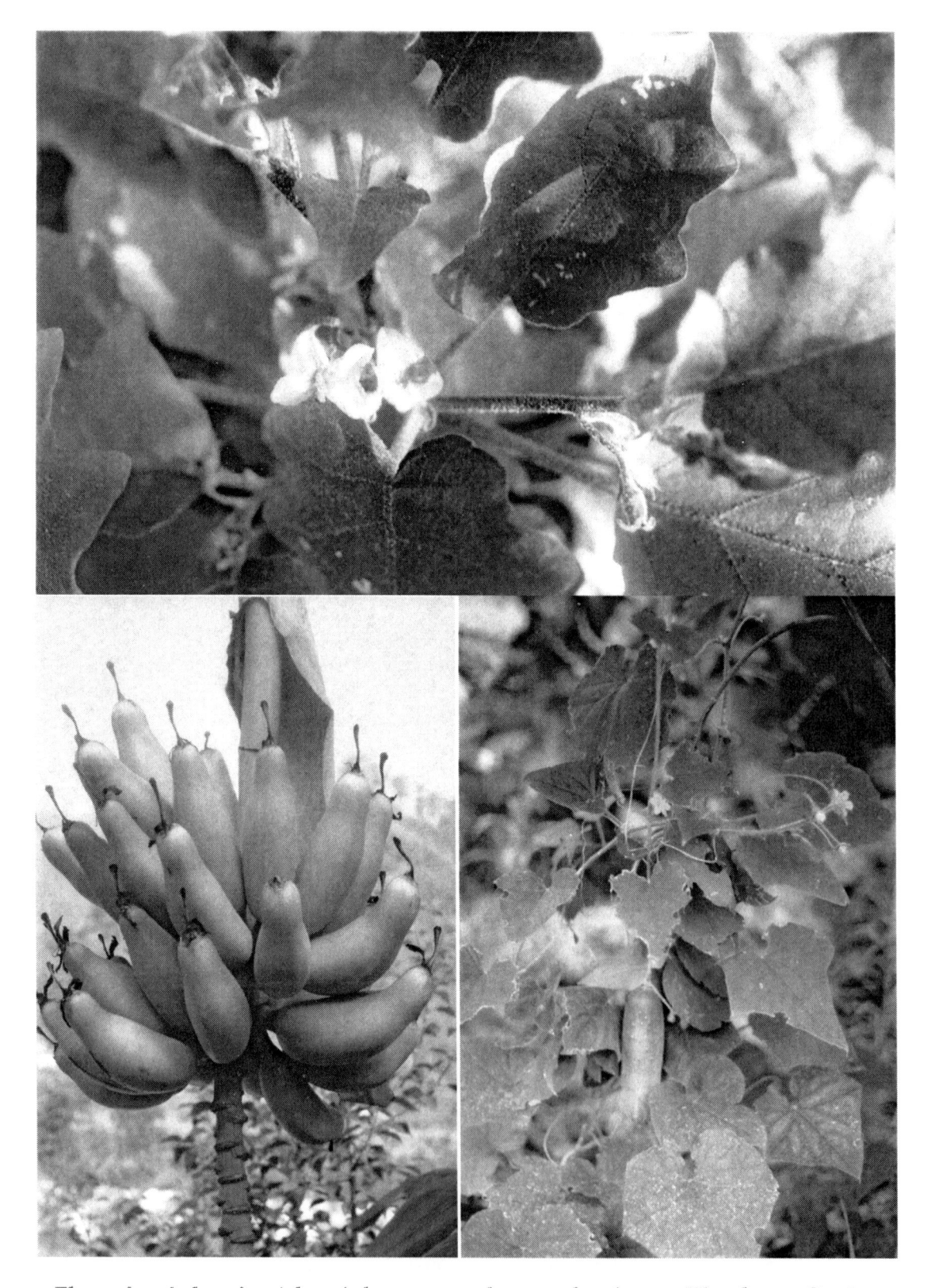

Flowering Aubergine (above), bananas and cucumber in our Himalayan Centre

APPENDIX

There are two reasons for me to write this chapter. First, there are many aspects of Ayurvedic food culture, which are either not considered significant enough or are thought to be universally 'understood', but in realty are ignored. Ayurveda lays great stress on some of these factors. Eating food while under stress or amidst unpleasant environment, over a certain period of time, may cause stomach ulcers. Then, at times people are in dilemma about what type of products they should buy as there are hundreds of brands in the market even of simple, everyday food like milk, butter, curd, cooking oil etc. The same is true for commonplace things like salt and sugar.

Second, under the name of Ayurveda, there is a lot of misinformation disseminated by charlatans and self-appointed gurus. I am aware of this through my students who quote these 'Ayurvedic prescriptions', if actually applied, would do more harm than good.

Ayurveda is much more complex than modern medicine, since in addition to preventing and curing ailments, it deals with every other aspect of life. The meaning of the word *Ayurveda* (science of life) itself suggests that. It includes cosmic philosophy, social behaviour, the environment and all other aspects of the human existence besides therapeutics. Sages say that one life is not enough to learn all about Ayurveda. Therefore, it is not possible to 'learn' Ayurveda by attending a few seminars or to study it for a brief period and then trying to be a doctor or adviser in this field. Taking all this into consideration, I have made a list of the most frequently asked questions (FAQ) about Ayurveda. Besides questions regarding erroneous information, I have also dealt with some of those aspects which many have difficulty in understanding. Along with this, I have provided information on vegetarianism from the point of view of Ayurveda.

Eating according to *Desha* and *Kala*

I have discussed about the relationship of time (ka*la*) and space (*desha*) to our nutrition. I will now dwell on two specific themes. The concepts of the five elements, the three energies, prakriti, vikriti, rasa theory etc. constitute the basic and eternal wisdom of Ayurveda, which is not bound to space and time. However, food and medicine are bound by space and time. According to the different geographical locations of the world, the vegetation and the availability of the nutrients vary. By applying the principles of rasa theory, we can use different products for making balanced nutrition and various remedies. For example, something bitter is good for taking excessive heat out from the body.

Appendix

Different plants in various parts of the world provide the bitter rasa. A person living in southern India or in Europe does not have to go to the Himalayan Mountains to get a particular plant. Nature provides us with all the rasas in our surroundings.

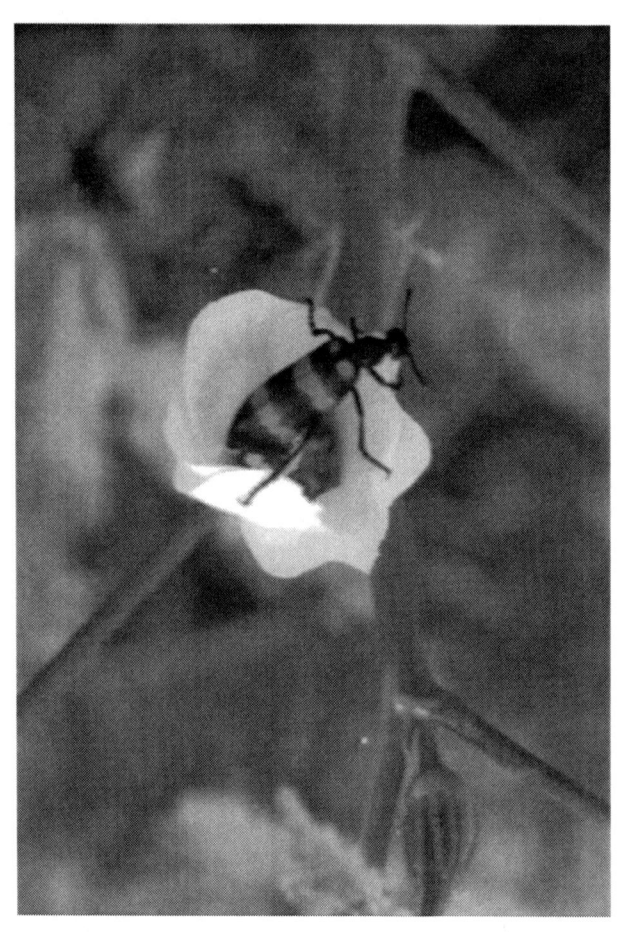

I have observed that people from Europe go to southern India or Sri Lanka to learn Ayurvedic wisdom and then come back with fixed ideas, which are not suitable in the cold climate at home. The application of coconut oil on the head, eating rice with every meal and some other cold nutrients are some of the examples I come across fre-quently. In a cold climate, it is better to use sesame oil for the head massage than coconut. Rice is cold in nature, and in cold countries it should not be eaten too frequently. I have already mentioned that one should avoid eating rice in winter for dinner. If you wish to benefit from the Ayurvedic wisdom for good health and harmony in your daily life, you should use understanding and judgement to avoid such mistakes.

Okara Flower

Obesity is in one way also related to *kala* or time. In former times, people did an enormous amount of physical labour, and their eating habits were formed accordingly. Now, the amount of physical work most people do has decreased considerably. Yet, eating habits have not changed accordingly or, in Ayurvedic terms, people no longer live according to *kala*. On the contrary, it has become a norm to eat too much and then to go for a work out in a gym. However, working towards the fundamental equilibrium of the body is something entirely different.

You should follow a diet which is in accordance with the nature of your work. Going for a walk twice a day and doing yoga exercises regularly is recommended. If you stick to the principles of Ayurveda you are not likely to become overweight: never fill your stomach more than two thirds with all the solids and liquids, never eat before the previous meal is digested, never eat between meals and leave two hours between going to bed and dinner.*

Many diets for losing weight may actually create an imbalance of the three energies, thus leading to various ailments. I have seen people eating only spinach or only pineapple for several days to lose weight. Such diets can be dangerous for the digestive fire (agni) of the body and may cause ailments. Dieting without fat is also very harmful, because it leads to vata imbalance and related disorders like dry skin, rough appearance, disturbed sleep or constipation and so on. Similarly, fasting also gives rise to vata related disorders. Therefore, if you wish to reduce weight, do it very gradually by altering your diet and eating less. Do not shock your system by losing weight suddenly. Think about your diet carefully, and never eat or munch things habitually. You should develop a control over your senses. That is what yoga teaches us.

In the United States, you often hear: **All good things in life are either illegal, immoral or fattening.** I tried to analyse this saying and reached the conclusion that it is not true. In fact, this statement is just another way of saying that people lack the wisdom of controlling their senses. The moment people think something is good, they want it in excess and later they suffer, so societies have always tended to prohibit such things or at least tax them. **Remember that excess of all that is good is bad.**

Calmness and Aesthetics

According to the Ayurvedic principles, the modern concept of fast foods is detrimental to health. Food should never be consumed in a hurry or while standing. You should sit down properly and bring your mind to a calm and quiet state. This is neither difficult nor does it take long. One just has to take a few deep breaths or say a short prayer.

Food should be prepared and served in a manner that it is appealing to the eyes and the heart. In my cooking classes in Europe, whenever I showed the preparation of mixed vegetables or vegetable rice, students invariably commented that the food looked beautiful. Obviously it looks more appealing than a piece of fried pork with french-fries. Vegetables and fruits contain different rasas, and with a variety of fresh things in a meal, you can prepare meals, which not only look good but are also rejuvenating.

---

* For more details of this theme, see my book *Losing and Maintaining Weight with Ayurveda and Yoga*, 2007, Gayatri Books International, available at www.amazon.com

Appendix

Serving on nice plates and in an aesthetic way is also very important. In Southern India, the food is sometimes served on banana leaves, which is both simple and beautiful. The idea is not that you buy the most expensive plates available, but to choose soothing colours and designs for your kitchenware.

Holistic and Organic Products

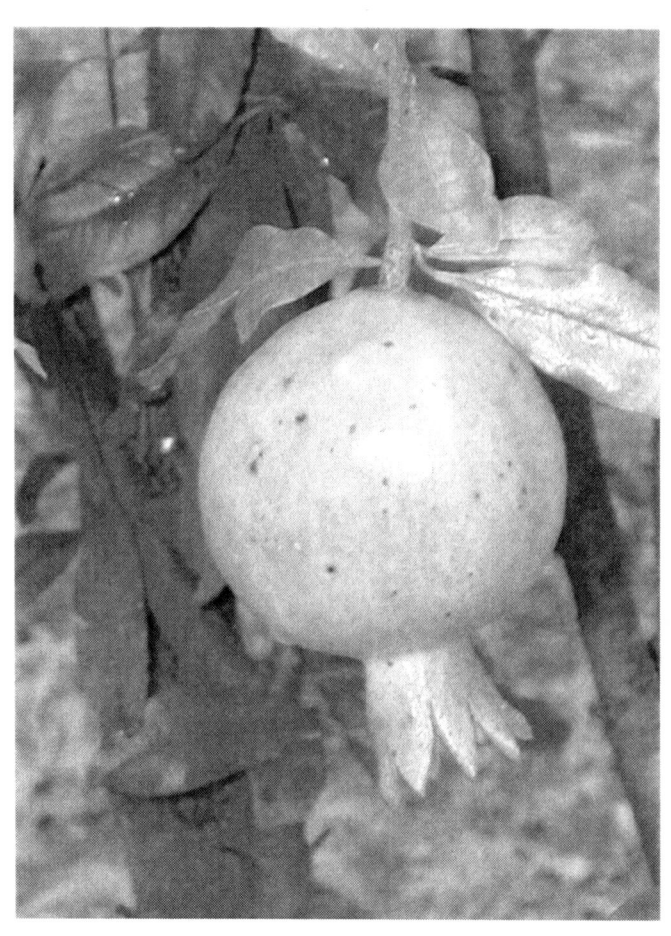

As I have mentioned earlier, it is advisable that you consume less food and use only wholesome products. It is recommended to eat organically grown food and no fat-free dairy products, synthetic sweeteners or other food replacements. With so many synthetic fertilisers and pesticides, we slowly poison ourselves. Therefore, as far possible, buy the organically grown products. Some people argue that the atmosphere is so polluted that even organically grown vegetables are not healthy anymore. I suggest that people should get together and should grow their own green vegetables and herbs.

The negative effect from chemical substances and its severity also depends on our basic energy level and constitution. With an Ayurvedic way of life, we can certainly reduce the impact of such dangerous materials. This is best done by taking rasayanas to enhance ojas in the body, following six monthly purification practices (pancha karma) and a regular purification of the blood through the intake of various blood-purifying substances.

Always buy full cream yoghurt (curd) with active bacteria or, preferably, make your own. For fruit yoghurts, it is better to add fresh fruits into the yoghurt or homemade jams. The milk you drink should be full cream and always fresh. Preserved milk or any other product with a long conservation period is heavy to digest and vitiates vata. Never buy anything ready-made (sauces or other things). Know what you are eating!

Processed cheese should not be consumed in excess and never taken more than once a day. Meat and cheese should never be eaten together. This would make the meal too heavy. Replace cheese with paneer from time to time, especially if you wish to eat cheese for the second time in one day.

Use different grains and always buy whole-grain flour, although in some recipes, it is essential to use white flour. There is no need to become fanatic about it as long as the entire meal does not consist of white flour products. For example, pasta made from white flour with only little tomato sauce is not a good idea. If you wish to eat pasta made of white flour, add different vegetables, herbs and spices to the sauce. This way, you will automatically eat less pasta.

Most people are in dilemma as how much salt and sugar they should take. I already mentioned earlier that a lot of sugar and salt is consumed in the readymade foods. Simply reduce your consumption of anything pre-prepared and readymade. While eating chocolate, keep in mind that there is about 50% sugar in it. A 100 gm chocolate bar contains the equivalent of 10 teaspoons of sugar. Cakes and pastries generally contain 25 % sugar.

Avoid eating white sugar; candy sugar is much better. Brown sugar, raw sugar and jaggery are also good. It is always better to alternate and use several different kinds of sugars. Honey is recommended in winter, but only in cold or warm things and never in hot drinks or for cooking or baking. Heated honey is toxic. Preferably, have fruit salads rather than desserts with large amounts of sugar.

Salt should always be taken in a very moderate quantity. In Europe, some products like olives or other preserved vegetables, certain varieties of cheese from Greece and Turkey and various preserved Italian salads and meats contain excessive amounts of salt. In India, some people eat excessive amounts of chilli and then balance the hot taste with too much salt. This is bad for health, as any rasa, taken in excess creates imbalance.

In my recipes, I have suggested certain quantities of sugar and salt, but you can always reduce them according to your taste and need. The use of chilli is always optional, and one may add a limited amount of them, but never in excess. The best way to use chilli is to partially crush it and soak it in olive or sesames oil. Gradually the chilli leaves its sharpness in oil and use this oil in small quantity to add the chilli taste in your cooking. Go on adding more oil in your container with chillies.

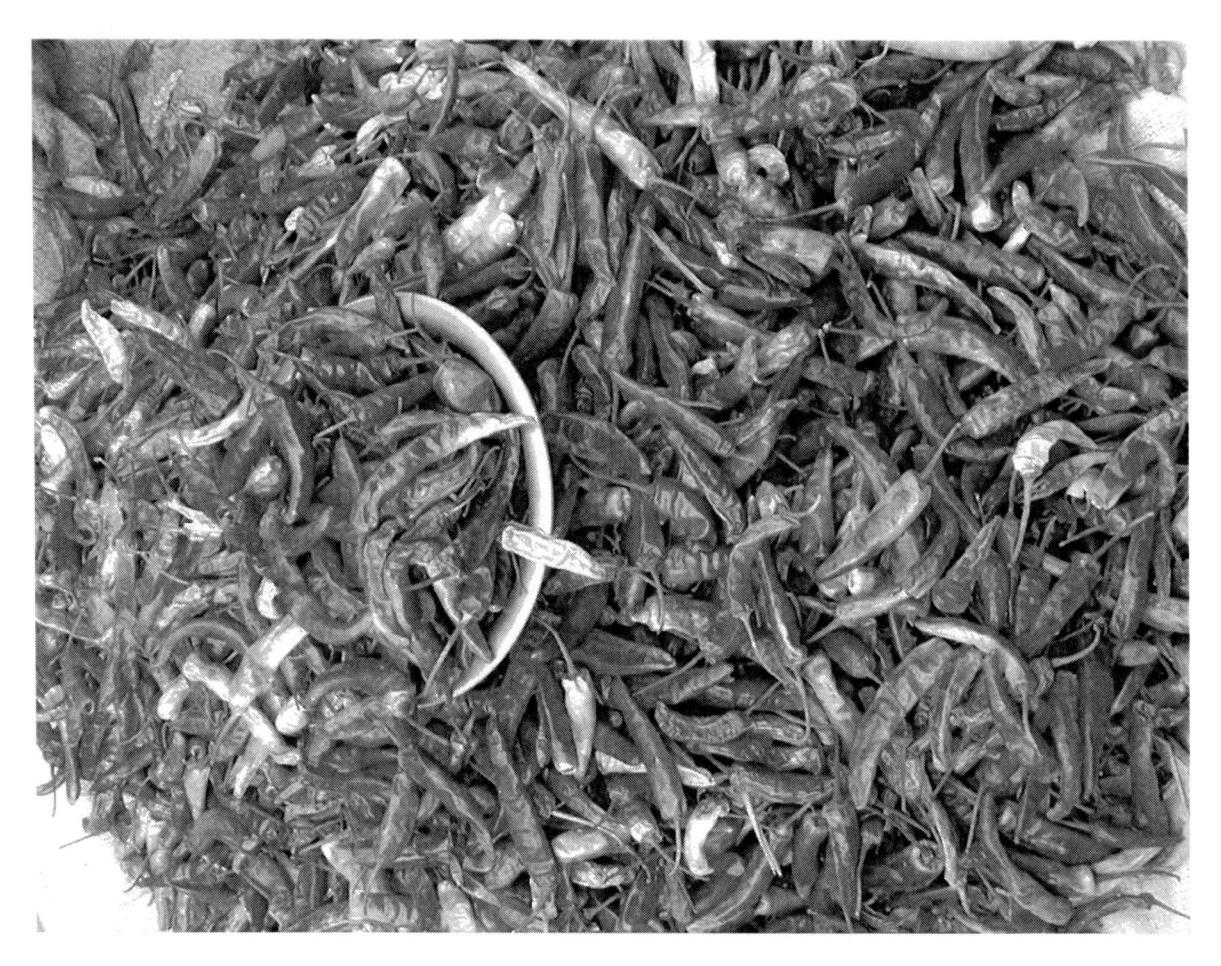

Refined oils are not healthy. Use cold pressed sesames oil or olive oil. Avoid getting influenced by media reports of things being healthy or unhealthy. Remember that the traders have to sell and there is a lot of misleading information behind all aggressive publicities.

Combinations of Food

I have seen that people eat strange combinations of food and then suffer from one problem or the other related to digestion. For example, for breakfast, many people eat fruits and yoghurt, and along with that they have coffee or tea. Some have everything for breakfast: bread, cheese, yoghurt (curd), tea, coffee and even more. They do not realise that coffee or tea with cold yoghurt is antagonistic. Yoghurt and fruits by themselves are all right and in this case, tea or coffee should be taken half an hour earlier. Bread and cheese along with fruits and yoghurt are heavy to digest. Generally, people put butter on their bread and then cheese, which is also a concentrated food. The further addition of yoghurt makes the combination too heavy to digest, since all these dairy products are kapha-promoting. Obviously, the excessive kapha depresses the *agni* or the digestive fire of the body. Therefore, it is better to have either bread, butter and cheese along with coffee or tea or only fruits with yoghurt.

At times, for lunch and dinner, many people eat strange combinations of food items. One should strictly avoid taking cold drinks with hot food. Once you finish eating, do not continue to drink alcohol or other things. Too much liquid will overfill your stomach and vitiate the three energies. Sit down and eat peacefully in one sitting. If you are eating your meal in courses, eat each course moderately. In case you have already eaten two thirds of your stomach full and you have no place for dessert or any other course, then leave them. Never eat heavy desserts like cakes or other things which are made with grains, eggs and a lot of butter. Sometimes, people say that they are full and will have the dessert after some time. According to the Ayurvedic principles, one should never eat like this, because it means that we are already eating again when our stomach is still digesting the previous meal. It is strenuous for the stomach and leads to an imbalance of the three energies. If done repeatedly, it may even give *amadosha*. That means that part of the undigested food will remain in the stomach, resulting in indigestion as well as other disorders like skin infections and allergies.

Respite from Food

A complete fast is not recommended in Ayurveda, since staying hungry vitiates vata. However, partial fasting with a special dietary regimen is a part of the Ayurvedic way of living, and it is meant to give rest to the stomach. For example, one can choose one day a week to eat less and to have only food without salt and without grains; in other words, the sattvic food a yogi eats. Sattvic food does not excite the senses or give excessive sleep. For example, garlic, onions, most spices and heavy, fatty and oily foods are not sattvic. Garlic and spices are rajasic foods, which excite senses; onions and fatty and oily foods are heavy to digest and induce sleep. They are tamasic, whereas rice, milk, yoghurt, sweet fruits, balanced vegetables like courgette, carrots and turnips are categorised as sattvic food. In your weekly fast, you should also leave out rice in order to purify the system. For breakfast, you can have sweet fruits, nuts or dairy products. If you need a lunch, eat one of these things again. For dinner, prepare a meal without salt and grains, preferably mixed vegetables and potatoes. Spice only with cumin and coriander and add some herbs. To accompany your vegetables, you can make some potatoes on a non-stick pan with a little ghee. You may add some raisins in your potatoes. This meal tastes very good, but it is very different from your normal meals.

Appendix

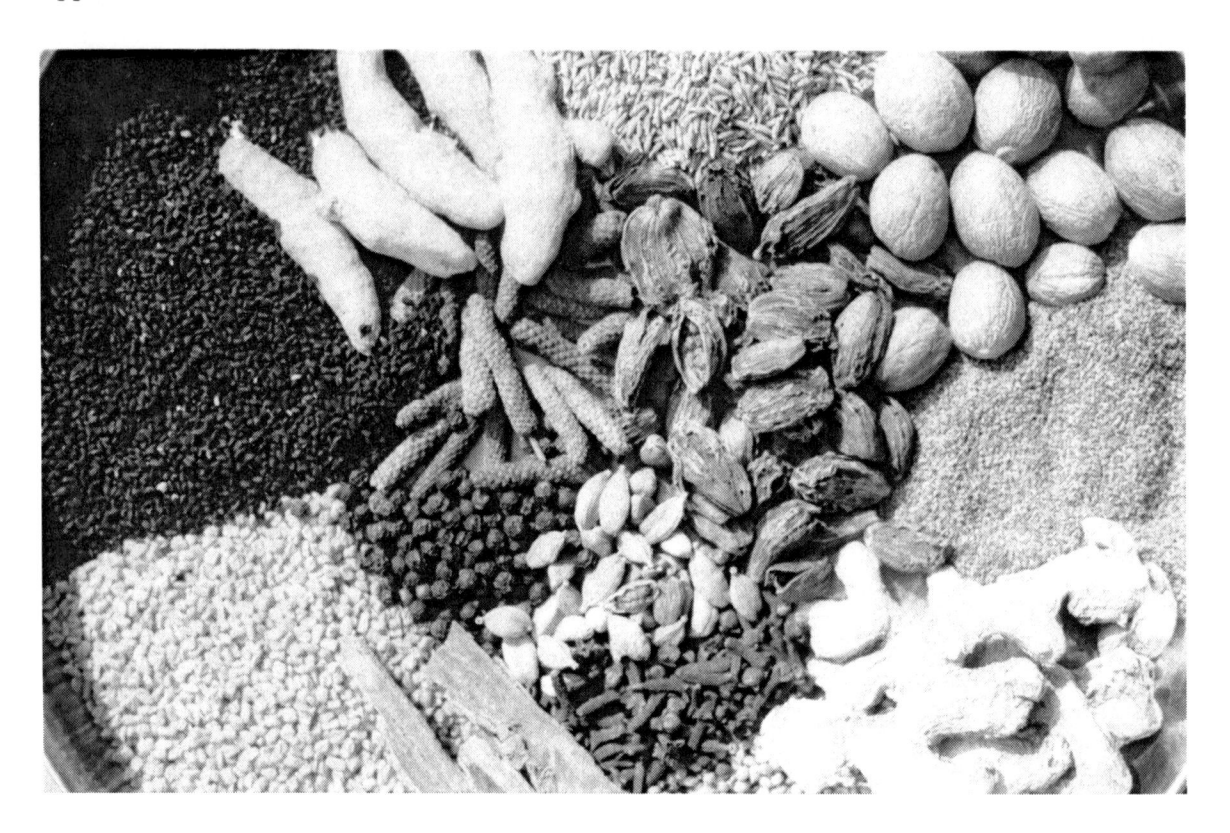

Your Food and your Appearance

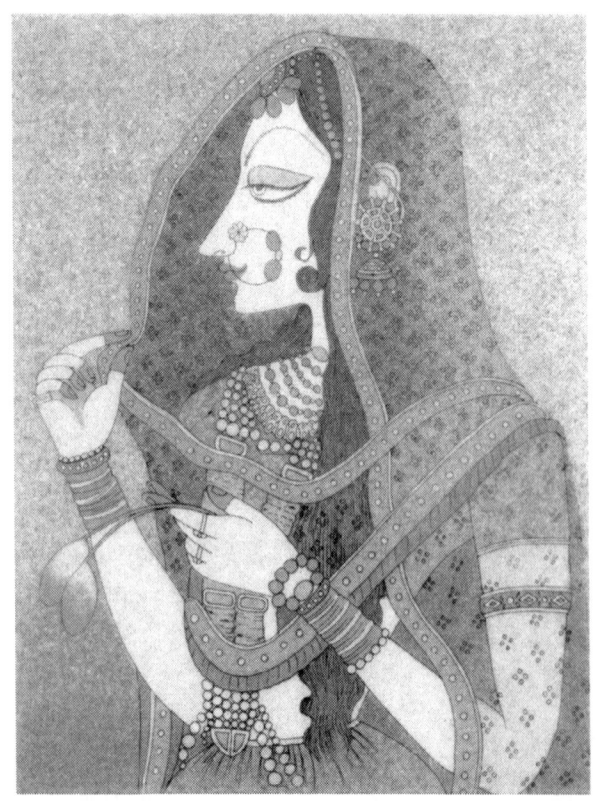

A balanced Ayurvedic diet can change your appearance. It is through the things you eat that you can change vikriti to parkriti. For example, strong body odour indicates a pitta imbalance, and you should eat cooling things or observe a sattvic diet as described above. Blood purifiers like turmeric and substances with bitter rasas will also help to get rid of body odour. Trying to mask it with deodorants or perfume is not a real solution to the problem.

If your skin is dry and you feel that despite all care, your hair and nails have a rough appearance, your vata is vitiated. In addition to the external application of oils with massage, you also need to eat more ghee and substances with sweet rasas.

A state of laziness, heaviness and feeling sleepy frequently is often due to vitiated kapha, and you need to eat spicy food for counterbalancing. Enhance the use of ginger and garlic in your meals and reduce sweet and fatty things. You will see that with the altered diet, your disposition will also change.

The effect of diet on beauty, sexuality and other aspects of life has already been described in my various books.

Frequently Asked Questions about Ayurvedic Nutrition

I have been teaching Ayurveda and holding seminars on Ayurvedic nutrition for more than two decades now. In each seminar on Ayurveda, nutrition is one of the most important themes. From my European students, I often get this feedback, 'Oh, my grandmother used to say the same'. This shows that the basic human wisdom about nutrition is the same the world over. In Middle Eastern countries, people use a sesame seed purée called Tahini for making different sauces. Sesame is good for the complexion and for the bones. But Tahini is heavy and hard to digest. Therefore, for making the sauce, lemon or something else that is sour is generally added. In addition, Tahini sauce has garlic and other spices and herbs in it, which promote digestion. Pasta with tomato sauce is another example in this direction. We can therefore conclude that the world over, traditional knowledge about nutrition follow the same principles.

A worrying feature is the number of different theories on food going around. While some say that one should not eat fruit after midday and others insist that eating only fruit cures all your ailments. There are others who say that fat is bad and sugar and salt are also harmful. It seems more rational to me to think that nothing is good or bad as such; rather, it is time, place and our constitution one should take into consideration while eating. Think of balance and equilibrium and do not go by personal experiences of people. Think cosmic, global and holistic.

Here are some frequently asked questions and my answers.

Does Ayurveda advocate vegetarianism?

When I teach, I give examples of hot, cold and balanced foods according to their Ayurvedic properties. As I assume that in my groups at least some students are meat eaters, I give examples of both vegetarian and non-vegetarian foods. Many students are quite surprised then, because they are convinced that everything healthy ought to be vegetarian, and they usually ask 'how come that Ayurveda allows eating meat?'

Appendix

Ayurveda is a science and does not take a moral stand on issues. It takes into consideration that there may be some parts of the world with less vegetation, where it could be necessary to eat meat. Charaka Samhita, which was compiled 2600 years ago by the sage Charaka, gives the Ayurvedic properties of a large number of edible substances from both the plant and the animal kingdom. The description of wild and domesticated animals and their different meats is also included. This indicates that Ayurveda does not insist that you be necessarily vegetarian for reasons of good health. Whatever one may eat should be taken according to time, place and one's parkriti. For meat eaters, it is extremely essential to consume different vegetables, and meat should not be taken in large quantities or too frequently. For vegetarians, it is essential to consume nuts, beans, lentils and cheese or other milk products.

Is it better to consume indigenous or locally grown products and not the fruits and vegetables which come from foreign countries?

There is no harm in eating products from foreign countries, but you should always keep in mind the principles of hot and cold. Even indigenous products are sometimes grown in artificial climatic conditions to make them available all year round. For example, papaya is a balanced food, but it does not grow in Europe. It is perfectly all right to eat it in Europe. Asparagus grows in Europe but it is very cold in its Ayurvedic nature. It is a summer vegetable, but now they cultivate it also in other continents and make it available in Europe throughout the year. It is not a good idea to consume it in autumn or winter. However, if you do, take care that you do not eat too much and add some dill seeds when you prepare a sauce for asparagus. Do not eat asparagus with ghee or butter, as both are cold. Sauce Hollandaise or Béarnaise, which is made of oil and eggs make a balanced diet with asparagus.

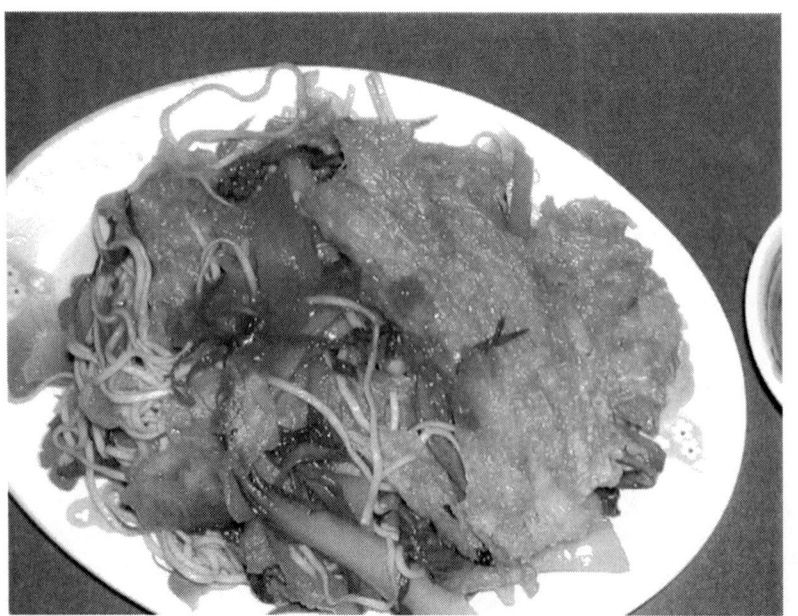

You can always determine the Ayurvedic nature of foreign products by eating them alone without any accompanying substances. Then carefully observe their effect on your body. Cold products have a diuretic and hot ones an anti-diuretic effect. However, juicy fruits eaten in excess always have some diuretic effect. Dill seeds, garlic and other spices that are hot in their Ayurvedic nature, are all anti-diuretic. Then there are spices with a cold nature like coriander, anise, fennel, clove, and so on, with diuretic effect. With new products, you have to learn how to improvise your own recipes.

Different books and different teachers give diverse opinions about the rasa with which one should start the main meal. Some say sweet and others say sour. What is right?

Normally, one should begin the meal with a predominantly but not excessively sour and bitter rasas. However, if you have been very hungry for a long time, you should eat something sweet before, in order to avoid consuming the meal in vata state. Staying hungry for a long time disturbs vata and vitiates it. In normal circumstances, if you have something sweet in the beginning, it will suppress the appetite, as sweet is kapha-promoting. To understand it easily, imagine the five elements: digestive fire or agni is a part of pitta, the fire element; kapha is water and earth. If you put water or earth on fire, it extinguishes. Therefore, eating sweet in the beginning of the meal will reduce the appetite or even cause indigestion. However, you should always end your meal with something sweet.

We are told by different teachers to boil drinking water for a long time, varying from 15 minutes to one hour. Which is correct?

In Switzerland, I learnt from my students that someone from Germany was lecturing on Ayurveda in Switzerland and telling people that according to Ayurveda one should boil water for one hour to change its properties. This is a very strange statement about Ayurveda. It is a pity what some people misleadingly say or claim on the name of this ancient wisdom for which they are not trained and qualified. Boiling water for one hour will make the concentration of the minerals and salts very high and will do you harm. There are regions where water has high concentrations of calcium salts and other salts. Water boiled for so long tastes awful and will also disturb the energy equilibrium in the body in one way or the other. Thus, be very careful about such wrong information.

You need to boil your water for 15 minutes if there is a fear of some biological contamination. For example in Delhi or in Cairo, it will be better to do this to save oneself of waterborne ailments. However in Europe, the United States and some other countries, tap water is mostly perfectly safe. As I said in the recipes of drinks, water should be boiled with a few cardamoms. With the 'safe' drinking water, you simply need to bring the water to boil.

Appendix

Are dals good for health? Should one take them every day?

I was told that in one of the popular books on Ayurveda, it is recommended to eat dals for dinner every day. As I said earlier, most books on Ayurvedic nutrition and cooking are simply Indian cookbooks and present the most common Indian food habits. A large majority of Indians eat dal and rice for lunch, and people from Punjab have dal at night. The concerned writer is a Punjabi and therefore he recommended eating dal for dinner.

According to Charaka Samhita, dals are heavy to digest and therefore should be eaten with spices and ghee. Many dals are highly vata enhancing, and therefore it is essential that ghee is added. Dals should not be eaten for dinner, as they are heavy and long to digest. During the day, due to various physical activities, they are well digested. At night, the bodily functions slow down, and therefore dals or any other heavy foods should be avoided.

Dals of different varieties or peas and beans are essential for vegetarians. But it is not necessary to consume them everyday. Vegetarians can also eat various kinds of nuts. People with weak digestion should take mung beans or mung dal and better avoid other beans and dals.

We have read in some Ayurvedic books that mustard oil is good for health and should be used for cooking. Why?

First of all, you should forget the notion of things being good or bad for health. According to Ayurveda, all that brings harmony is a remedy and all what brings imbalance is anti-health. Depending upon time, place and your prakriti, the same things may be used as remedies or they may be harmful.

Mustard oil has a very strong taste and flavour and has antibiotic qualities. It has also pain-relieving properties. It is used as a base for certain remedies to cure skin ailments and for pain relieving oils. It can be used for cooking but is extremely hot in its properties and, because of its strong taste and flavour, it is not a fine cooking medium. The traditional Ayurvedic texts recommend sesame oil for cooking, whereas mustard oil is said to be more suited for medicinal purpose than food. In certain parts of India, it is used in some food preparations, but it should not be used too often. It is better to use both ghee and oil for cooking. If you make one preparation with ghee, make the second one with oil. Rapeseed oil should not be taken as some recent studies show that it has harmful side-effects. Use olive or sesames oil for cooking.

Some nutritionists recommend eating different food items separately for better health and longevity. How would this be considered in the light of Ayurvedic principles?

It is essential to avoid eating foods that are antagonist in nature. It is also very important not to eat odd combinations of foods that are heavy to digest. Other than that, there is no need to separate different food items. On the contrary, since Ayurveda recommends taking all rasas in every meal. It is necessary that you combine diverse food items and enrich them with various spices. Therefore, separating different foods is not to be recommended from an Ayurvedic point of view. Neither does it support health care by way of eating insipid food. Sensuous fulfilment and pleasure is very important from Ayurvedic point of view.

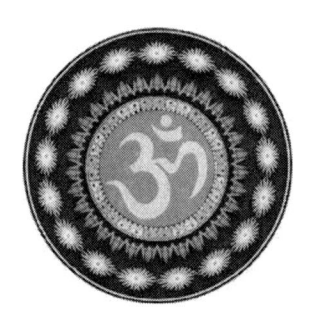

AUM SHANTI

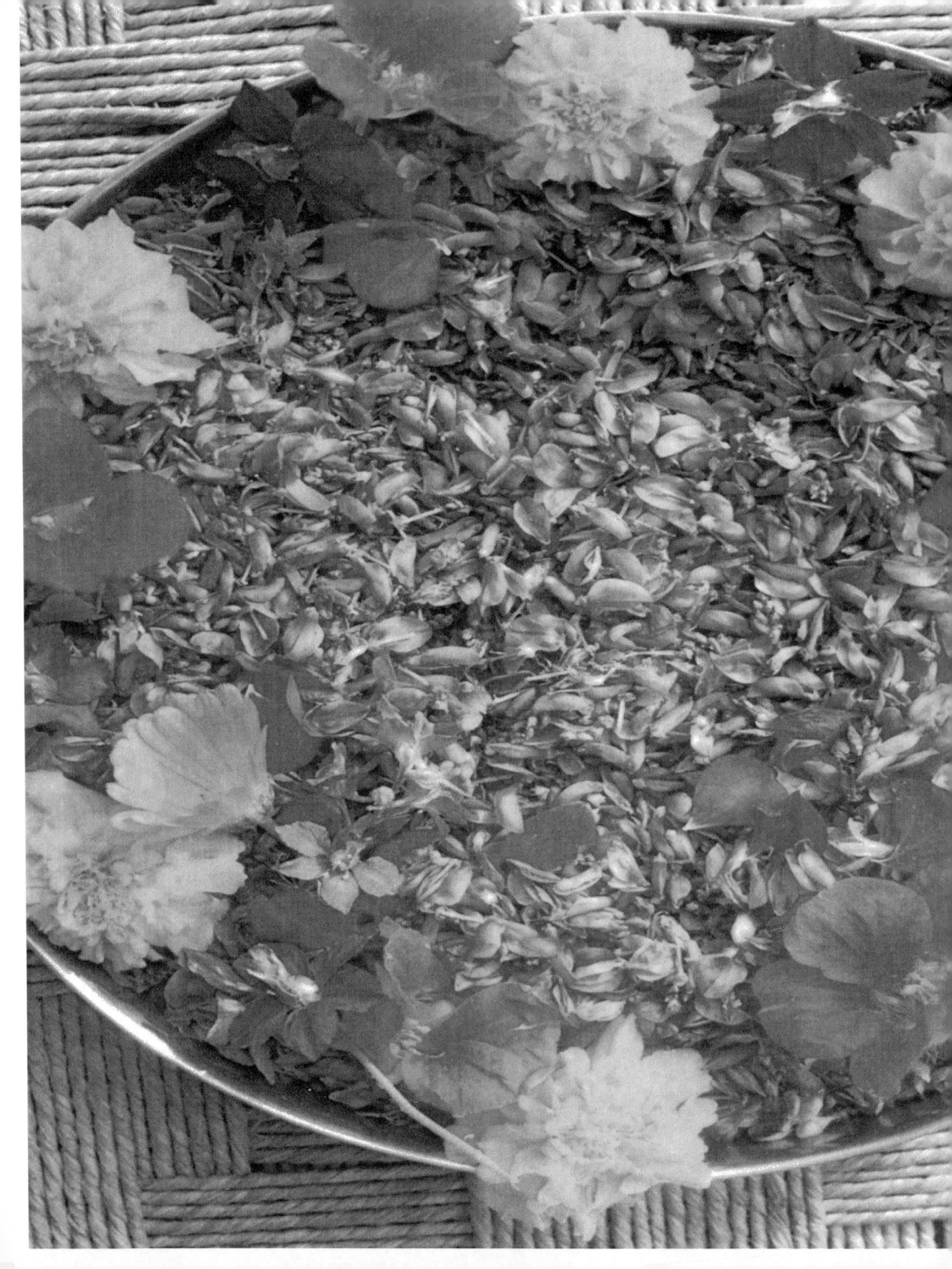

About the Author

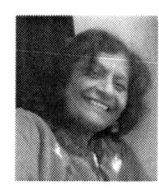

Along with a doctorate degree in reproduction biology in India, Dr. Verma studied Neurobiology in Paris University and obtained a second doctorate. She pursued advanced research at the National Institutes of Health, Bethesda (USA) and the Max-Planck Institute in Freiburg, Germany. At the peak of her career in medical research in a pharmaceutical company in Germany, she realised that the modern approach to health care is basically fragmented and non-holistic. Besides, we are directing all our efforts and resources to cure disease rather than maintaining health. In response, Dr. Verma founded The New Way Health Organisation (NOW) in 1986 to spread the message of holistic living, preventive methods for health care and to promote the use of mild medicine and various self-help therapeutic measures.

Dr. Verma grew up with a strong familial tradition of Ayurveda with a grandmother who had enormous Ayurvedic wisdom and was a gifted healer. She has studied Ayurveda in the traditional Guru-shishya style with Acharya Priya Vrat Sharma of the Benares Hindu University for 23 years.

Dr. Verma is an ardent researcher and is working hard to compile the living tradition of Ayurveda and spread it in the world through her books and other activities. She has published twenty three books on yoga, Ayurveda, Women and Companionship. The books are published in various languages of the world. Besides, she has published numerous scientific articles. Several other books are in preparation. She lectures extensively, teaches in Europe for several months a year, trains students at her two centres in India and gives radio and television programmes. A film on Ayurveda with her was made by German television in 1995 and was shown in 100 countries, in 130 languages. It was the first film on Ayurveda.

Dr. Verma has founded Charaka School of Ayurveda to train interested people with genuine Ayurvedic education so that they can further impart the knowledge of Ayurvedic way of life and save people from becoming a victim of charlatanry in Ayurveda. She is doing several research projects on medicinal plants and their combination in the form of remedies. She is the founder and chairperson of *The Ayurveda Health Organisation,* which is a charitable trust for distributing and promoting Ayurvedic remedies and yoga therapy in rural areas of India. She does regular lectures and workshops for school children in the rural and remote areas of the Himalayas to promote wisdom of traditional science and medicine. Dr. Verma gives seminars, lectures and teaches in the *Charaka School of Ayurveda* with guru-shishya tradition. She is the Academic Director of the *Charaka Ayurveda and Yoga Academy and Cultural Centre (CAYACC).*

For more information and contacts for Dr. Verma's school and teaching programme see www.ayurvedavv.com and www.drvinodverma.com

Dr. Vinod Verma's Publications

1. *Patanjali's Yoga Sutra: A Scientific Exposition* (Published in English, Hindi and German).
2. *Ayurveda for Inner Harmony: Nutrition, Sexual Energy and Healing* (Published in English, German, Italian, French, Romanian and Hindi).
3. *Ayurveda a Way of Life* (Published in English, German, Italian, French, Spanish, Czech, Greek, Portuguese, Slovenian and Hindi).
4. *The Kamasutra for Women* (Published in English [America and India], German, French, Dutch, Romanian, Italian, Portuguese, Slovenian Hindi and Malayalam).
5. *Stress-free Work with Yoga and Ayurveda* (Published in German, English [America and India] and Hindi).
6. *Patanjali and Ayurvedic Yoga* (Published in English, German and Hindi).
7. *Programming Your Life with Ayurveda* (Published in German, French, English, Slovenian and Czech).
8. *Ayurvedic Food Culture and Recipes* (Published in English, German, Czech and Hindi).
9. *Yoga: A Natural Way of Being* (Published in English, German, French, Italian and Hindi).
10. *Companionship and Sexuality (Based on Ayurveda and the Hindu tradition)* (Published in English and German).
11. *Natural Glamour: The Ayurveda Beauty Book* (Published in German, Spanish and English)
12. *Losing and Maintaining Weight with Ayurveda and Yoga* (Published in English, Slovenian and German).
13. *The Timeless Wisdom of Ayurveda: A Scientific Exposition* (Published in English and German)
14. *Prakriti and Pulse: The Two Mysteries of Ayurveda* (Published in German)
15. *Good Food for Dogs: Vegetarian nourishment based on Ayurvedic wisdom* (Published in German and English)
16. *Diet for Losing Weight* (published in German and English)
17. *Aum: The Infinite Energy* (Published in German and English)
18. *Pulse Diagnose in Chinese and Ayurvedic Medicine* (co-author for TCM Dr. Florian Ploberger) (published in German)
19. *Shiva's Secrets for Health and Longevity* (published in German and English)
20. *Healing Hands: The Ayurvedic Massage workbook* (in press)
21. *Prevention of Dementia* (published in German and English)
22. *Ayurveda for Dogs* (published in German)
23. Ayurvedic Cuisine: God's own Apothecary— Simple Healing Remedies from Ayurvedic Herbs and Spices (in press)

The Charaka School of Ayurveda and Patanjali Yogadarshana Society (Himalayan Centre)

The Charka School of Ayurveda (CSA) has been founded by Dr. Vinod Verma to spread the genuine classical tradition as well as the living tradition of Ayurveda in the world for promoting healthy living and preventing ailments. Its aim is to teach people a healthy lifestyle which enhances immunity and vitality and enables them to live a life with an optimum level of energy. For minor ailments, people should be capable of using home remedies, appropriate physical and mental exercises and nutrition.

CSA aims to bring genuine and practical aspects of Ayurveda to people and save them from Americanised and Europeanised distorted versions of Ayurveda and other forms of charlatanry that do more harm than good.

To achieve this purpose, CSA organises to train students in Europe who can further spread the message of Ayurvedic lifestyle and help people with genuine massages, purification practices, nutrition and other practical aspects of Ayurveda. The school is in association with the most learned persons of Ayurveda in India and several exclusive persons involved in health education in Europe.

The object of Patanjali Yogadarshana Society is to spread the message of Patanjali in the world. The wisdom of the Yoga Sutras is not only beneficial for the yogis but also for our day-to-day normal life. Its aim is to enhance *sattva* or the inner stillness and peace in the world as well as in the individual minds. With years of research on Yoga and Ayurveda, Dr. Verma has founded the Ayurvedic Yoga and has written a book on the subject.

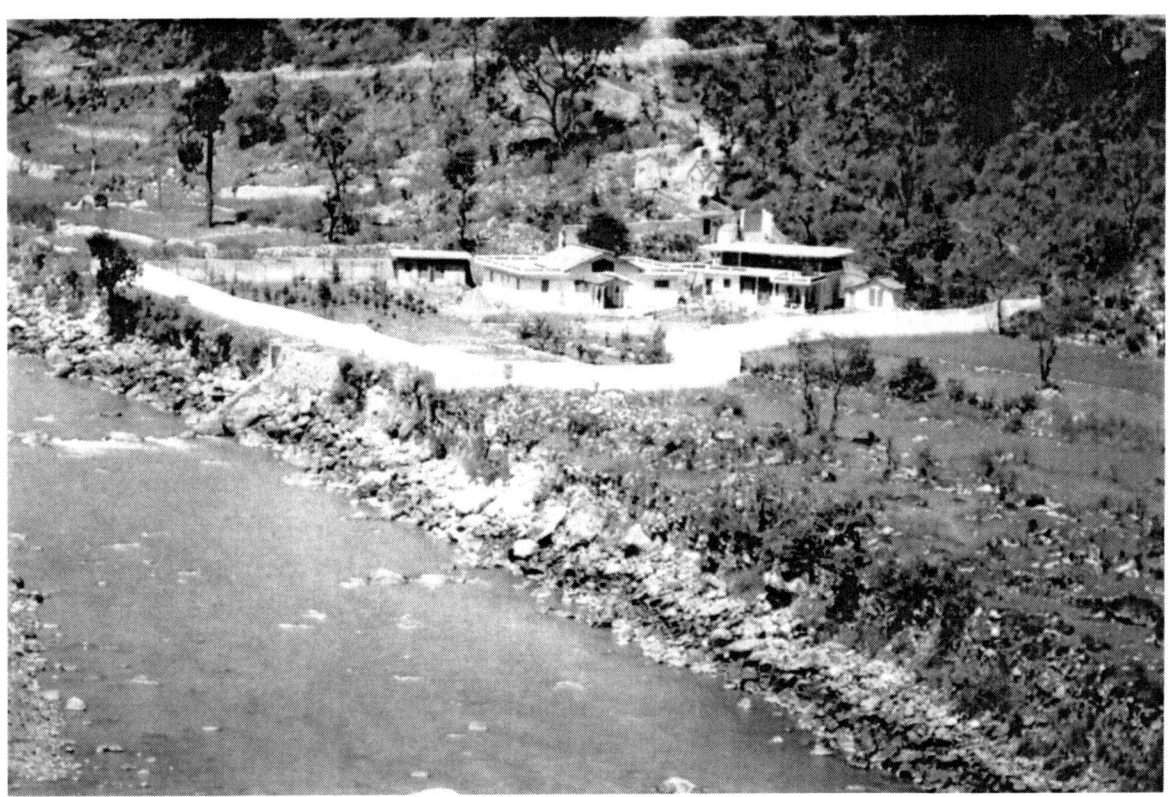

Himalayan Centre

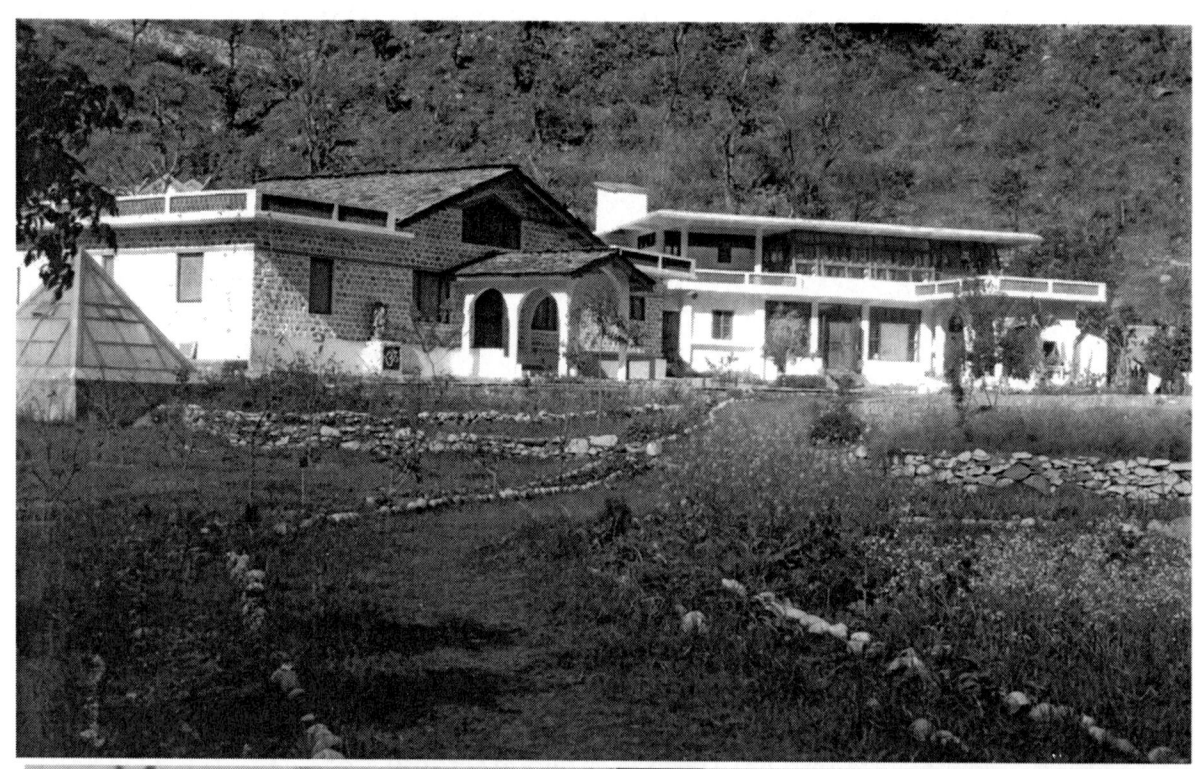

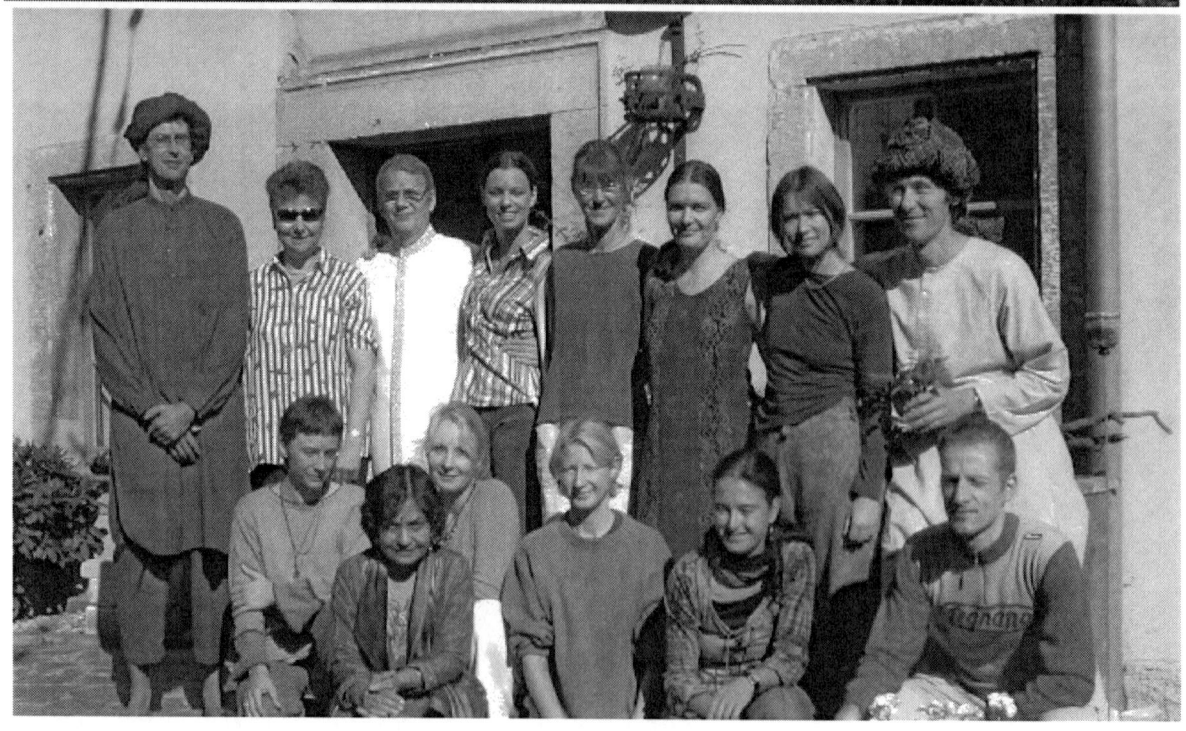

Lectures, Seminars and Training Programmes

To get detailed information on the Charaka School of Ayurveda as well as our other programmes in India and Europe, visit our website or contact us by email.

The New Way Health Organisation .NOW.
A-130, Sector 26, Noida 201301, U.P., India
Tel. 0091 (0)120 2527820 or (0) 9873704205 or (0)9412224820
www.ayurvedavv.com   www.drvinodverma.com
Contact at: ayurvedavv@yahoo.com

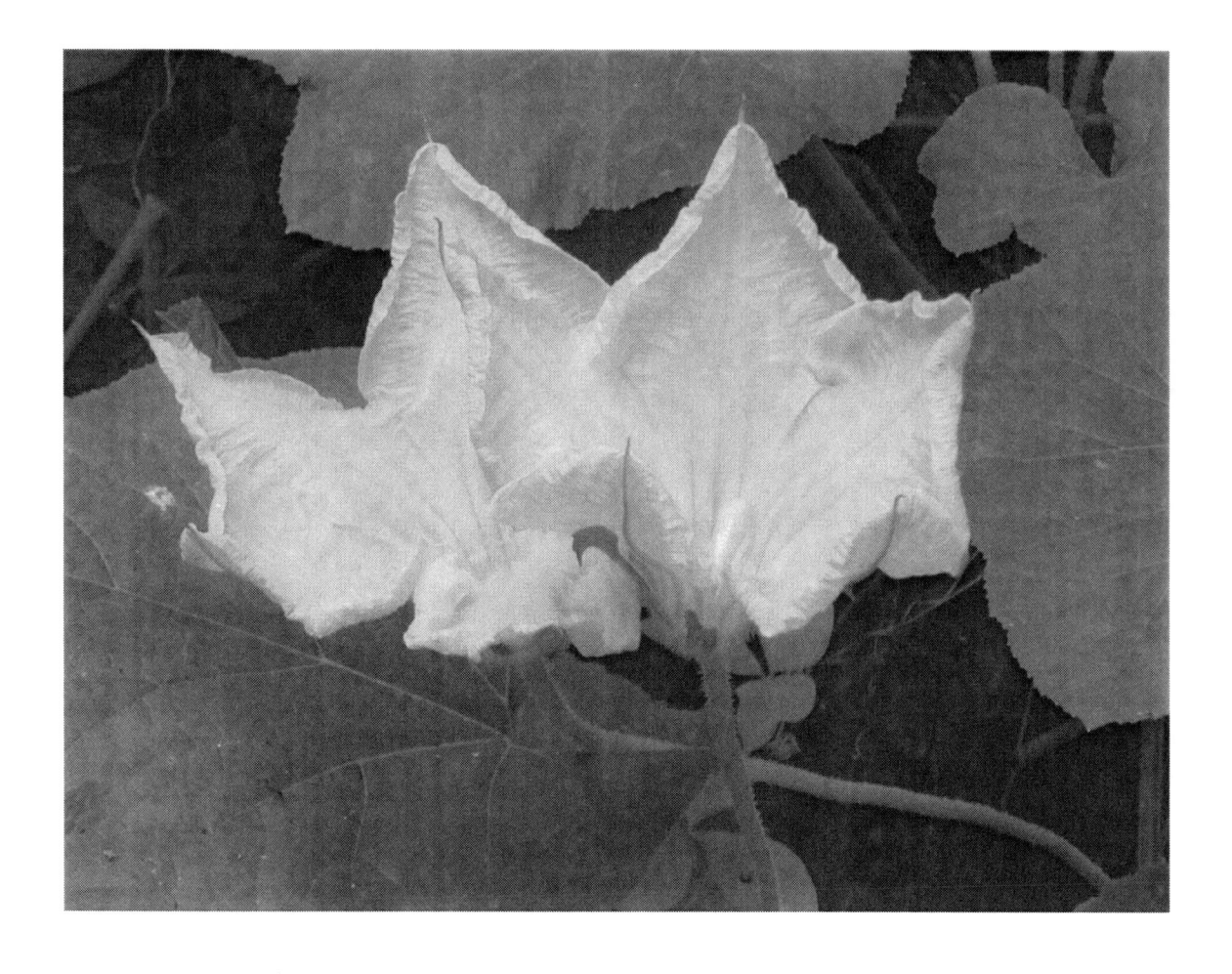

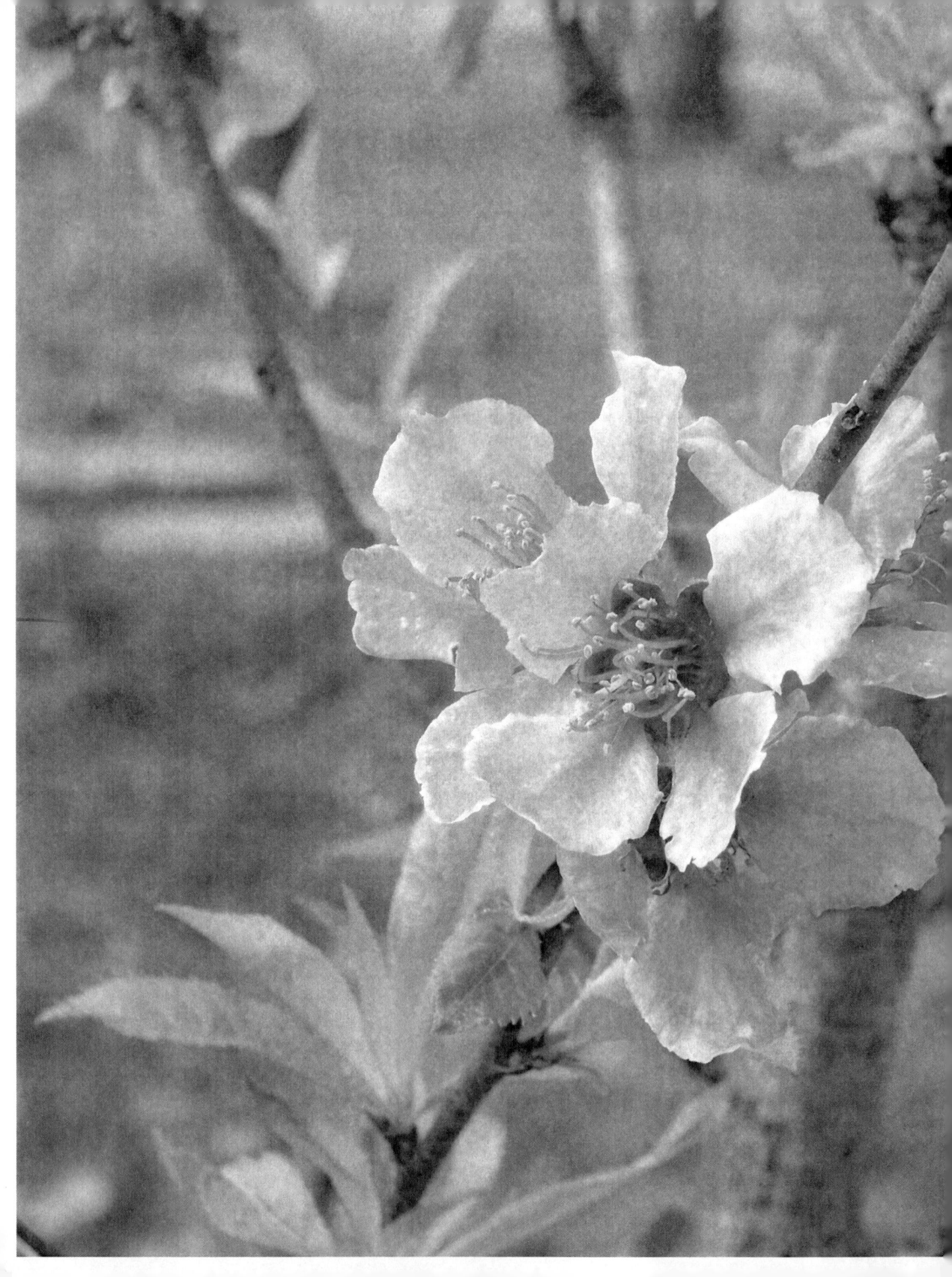

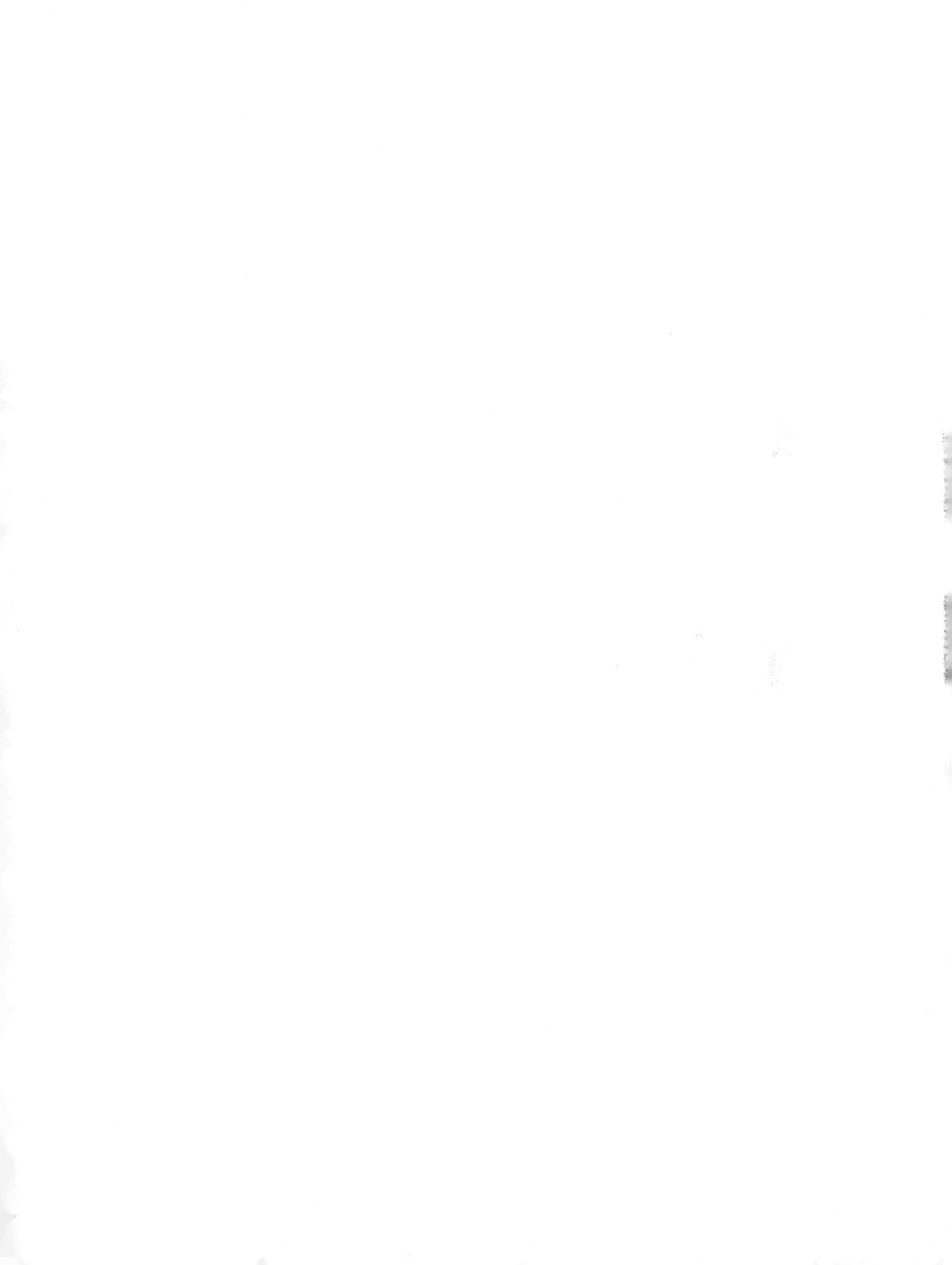

9 788189 514235